GET WELL AT HOME

Complete Home Health Care for the Family

Richard A. Hansen, M.D.

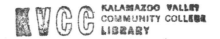

Copyright © 1980, 1995

by

Richard A. Hansen, M.D.

Published by:
Shiloh Medical Publications
RFD 1, Box 4035
Poland Spring, Maine 04274

Library of Congress cataloging information
Hansen, Richard A.
   Get Well at Home
   Includes index.
   1. Therapeutics—Popular works.
   2. Medicine, Preventive—Popular works.

RM122.5.H36   616.02'4   81-117423

ISBN 0-9643914-1-4

Printed in the U.S.A.
at
BookCrafters

DEDICATION

To my loyal and talented wife, **Ulla**, and three devoted daughters, **Ingrid**, **Luvon**, and **Maria**, who all have enriched the author's life with a beautiful demonstration of love, patience, and encouragement.

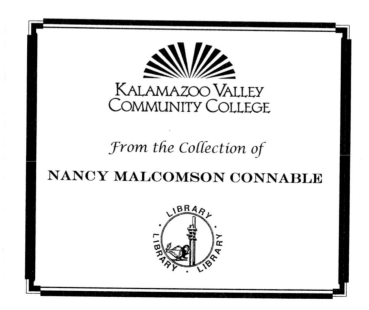

ACKNOWLEDGEMENTS

The preparation of a comprehensive book of natural therapies and preventive medicine involves many individuals. Much of the background for this project came from experiences in patient care and teaching at the **Wildwood Lifestyle Center and Hospital**, located in Wildwood, Georgia. Special appreciation must be paid to Doctors Bernell and Marjorie Baldwin—physiologists, scientists, researchers, medical mentors and friends. W. D. Frazee, founding president of the above institution, has been a great inspiration to me, and deserves much credit for the incentive to write this book.

For over fifteen years, the staff of the **Poland Spring Health Institute**—located in Poland Spring, Maine—have skillfully served the many patients admitted under my medical care. Each nurse, cook, therapist, secretary, health educator, administrative leader and teammate contributed to the healing experience from which this volume is written. Faithful secretaries and nurses—Candace Ledoux, Jeni Brown, Melody Newcomb, Ingrid, Luvon, and Maria Hansen, Dorothy Hall, Rosemary King, Kathy Gilman, and Darrell Atwood—typed diligently, assisting in preparing this manuscript for publication. **Chad Verrill**, a talented young artist, contributed most of the drawings and illustrations. Craig and Lynette Wilcox assisted with final editing, proofreading and the ultimate cover design. Bill Gross from IMAGESET provided the color film. Tom Plain and others of BOOKCRAFTERS helped with many vital decisions as this manuscript went to press.

Especially, however, it is to the Lord, that my highest gratitude belongs—for the strength and wisdom and health, without which it would be impossible to practice the healing arts, write coherently, or devise new and rational methods to approach in a physiologic manner the needs of patients, students, and families. To this great and merciful Creator, all true thanksgiving and praise ascends.

R. A. Hansen MD

PREFACE

There has never been a time in history when greater need exists for true preventive medicine and lifestyle changes to transform our society. New and mysterious diseases appear on the horizon each year. Preventable killer diseases, such as heart attacks and cancer, must be addressed and the death toll modified. *Get Well At Home* has been published to help husbands, wives, fathers, mothers, children, physicians, students, and people everywhere to understand common symptoms, to learn to administer simple home remedies, and cooperate better with nature and their physicians in the treatment of common diseases.

It is not with any desire to criticize conventional medicine that *Get Well At Home* was written. Rather, it is to inform average individuals, laymen as well as homemakers, in the art and the science of medicine, thereby saving not only needless medical expenses, lost time with unnecessary illnesses, but possibly many lives as well. Careful application of the preventive principles in this book will, without doubt, produce better health at home and offer more intelligent approaches to disease.

When using this book as a ready reference, please consult the table of contents and the index frequently. Both of these, as well as other tables, charts, and appendices will make *Get Well At Home* even more valuable as a handbook for emergencies, a reference for study, and a guide to health and healing in your home. Remember nevertheless, to consult your physician. Seek professional advice for a detailed diagnosis in cases of serious accident, or any prolonged illness, especially in children.

Get Well At Home has been written, not only for laymen, but also for those special physicians and nurses who are seeking rational and natural approaches to common diseases. Together with detailed and systematic study of the medical literature, this introduction to simple remedies contains knowledge with which every medical practitioner should be familiar. This author anticipates that *Get Well At Home* will become one of the most valued health references in every family library. It is to the health and happiness of you, dear reader or patient, that time has been devoted in translating a unique medical education into terms understandable by everyone.

R.A.H.

TABLE OF CONTENTS

CHAPTER ONE

INTRODUCTION

TO

HEALTH

AND

DISEASE

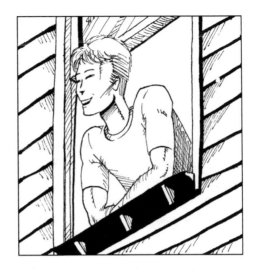

It is possible for you and your family to be healthy. You, my friend, may **choose** to enjoy better health. However, that means much more than the mere absence of illness. True health involves physical, mental, emotional, and spiritual dimensions. It does not come by accident; vigorous health is a positive **achievement**. This book will introduce you to the exciting adventure of really knowing your body. The proper understanding of physical and mental health, and its mortal enemy, disease, will safeguard you against many worries. **Fear** of illness, disability, or suffering is a major destroyer of peace. Welcome now to the greatest adventure. We will become good friends in the exploration of true healing, jointly in partnership with our bodies.

Sickness in the home always presents numerous problems. There is usually anxiety in the heart of every family member, when a loved one becomes ill. Naturally, we harbor uncertainty concerning the diagnosis. Moreover, there is our built-in fear of death to be understood, as well as the frequent frustration experienced just caring for a sick person. Sometimes the numerous symptoms that characterize our health problem can be misinterpreted. They may be either trivial and self-limited, or much more serious than they really appear. All this must be studied.

Looking at illness from the viewpoint of home treatment, you must first consider the various possible **causes**. One author defined disease as an *effort of nature* to free the system from conditions that result from violation of the laws of health. That definition looks at the various symptoms as evidences that the body is trying to rid itself of poisons, toxins, or foreign invaders. In fighting for a speedy return of health, your body generates numerous symptoms and signs— for example, fever or pain.

Approaching disease from this vantage point, we must first endeavor to **ascertain the true causes**. The cause may be *infectious* in nature, or it may be related to various *degenerative* processes of the body. Disease can in addition result from an *accident, injury*, or another form of *trauma*. The accumulation of toxins or foreign *viruses* may result in the development of a growth, usually referred to as a *neoplasm* or tumor. Other causes of common diseases include *allergic* reactions, *emotional* problems, *hormone* imbalances, *nutritional* disorders, and occasionally *inherited* tendencies.

Correcting wrong personal habits that have contributed to the cause of an illness may require a major dietary change. Exercise often needs to be encouraged, or sometimes curtailed, depending upon the type of illness. Specific treatment recommendations will be presented in subsequent chapters as we consider individual diseases. Simple treatments in the home, such as water taken internally or applied externally—the use of hot or cold baths and showers—as well as simple poultices or herbs, may be therapeutically employed in any home setting to combat numerous ailments.

Most of the following natural methods *assist* "Nature" in her effort to restore right conditions and re-establish a normal balance to all of the body's processes. It naturally follows then, that a proper understanding of physiology and some knowledge of the structure of our bodies, especially our anatomy, is crucial to a person seeking assistance to combat disease in a home–like, natural setting. Wise progressive physicians today encourage more independent judgment on the part of their patients, while teaching modern mothers how properly to care for their children. This **self–help trend** became increasingly important in the recent decade as medical costs skyrocketed. It could be even more vital in the future when specialized health care becomes unaffordable.

RATIONAL APPROACHES to ILLNESS

In dealing with any disease, the first step toward diagnosis is found in the **health history** and its interpretation. All facts of significance in the lifestyle of the individual up to the time of illness should be evaluated as possible contributors to the present problem. **Allergies** to drugs, foods, or environmental factors should also be evaluated in the face of present illness.

Second, the careful analysis of the illness under question with all of its various symptoms, including other factors that have ensued from the first onset to the present need to be considered. Most diseases fit certain patterns. As organ systems and their disorders are discussed, these patterns will become obvious. Thus, the intelligent interpretation of a medical history provides one of the most valuable clues to understand illness and its proper diagnosis.

Remember this one caution in the proper interpretation of health history. Accurate recall for the patient is very important. However, most sick individuals color their subjective awareness of symptoms with substantial concern over the consequences of illness to their families. **Fear** of disease, disability, and even death may affect the person's response to the otherwise clear question or stimulus. Although the story of every illness is extremely important, in most cases, it is not definitive, but rather narrows the number of diagnostic possibilities, and thus guides any subsequent investigation. A physician's skill, knowledge, wisdom, and experience is most clearly evidenced in his history taking. Likewise, the thorough analysis of symptoms in home health care will provide your best clues toward understanding disease.

COMMON SYMPTOMS and THEIR INTERPRETATION

Some generalizations are in order to help you evaluate the most common symptoms of disease. These questions may be asked: When did it begin? What were you doing when the problem started? Have you ever had such a problem before? What measures seem to give relief? Has the disease progressed; or, is it getting better? Are there measures that promote comfort? Where does the primary problem seem to be located? Are there other symptoms that appeared to begin at the same time?

This approach to history taking, whether applied to pain, headache, stomach ache, and many other common symptoms, will help you elicit the true story of illness in a direct and constructive manner.

Loss of Appetite

The medical term for this is *anorexia*. This symptom may be associated with a disease of the digestive system, such as an ulcer, or some problem located elsewhere in the body, such as an infection or emotional reaction.

Nausea and Vomiting

Nausea is a feeling of discomfort in the region of the stomach, often associated with loss of appetite. When vomiting occurs, the patient throws up the contents from the stomach through his mouth. This action results from a sudden strong contraction of the diaphragm and stomach muscles. Strong emotional reactions, effects of drugs or their withdrawal, excessive fatigue, and many diseases such as ulcer, appendicitis, gallstones, even brain tumor, are examples of diseases that produce nausea and vomiting.

Diarrhea

An increased number of loose or watery stools is known as *diarrhea*. The frequency may vary from one or two, to thirty or forty per day. Usually diarrhea is a symptom of irritation in the bowel and not an actual disease. The body tries to rid itself of this irritation by increasing the movements of the intestines. Because of the rapid passage of the intestinal contents, there is more fluid in the stool, and sometimes its passage is associated with abdominal pain or cramping. In severe cases, dehydration may occur, resulting in thirst and dryness of the mouth and skin. A sudden and excessive loss of fluid is especially dangerous in infants and small children.

There are many causes of diarrhea. Nervousness may produce this condition. Many types of laxatives produce an increased number of loose stools. Spoiled food, over-ripe fruit, contaminated canned foods, all irritate the intestines. Diarrhea may also be a symptom of intestinal obstruction, infection of the intestine, or inflammation of the colon, called **colitis**. Microorganisms, such as the amoeba, typhoid bacillus, and other bacteria may cause diarrhea.

Constipation

The individual who produces fewer stools than usual has constipation. The fecal material may be hard and dry. This condition may be a symptom of organic disease, such as an obstruction in the bowel or just increased muscle tone. Nervous conditions can also cause constipation. In such a situation, the colon becomes spastic, preventing normal elimination. Lack of exercise may result in constipation, as does a diet low in roughage, fruits, and vegetables. Drinking an insufficient amount of fluid or taking narcotic drugs for pain may inhibit intestinal contractions (*peristalsis*) and trigger this symptom.

Dehydration

This results from the loss of water within the body's tissues. Normally water makes up over 75% of your body's weight. Replacement of water is the body's most urgent dietary requirement. A patient who is dehydrated has extreme thirst, dry tongue, parched lips, dry skin, and reduced amount of urine. If this disturbed water balance is not corrected, particularly in the infant, the patient may lose consciousness or die. Loss of fluid may result from excessive perspiration, from diarrhea or excessive urination, from hemorrhage, or persistent vomiting. Inability to drink fluids occurs in unconscious patients, and in those with nausea and vomiting, and severe loss of appetite. Complications in the aftermath of surgery, may result in slight dehydration due to fever or vomiting.

Edema

Fluid retention in the cellular tissues results in swelling. *Edema* is the medical term for *dropsy*. It way be a symptom of heart disease, kidney disease, or a local obstruction of lymphatic or venous circulation. Edema usually occurs in the part of the body that is closest to the ground and tends to settle by the action of gravity.

Chills

When a patient has a chill, he feels cold, and shivers and shakes. This increased muscular activity raises the body temperature. It can be compared with the shivering that occurs when a person is cold and trying to get warm. When the chill is the result of nervousness, the patient generally does not have a fever. However when chills are symptoms of infection, fever commonly results.

Fever

A patient with a fever has a body temperature above normal. The average normal temperature varies in different parts of the body, but in the mouth it is 37° Centigrade or 98.6° Fahrenheit. The rectal temperature is slightly higher at 38°C. or 100.4°F. Fever is usually a symptom of infectious disease. However, strenuous exercise, heat stroke, and dehydration can also cause a fever. This is one of the most important defenses of the body against infection. Measures to reduce fever should not be used too frequently, except in cases of extreme temperature elevation.

Cough

Coughing is a violent expulsion of air following a deep respiration, as a rule occurring involuntarily. Usually it is a symptom of irritation in the respiratory tract, but it may be a nervous habit or a means of attracting attention. A cough usually, however, is a symptom of a disease. Sore throats, tuberculosis, whooping cough, bronchitis, pneumonia, or lung tumors can all cause coughing spells. Inhalation of food particles, or irritating substances, such as tobacco smoke, dust, or other toxic gases, can trigger a coughing episode. At times blood will be present in the sputum. This alarming event, called *hemoptysis*, may occur in patients with heart failure or diseases of the lung, such as pneumonia, cancer or lung abscesses. When a chronic cough causes persistent respiratory distress, the cause should promptly be identified.

Shortness of Breath

A patient who has difficulty breathing may be showing signs of obstruction in the respiratory tract or of lung disease, heart disease, or some blood disease, such as anemia. Medically, this condition is called *dyspnea*, and basically refers to shortness of breath.

Cyanosis

When the skin around the mucous membranes, the lips, or the nail beds turn bluish in color, the patient has *cyanosis*. This is a sign of inadequate oxygen transport in the red blood cells. Sometimes in lung disease an insufficient supply of oxygen is obtained from the air. In other conditions the circulation becomes stagnated and cyanosis is seen.

Nose Bleeds

Bleeding from the nose usually occurs from injury. A delicate blood vessel within the nostril gets ruptured. Seen particularly in children, this may be secondary to picking the nose. Medically this condition is called *epistaxis*. Nosebleed may also be a symptom of certain disease conditions, such as high blood pressure, rheumatic fever, measles, influenza, or a disorder of blood clotting mechanism. Injuries, trauma to the face, and the excessive use of certain drugs, such as aspirin, may cause nosebleeds.

Variation in Heart Rate

Sometimes the heart can beat exceptionally slowly. This may be a symptom of disease and is medically termed *bradycardia*. Kidney failure, underactive thyroid gland, heart disease, or overdosage of certain cardiac drugs, such as digitalis may produce slowness of the heartbeat.

At times the heart beats too rapidly. This is called *tachycardia*. This may be associated with fever, an overactive thyroid gland, emotional excitement, hemorrhage, heart failure, or just a normal effect of exercise. When the heart beat is irregular, the diagnosis is more difficult. This may be the result of aberrant contraction in the heart or a complete instability of heart rhythm. An electrocardiogram is usually needed to establish the precise diagnosis.

Pain

Pain is one of the most common symptoms that prompts an individual to receive therapy. It results from irritation and stimulation of nerves that carry the feeling of pain to the brain. Actually, pain is a protective mechanism of the body. It is usually a warning that certain parts of the body are either diseased or injured. Sometimes, however, pain may be felt in an area of the body that is not diseased. This is called *referred pain*. Study the next chapter for a more comprehensive outline to various causes of pain and their rational treatment.

Convulsions

Convulsions are sometimes called spasms or fits. This usually is a sign of serious disease in the body. Such problems as epilepsy, a brain tumor, brain injury, stroke, or high blood pressure can cause convulsions. Some poisons, and drug overdoses (such as Insulin), may also produce seizures. First aid requires the patient's protection from injury. A rapid and careful diagnosis, then, is important to understand the mystery of these seizures.

These symptoms and many others comprise the signs of diverse disease states. It is easy to see how complicated actually determining the cause may become. Nevertheless, an important review of these signals, and their interrelationships, may provide the missing link to understanding the real causes of illness.

EXAMINATION OF THE BODY

Generally, the examination is called the **physical**. This involves a look a the patient, his skin, his eyes, his level of alertness, and any defects visible in any part of the body. It is important to touch and feel certain areas where there is pain, to see if it is due to afflictions in the skin, the muscles, or deeper structures. At times percussion is used to elicit areas of deeper tenderness. Tapping skillfully over an organ, such as the heart or liver, serves to outline its size, as well as compare that area with others for tenderness or distention, as when the bowel is obstructed and there is accumulation of gas.

Finally, the use of a *stethoscope* has achieved a degree of prominence in medical diagnosis and many uses of this may be learned by the layman, with a little practice. This instrument, invented by Laennec about 1816, has gone through many refinements in recent years. The stethoscope is commonly used to take the blood pressure. This measurement is extremely important in a physical examination, and can be done by anyone who understands the physiology involved and has practiced to attain proficiency.

The **blood pressure** is measured by wrapping the inflatable cuff, connected to a measuring device, around the arm, or sometimes the leg. Usually this is done with the patient in a sitting position, but it an also be done lying down or standing up, if the position of the patient is noted and the blood pressure compared with other postures. The standard of measurement is that of mercury barometer. Usually the pressure is measured in millimeters of mercury. The pictured instrument measures the blood pressure on a round dial. It is called an *aneroid*–type device, or *sphygmomanometer*.

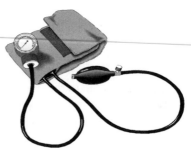

**The blood pressure cuff,
or *sphygmomanometer***

The blood pressure cuff, after being calibrated, is inflated by closing the screw knob on the blood pressure cuff. Careful listening over the artery detects the beginning of a sound. This is intermittent and corresponds to the beat of the heart, pumping blood through the now opened vessel. The pressure continues to drop; where it just begins to fade, a second muffled sound occurs, termed the diastolic pressure. The two figures are conventionally recorded as a fraction, i.e., 120/80. This is called the blood pressure. It is felt that although the pressure increases with advancing age in most people, a pressure higher than 140/90 is abnormal. Usually the lower values correlate with a lessened risk of cardiac disease or stroke.

The **pulse** is also an important measurement. It can be obtained by counting the pulsations in any artery of the body. The radial artery on the thumb side of the wrist, the carotid arteries in the neck, the femoral arteries in the groin, or small vessels in the forehead can also be used to measure the number of beats per minute the heart makes. More skill is required to assess the character of the pulse.

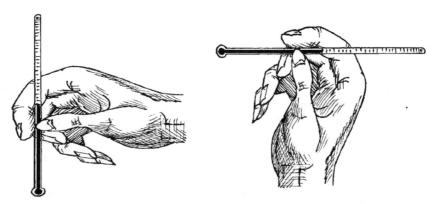

The *thermometer* should be held between two fingers only, shaking it down with a quick thrusting motion before taking the temperature. To read the thermometer, hold it at eye level and rotate it slightly until the mercury column becomes visible behind the scored degree markers.

Recording the **temperature** of the body is a useful marker of physical health. After the patient holds the thermometer under his tongue for three or more minutes, a careful reading of the thermometer usually gives the accurate temperature. If water or cold liquids have been taken just before the measurement, it will not be accurate until the mouth has returned to its

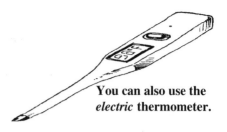

You can also use the *electric* thermometer.

previous temperature. Rectal temperatures can be taken and should always be used in children under four years of age. A patient who is comatose or unable to hold a thermometer in his mouth, and conditions where extreme shortness of breath prevents the taking of the temperature orally likewise require a rectal or axillary approach. Newer electronic thermometers are useful and safe in children, though more expensive. Most thermometers are available with directions that explain how they can be read. Disinfecting the thermometer in alcohol between patients is important for household hygiene.

Examination of the **head** can detect many health problems. The nose should be inspected to see if one side or the other is blocked, and if the blockage is due to mucous, blood, or some foreign material. Symmetry of the organs of the face, including eyes, ears, nose, and mouth, as well as the facial muscles, smiles and grimaces, can also be a helpful sign.

Inspection of the **ear** canals can be done with a flashlight or even better with an *otoscope*. This instrument has a small light, operated by batteries, attached to a speculum— a tiny plastic cone— that is inserted carefully into the ear to visualize the drum.

Shine a light into the **eyes** to reveal if both pupils are of equal size. Both should constrict when the light is beamed on them. The eyes should both track back and forth, and up and down in a normal direction.

The **teeth** should be in good condition with no inflammation, redness, or swelling of the gums. The tongue should be a healthy pink color. Redness of the **tongue** may indicate an inflammation, such as scarlet fever or a B vitamin deficiency. If the throat contains pus or a material resembling cottage cheese, infection with *Streptococcus* or yeast is quite likely. In children the tonsils protrude and could actually block the oral cavity, hindering swallowing or respiration. Unusual coating of the tongue is seen in certain disease states, particularly in tobacco users and in those who are dehydrated.

Careful palpation of the **neck** to estimate the size of the thyroid gland, to assess the quality of the pulses in the carotid arteries, and to detect any enlargement of the lymph nodes is advisable. At times stiffness in the neck, in association with high fever may be the first sign of meningitis, a serious infection in the lining of the brain and spinal cord.

Respirations should be free and unhindered. Both sides of the chest should expand equally and there should not be unusual retractions of soft tissues between the ribs during the phase of inhalation. Listening with the stethoscope over the lungs may disclose the presence of *wheezes*. These musical sounds are caused by bands of mucus in the bronchial tubes and may be associated with asthma, emphysema, or pneumonia. *Rales*, or crackling sounds, resemble the rubbing of hair between the fingers. They may indicate fluid in the small air sacs of the lungs. This is often found in pneumonia, and sometimes can also indicate congestion from heart disease.

The **heart sounds** are of particular interest and the "lub dup" sounds are familiar to anyone who has listened to the heart. The chest usually does not rise markedly, although a thrust may be felt with the hand on the left side of the breast bone, during heart contraction. Listening with the stethoscope should disclose a regular rhythm. Murmurs are sounds produced by damaged valves, where blood is flowing either in the wrong way or under difficultly, and may sound like the rushing of water through a pipe that is narrowed. These murmurs should be brought to the attention of a physician.

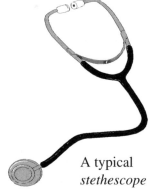

A typical *stethescope*

The **abdomen** should be soft. The liver edge is sometimes felt below the right rib margin. Tenderness in the right lower corner of the abdomen should be observed for possible appendicitis. Unusual bulges in the lower abdomen or groin may indicate a *hernia*. This rupture sometimes requires surgical repair. Listening with a stethoscope over the abdomen should disclose the presence of bowel sounds. These occur intermittently and are a gurgling or rushing in nature. The abdomen should not be unusually drum–sounding (*tympanitic*), as when distended by air, or completely dull–sounding to percussion, as when there is an excess of fluid accumulation.

The examination of the external *genitalia* may give some clue to disease. Female disorders will be covered in the chapter on obstetrics.

The **extremities** should move freely with a normal range of motion. *Varicose veins* are dilated blood vessels in the legs. These may be troublesome. Occasionally thrombosis or clotting occurs. The calves of the legs should not be tender and the ankles should move freely. Stiffness in the ankles or pain in the calves when the foot is raised may be an early indicator of a clot in the veins, called *thrombophlebitis*.

Reflexes may be assessed by stroking the abdomen to elicit a muscle contraction. Tapping just below the knee cap, with the leg hanging in a relaxed position, should elicit a kicking motion. The Achilles' tendon behind the heel can be tapped briskly with a small blunt object to provoke a foot contraction in a downward direction. The *Babinski sign* is an abnormal reflex, except in infants, and involves a spreading of the toes with raising of the great toe when the bottom of the foot is stroked with a sharp object. This indicates central nervous system disease, and is often seen after a stroke or in multiple sclerosis.

The gait is evaluated by having the patient walk, noticing if there is tremor, unsteadiness, limping, or lack of coordination. Balance can be tested at the same time. Coordination of all the extremities is important in evaluating a person for neurological disease.

LABORATORY TESTING

Most laboratories today require requisitions from a physician to run various tests. New self-care home kits are now available for many screening tests, which can be done at home. Some of these are as follows: pregnancy test, blood cholesterol, blood glucose, and stool testing for occult blood. The latter is useful to periodically evaluate possible blood loss, as well as causes for anemia. Urine testing for protein or sugar, and fasting blood sugar measurements, are good screening tests for diabetes. These tests can be done on a group basis at health fairs, and for a considerably reduced cost.

Cholesterol and **triglyceride** evaluations are periodically performed in coronary screening programs, and occasionally, it is possible to secure chest x-rays, electrocardiograms, and even treadmill tests from public health groups or private groups screening for cardiovascular disease. Sometimes the YMCA, religious camp meetings, or special health fairs in shopping centers will provide these tests at a very reasonable cost. Cooperative physicians may provide other laboratory determinations in the case of acute disease.

TYPES OF THERAPY

In the privacy of your home, there are several types of therapy that deserve particular attention. Naturally, it is our instinctive tendency to look for the simplest way of getting well. Often people resort to **drugs** in an attempt to cure themselves, only to find that the drug has changed the form and location the disease, producing new symptoms or complications that might even be worse than the original disease. Furthermore, the expense of drugs, together with their long term risk are reason for great caution in their use by the home health practitioner.

Diet is an extremely important type of home treatment. In case of illness, the patient's diet should be more simple than is usually eaten. Sometimes a fruit fast for a few days will help a person recover without a grain of medicine. Juices have a more limited place. Sometimes skipping a meal and drinking water or fruit juice will allow nature a chance to build up defenses against the invader. This should be done at mealtimes, not drinking juices all through the day.

Herb teas have a valued place in healing. Hence, a special chapter is being devoted to their use. Medicinal teas are usually prepared by mixing one teaspoon of the herb in a cup of boiling water and allowing it to steep for three to five minutes, until the tea is ready. The herb is strained out before drinking. Other herbal beverages made with parsley or comfrey, create the so called "green drink," which is popular in health food stores today. There are many common symptoms that can be treated safely with herbs, making it unnecessary to consult a physician nearly as often as we do these days.

Hydrotherapy seems to be the most neglected home remedy. These treatments involve the use of water, and include such remedies as the hot half bath, cold shower, cold mitten friction, contrast bath, the heating compress, and other therapies discussed in chapters devoted to the specific treatments. Hydrotherapy offers a powerful technique of shifting the circulation in your body. Its purpose is to decongest certain areas, then improve the ability of an organ to fight infection and overcome any invasion of germs. *Perfect health depends upon perfect circulation.* Water therapy is one of the most valuable ways to achieve this goal.

Exercise is also a valuable remedy in the treatment of many diseases, particularly those of degenerative nature. The chapters on heart disease, vascular disease, respiratory problems, and nervous disorders will particularly contain advice in regard to therapeutic exercise.

Sunlight, fresh air, abstinence from harmful substances, **rest**, and the mind healing influence of **trusting in Divine power** are also powerful remedies that one can use in the home to combat disease and restore right conditions within the system. We will apply these in the next chapter to approach the subject of pain, one of the most common symptoms that afflicts mankind.

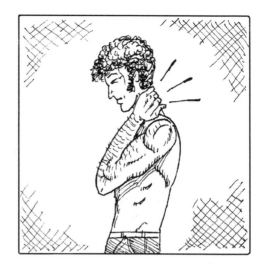

CHAPTER TWO

CAUSES,

TREATMENTS,

AND

REMEDIES

FOR

PAIN

Pain, it has been said, is one of nature's first signs of illness. Most will agree that *pain* stands preeminent among all unpleasant sensory experiences by which people perceive disease within themselves. There are very few illnesses which do not have painful phases. In many conditions, pain is characteristic of the illness, without which the diagnosis must remain in doubt.

In order to understand the subject of pain, every individual should understand normal *anatomy*. Pain is perceived as an unpleasant sensation, because of the stimulation of certain nerves in the skin or internal organs. These electrical messages are carried through our nerves to the spinal cord, then up specific pathways to the brain. An unpleasant sensation is first perceived in a portion of the brain called the **thalamus**. A rendezvous with nerve connections to the highest nerve centers, finally sends a message on to the cortex, our outer covering of the brain. There it is interpreted as to location, type, intensity, and integrated with past experiences and avoidance mechanisms that will protect your body from damage.

Pain may be perceived from any of your nerves. Cold, heat, pin prick, pressure, muscle spasm, distention of hollow organs, lack of oxygen to certain areas, and other stimuli may be perceived as pain. Some types of pain, such as phantom pain, occur after an amputation, following less known pathways, but presumably they result from irritation of nerve endings. Direct pressure on a nerve, as in degenerative disc disease of the spinal column or other conditions where peripheral nerves are compressed can also be painful. Infections of the nerves, such as that produced by the *shingles* virus may produce severe unrelenting pain. So, there are many mechanisms, many syndromes, and a most careful study is necessary to understand the causes of the pain response.

Several **types of pain** can be confused. The stimuli that arouses pain varies from organ to tissue. For example, the intestinal tract is not responsive at all to pin prick, burning, cutting or pressure. But it responds with exquisite pain to the distention produced by stretching, as in an obstruction or the mere presence of excessive gas. In contrast, the skin is exquisitely sensitive to pin prick, burning, freezing, and cutting. Each of these sensations is carried through separate nerve receptors. The nerve impulse is mediated by specific chemical agents. Such substances as acetylcholine, serotonin, histamine, and bradykinin are released by tissue injury, and have been found to elicit pain when applied to the base of a blister.

It is felt that the **threshold** for perception of pain is approximately the same in all persons. This threshold is lowered by inflammation, in alcoholics, and is influenced by certain other analgesic drugs as well as strong emotions, such as fear or rage. Greatly varying, however, is the degree of emotional reaction, and the verbalization (or complaint) in response to pain. The personality and character of the individual influences this reaction greatly.

Superficial Pain

The largest pain fibers are used in transmitting a pricking type of pain. Sharp sensations are conducted much more rapidly than a sense of burning. Most normal individuals can localize instantly such pains with precision. This surface sensitivity to the place where a stimulus is applied helps us distinguish superficial pain from deeper types.

Visceral Pain

Deep pain, including that of the internal organs and skeletal structures, has basically the quality of severe aching. However, intense, visceral pain may also be sharp or knife-like. Occasionally there is a burning type of deep pain, as in the case of heartburn from esophageal irritation, and rarely, in the angina pectoris of heart disease. These pains are felt beneath the body surface. Localization is poor and the margins of pain are not well outlined, presumably because of the scarcity of nerve endings in these organs.

Deep Musculoskeletal Pain

The same common nerve system transmits the impulse of both deep skeletal pain and visceral pain. Hence, their characteristics as to type, localization, and referral are similar. These pains are usually corresponding to the nerve roots coming from the spinal cord. A knowledge of nerve anatomy helps to localize these pains as to origin, although the exact origin is often obscure.

Referred Pain

Deep pains within the body organs tend always to be referred to the surface structures within the similar and corresponding spinal segment. In the case of pain from the heart muscle, these nerve impulses refer such pain primarily to the chest wall overlying the heart. Sometimes this extends up to the shoulder and the neck, most commonly on the left side. Pain from the rectum, prostate or female organs is usually referred into the low back. Sometime the back of the neck is involved in the referral from pain in the sinus region. Since a similar nerve innervates the shoulder and the diaphragm, irritation under the diaphragm as in a liver or gallbladder condition, or upper abdominal abscesses can be felt near the shoulder blade.

Radicular Pain

This type of pain usually refers to the shooting extension of pain from the neck or low back. A disc that is pinching part of a root of the sciatic nerve usually sends a shock-like sensation down the nerve along the side or the back of the leg. This may coexist with numbness in the involved extremity, and, at times, weakness or lack of reflexes can also be seen. Similar types of radicular pain are present in the upper extremities from disease in the spine at the neck.

Psychological Aspects of Pain

The emotional state can influence greatly the perception of pain and its effect upon the body in general. Ambrose Paré, a French Huguenot barber and surgeon, remarked, "There is nothing that abateth so much the strength, as pain." Continuous pain can be observed to have an adverse effect on the entire nervous system. There are increased irritabilities, fatigue, troubled sleep, poor appetite, and loss of emotional stability.

Courageous men are sometimes reduced to a whimpering, pitiable state in their reaction to severe pain. They become irrational about illness and may make unreasonable demands on their family. This condition is sometimes called "pain shock," and, when established, requires delicate, but firm management. Depression is common, especially in chronic pain syndromes. At times unfortunately, the demands for and dependency on narcotic drugs often complicate the picture.

SPECIAL TYPES OF PAIN

Headache

The term *headache* encompasses all aches and pains associated in the head. Along with fatigue, hunger, and thirst, headache represents man's most frequent discomfort. It must always be kept in mind that headache is a symptom, not a disease, and its cause should always be ascertained. Some types of headaches are quite easy to diagnose. Infection or blockage of sinuses is usually accompanied by pain over the sinus area and in the forehead. It is often associated with tenderness of the skin in the same area. Sometimes the head seems to throb. Often headaches tend to return at the same hour of the day.

Headache originating in the eye is usually located near the eye or in the forehead. It is of steady, aching type and tends to follow prolonged use of the eyes in close work. Muscle imbalance is often involved. A careful examination of the eyes by your doctor is recommended.

Headaches accompanying diseases of the ligaments, muscles, and joints in the upper spine are usually referred to the back of the head and nap of the neck. Later in life, these pains are seen frequently in arthritis and also tend to occur after whiplash injuries. Massage very deeply in the area and you may disclose the presence of tender nodules near the insertion of the neck muscles. Moist heat, as well as skillfully performed massage are particularly helpful in relieving this type of pain.

The headache of irritation in the meninges or coverings of the brain, is usually of an acute onset and becomes severe, deep seated, and constant. Usually this occurs in conjunction with fever. Whenever the neck becomes stiff, immediate consultation with a physician is recommended. Both meningeal infections or brain hemorrhages can cause this type of pain. Lumbar puncture in about 20% of normal patients may produce a transient headache. Usually this is relieved in the lying position and subsides after a few days.

Migraine

The term *migraine* refers to periodic, throbbing headaches on one side of the head, which usually begins in childhood or adolescence, and occur with diminishing frequency during advancing years. Sometimes, along with the headache, nausea and vomiting may actually disable the affected individual for several hours each time the migraine occurs. Some variations are seen. Many are forced to lie down and to shun light and noise for what they call a "sick headache." Other milder forms do not require withdrawal from accustomed activities. Between attacks the migraine sufferer is essentially normal. In fact, the headache seems to be brought on during the "let down" period after many days of hard work or stress. Spasm in the blood vessels has been implicated and many powerful hormones are often released that perpetuate discomfort for several hours.

Tension Headache

This type of headache usually occurs over both sides of the head and often settles at the base of the neck. A fullness, tightness, or pressure is often described. Sometimes these headaches show the peculiarity of being continuous day and night for long periods of time. Sustained muscle tension, as well as vascular changes may be involved. Sometimes a similar headache may follow injury (auto accidents, head trauma) and gradually resolves over many months.

Simple remedies may be used with success in the treatment of headache. A person should lie down in a quiet area, apply a cold compress to the head, and seek to put the mind at rest. Often a drink of water or mild nerve-calming tea such as catnip or chamomile tea can relax the person until the headache passes. More severe types of headaches can be treated with the hot foot bath. This is described in the section on hydrotherapy. Adding mustard to the foot bath may also bring relief through acting as a *counterirritant* as well as pulling blood to the lower extremities (called *derivation*) to relieve congestion in the head. Extra hours for sleep, daily nature walks, or a change of pace may be needed. General hygienic recommendations for a more healthful diet, systematic exercise, and improved stress control are valuable preventives.

Chest Pain

There is very little parallel between the severity of chest pain and the seriousness of its cause. A frequent problem exists in distinguishing trivial disorders from coronary artery disease or other serious health hazards. It is important to avoid the long tradition now shown to be myth, that pain beneath the left breast or radiating into the left arm is always of cardiac origin. Such pain is often observed in patients who are tense, easily fatigued, or anxious.

Oxygen deficiency of the heart muscle can produce pain. This is the syndrome medically termed *angina pectoris*. When the oxygen supply is deficient in relation to the need, pain will develop in the heart muscle. This may be aggravated by exercise, or occur during a stressful situation, or after a heavy meal. Atherosclerosis (narrowing) of the coronary arteries is the most common cause. Spasms of the small cardiac vessels may also trigger this pain (*angina*), which usually subsides with a short rest. Further approaches to treatment are described in Chapter Four.

Pain in the esophagus usually results from acid irritation of the lining (mucous membrane) of the esophagus. Spasm of the swallowing muscles or the presence of obstruction can also produce this deep chest pain. Accompanying symptoms of difficult swallowing, regurgitation, and weight loss direct attention to the esophagus.

Pain in the pleura or the lining of the lung is very common. It results from stretching of the inflamed membrane and occurs in viral, as well as bacterial, pneumonia. Sometimes air in the chest cavity *(pneumothorax)* and tumors can mimic this type of pain. Inflammation of the outer covering of the heart *(pericarditis)* can also produce it. It is usually aggravated by coughing or deep breathing. Sometimes swallowing or a change in bodily position produces the same type of pain. Applications of moist heat and rest are important in the relief of these deeper pains.

Tension is also a common cause of chest wall pain. Usually the discomfort is experienced as a sense of tightness, sometimes called aching. It may occur on various occasions and in different areas of the chest, and is usually associated with fatigue or emotional strain. It is important to distinguish these and the above categories of chest pain from various abdominal problems, some of which are described below.

Abdominal Pain

The correct interpretation of acute abdominal pain is one of the most challenging demands made of any physician. Sometimes proper therapy requires urgent action. A great deal of experience and judgment is needed to elucidate the cause.

A number of mechanisms can produce abdominal pain. Inflammation of the lining of the abdomen *(peritoneum)* can produce pain of steady, aching character. This pain is usually located directly over the inflamed area and the area will also be quite tender. Release of a small amount of stomach acid will cause much more pain than even contaminated intestinal contents will when the appendix ruptures.

Another type of pain occurs in the distention or obstruction of hollow organs. This is usually intermittent or cramping in nature. *Colic* in the abdomen can be produced from obstruction of bile duct, the gallbladder, the ureters or the intestines. Since all of these may cause vomiting, the location of the pain and other related symptoms must be considered in arriving at a rapid diagnosis. Finally, it is important to consider the blood vessels in the abdomen as causes of potential pain. An out pouching of the aorta *(aneurysm)* may produce pain, developing slowly, increasing gradually, or in a sudden rupture, may become quite catastrophic. Abdominal angina occurs when the vascular supply to the intestines becomes clogged with cholesterol deposits and this pain, similar to the angina pectoris of the heart, occurs following a heavy meal.

Referred pain from the chest, the spine, or the pelvic organs, may also make diagnosis difficult. Compression or irritation of nerve roots in the spine is usually intensified by coughing, sneezing, or straining. Pressure on the genital organs will usually be very painful and show the origin immediately of this referred pain. Respiratory origin is usually indicated by obvious interference with breathing.

It is important to become acquainted with the clinical pictures of these various abdominal problems. A knowledge of anatomy of abdominal organs, as well as their function is essential in understanding abdominal pain. Some types can be treated safely at home. In these cases, moist heat and temporary abstinence from food is often helpful. There are conditions requiring surgical intervention. Basically keeping in mind these possibilities, will help an individual to seek a physician promptly at the appropriate time while avoiding unnecessary dependence on drugs or expensive diagnostic testing in the more self-limited and trivial conditions.

Back Pain

Pain in the lower back, as well as the neck is very common in America. Many related, but distinct conditions can produce discomfort here. Disease of the spine, although less common than other problems, is often related to injury. An auto accident or sudden fall, causing acute flexion of the back, may compress and fracture one of the vertebral bodies. It may be an early sign of osteoporosis, thinning of the bones due to calcium deficiency. X-ray is often necessary to diagnose this condition accurately. Immobilization on a straight board, with the avoidance of any flexion, standing, or walking is extremely important First Aid in dealing with these acute injuries. Braces which keep the back in extension are often worn for several months in the treatment of a fractured spine.

Local pain in the low back can be caused by any process which irritates nerve endings. Straining of the muscles, protrusion of a disc, rupture of a ligament, and many less common problems can injure the tissues and aggravate this pain. Tenderness is usually found upon pressure in the region involved. Associated muscle spasm may produce pain around the involved area. At times, the pain may be referred or projected into regions lying in the area of the associated nerve roots. For example, pain produced by diseases in the upper part of the lumbar spine is usually referred to the front of the thighs and legs. That from the lower part of the lumbar spine, is referred to the buttocks, posterior thighs, and calves. *Radicular* or root pain has some similar characteristics, but usually is much more intense and is often aggravated by a cough, sneeze, or strain. Any motion which stretches the nerve, such as straight leg raising, may have a similar effect.

Proper examination of the back is an art requiring considerable knowledge of muscle, nerve and skeletal anatomy. Often tenderness over the lumbosacral junction, the sacroiliac joint, the costovertebral angle over the kidneys, or a specific vertebra can help the examiner in accurate diagnosis. The usual testing of the blood, urine, and x-rays of the back are often adjuncts in understanding the cause. Appropriate exercises may then be used, together with rest or the use of moist heat in bringing relief to all but the most stubborn condition. Special problems may be treated effectively in a lifestyle center.

Musculoskeletal Pain

Pain involving the ligaments and muscles is often seen in athletic injuries. When the ligament is torn, the injury is called a *sprain*. This often occurs in the ankle, the knee, the low back, or shoulder. Muscles that are bruised often become painful and when the injury is considerable, that is called a *strain*. These small ligaments and muscle fibers may actually be torn, but heal without any residual weakness, after a short period of rest.

Inflammation of the bursa *(bursitis)* may occur as the result of trauma, arthritis, infection or other disorders. Common locations include the shoulder, hip, knee, elbow and heel. Severe local pain and tenderness is often present. Sometimes calcium deposits are seen on x-ray. Immediate application of cold in the form of snow or an ice bag is one of the most helpful remedies, followed by mild exercise and gentle hot and cold compresses, after the acute inflammation subsides.

The **tendon** sheath of the hand or wrist may become inflamed. Some of these are due to constriction of tendons or nerves, and may require surgery. In the wrist this is called carpal tunnel syndrome. Others are seen in conjunction with rheumatoid arthritis, discussed in chapter five.

A number of **metabolic** problems can produce, skeletal pain, muscle cramps, or deep visceral pain. The sudden restriction of oxygen supply, disorders of the adrenal glands, and the so-called *autoimmune* diseases, may produce severe weakness or muscle pain.

Three forms of **vascular** obstruction particularly deserve mention. Arteriosclerosis of the large and medium sized arteries is the most common vascular disease of man. This often leads to pain in the muscles, particularly in the legs induced by exercise *(intermittent claudication)*. Diabetic patients are particularly susceptible. Often the pulses in the lower extremities are reduced. Changes occur in the skin with hair loss, deterioration of the nails, and even gangrene. **Buerger's disease** *(thromboangiitis obliterans)* is a disease of young and middle-aged male cigarette smokers. This hypersensitivity to tobacco produces spasm in the small vessels of the hands and feet. Sometimes a smoker is so addicted to nicotine, that he continues to pursue the habit, in spite of progressive gangrene and amputation of fingers, feet, legs, and even hands. I have often seen these unnecessarily handicapped patients suffering the terrible sequels of nicotine addiction.

Raynaud's disease is often caused by cold. Women are most commonly afflicted. With exposure to cold, their fingers become white, then blue, and finally red. Pain and tingling are common during this crisis, due to the lack of blood supply. Exercising by whirling the arm in a windmill motion can help to bring blood to the involved areas. Another occupational complication of a similar nature may produce ulceration in fingertips or toes. These are more commonly seen in smokers and those with auto-immune disorders.

Obstruction of the lymphatic return may produce a type of edema, associated with pain. Also, *thrombosis* of the veins is usually painful, involving the overlying skin with redness and swelling. When larger veins are involved, the muscle and entire extremity is very painful.

Most of these pain syndromes can be approached effectively by the intelligent home health observer. With a knowledge of anatomy and physiology, and a few simple remedies, they can bring relief to many cases. It is important first to ascertain the *cause* of these pain responses. Wrong habits may need to be corrected. Then nature is assisted in her efforts to restore right conditions within the nerves, muscles, and other involved organs. The relief of pain will always evoke profound gratitude from chronic sufferers. Its study can challenge the layman or specialist for at least a lifetime.

CHAPTER THREE

COMMON
INFECTIONS

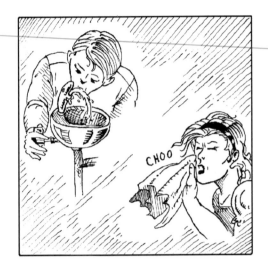

The majority of human illnesses with known causes are produced by infectious agents. In fact, some of the greatest medical discoveries in the twentieth century have resulted in the controlling of many contagious diseases through public health measures, sanitary engineering, immunization, etc. Although there remain some exceptions to this rule, infectious diseases as a class are more easily prevented and cured than any other major group of disorders. Yet, despite the elimination of certain infectious diseases and a profound reduction in the death statistics of others, man is by no means free of infection. Only a modest decrease in the total effect of disease has been produced through these control measures. I am thinking primarily of smallpox vaccinations and malaria control.

Additionally, numerous **new** infections have resulted from the widespread use of broad spectrum antibiotics, immune suppressive agents used in transplant procedures, the progressive longevity of people with chronic degenerative disease, and high-risk lifestyles such as drug abuse and homosexuality. Life threatening diseases that were never seen before this decade are now invading the immune deficient. These infections are termed *opportunistic*.

There is a very complex interaction between the microorganism and man when an infectious disease occurs. Much has been learned about the way microbes enter the body, the ways they produce injury to the tissues, and the resistance of a person (the host), as well as the mechanism of recovery. Unfortunately, though, it is often difficult to transfer much of this scientific information to help the individual patient with his infection. It is well known that microorganisms of different species or different strains of the same species, vary widely in their capacity to produce disease. Furthermore, we know that human beings are not equally susceptible to disease caused by a given bacterium or virus. Fortunately for us, the mere presence of an organism in the body does not always lead to clinical illness. Often there is a *carrier* state (like the story of Typhoid Mary) or a hidden *(subclinical)* infection. Several factors are involved in the mechanism of getting an infectious disease.

Most microorganisms that are capable of producing disease vary in several ways. Their *virulence*, that is, the degree of capability to produce illness, can be distinguished from their *invasiveness*, or their ability to spread and disseminate in the body. A few parasites produce *toxins* that account for their ability to damage body tissues. Some organisms tend to localize in certain cells or organs and produce their damage there. Most vital, we must try to understand the natural and acquired factors that can enable a person to not only resist the invasion of organisms, but also reduce our susceptibility to disease. The white blood cells, the antibodies, many enzymes, and environmental factors including nutrition, can affect a person's recovery from infectious disease.

There are general features that suggest infection. The **abrupt onset** of any illness, particularly associated with fever and chills, may well indicate an infection. Pain in the muscles, sensitivity to light, sore throat, swelling of the lymph nodes or spleen, and upset in the digestive tract, often constitute hallmarks of infections. Many specific infectious diseases can be recognized by the "story of illness", or medical history, in association with obvious physical findings. Blood counts, urine testing, x-rays of the chest, and more specific laboratory procedures can be helpful in confirming the diagnosis of more difficult cases.

Many organisms that cause disease can be demonstrated by a microscopic examination of properly stained preparations of sputum, spinal fluid, and other body secretions. The microscope is indeed a most helpful laboratory instrument in the diagnosis of infections. **Cultures** can be obtained from the blood, sputum, urine, and other discharges. Investigation by the microbiologist, who applies appropriate tests to the germs, while growing these cultures in his incubator, will usually yield the specific infectious agent, particularly in bacterial disease. The presence of **antibodies** may indicate the type of infection, and for contagious illnesses, such as tuberculosis, the skin test is very useful. All of these diagnostic procedures help to determine the cause, which then can lead one to specific therapy.

VIRAL ILLNESSES

By far, the majority of mild illnesses affecting people in their homes are caused by viruses. These conditions are usually self–limited, that is, our bodies overcome the infection and get well spontaneously. Recent advances in the science of microbiology, including the use of the electron microscope, have helped to identify most of these germs. Viruses are nonliving organisms, different from bacteria or protozoa (one-celled animals). The virus particle is a combination of proteins and nucleic acid. They enter the cell of the host, take over its specific enzyme systems, and rapidly multiply to produce disease. Some of the more common viral infections will be discussed below.

The Common Cold

More than one hundred types of viruses are known to cause the common cold. This explains why scientific attempts to produce a vaccine have been so unsatisfactory. Over 40% of respiratory illnesses in children and adults are caused by this family of organisms. Although colds occur throughout the year, there are peaks of incidence in the spring and fall. The disease is more severe in children, especially those under two years of age. Higher fevers, cough, croup, and occasionally pneumonia occur. Family infections are more often initiated by children. They spread like gossip in schools or any setting where close contact is found.

After introducing the respiratory virus into the nose or throat, congestion, symptoms of discharge in the nose, general aching, and mild headache result. There is usually no fever. Nasal secretions increase over the period of a day or two. After a week or more, the individual has completely recovered. A number of factors predispose to the common cold, including unwise ingestion of a large amount of sugar, and exposure to sudden changes in temperature, particularly with chilling. Negative emotions are thought to be related to host susceptibility through a change in the acidity of the nasal mucous membrane. Such reactions as hatred, anger, fear and frustration bring about the temporary deficiency of *lysozyme*, a potent enzyme capable of killing many germs.

The treatment for a cold should include the general health measures for respiratory hygiene, utilizing copious intake of fluids, especially water, increased rest, steam inhalations, hot packs over the congested areas, and the avoidance of close contact with other people who are susceptible to the same disease. Recovery is usually complete. Diet should be light with easily digested foods, especially fruit.

Influenza

A great deal of attention has been directed toward the prevention influenza, (an Italian word referring to the *influence* of heavenly bodies previously thought to cause disease). The disastrous epidemic of 1918 caused an estimated 20 to 40 million deaths from this viral disease. Vaccinations are available annually, especially recommended for the elderly and others with a chronic debilitating illness.

HOME REMEDIES FOR COLDS AND FLU

FRUIT, JUICES, extra WATER

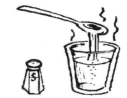

GARGLES with hot salt water, use 1/2 tsp. of salt per glass of hot water

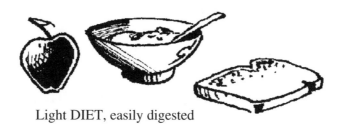

Light DIET, easily digested

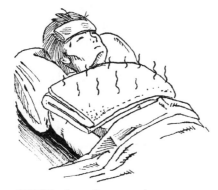

REST, chest fomentations

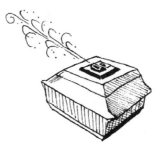

Steam VAPORIZER, Humidifier

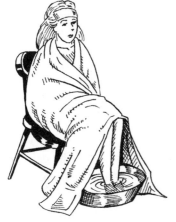

Hot FOOT BATH

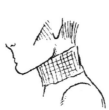

Heating COMPRESS to neck, for sore throat, laryngitis (see chap. 17)

Flu symptoms are of sudden onset, with headache, muscle pains, fever, and prostration. Often a discharge from the nose, sneezing, hoarseness, cough, chest pain, and shortness of breath and or gastric symptoms make the patient feel quite ill. The disease begins within one to three days after exposure. Like other common viral infections, antibiotics are completely ineffective.

Hot baths are very helpful and should always be followed by a cool shower, cold mitten friction (Chapter 17) and a period of bed rest. The avoidance of usual activities and the consumption of a light diet, such as fruit, juices, and increased water intake, will help your body fight these infections. Hot packs to the chest (as described in the chapter on hydrotherapy) and steam inhalations will relieve many of the symptoms of chest pain, and aid the fight for recovery. They help as well to control fever. Return to full activity should be gradual. Usually one infection confers immunity to that particular type of virus.

Polio

Poliomyelitis was a common acute viral infection; it occurs naturally only in human beings. Infection with the polio virus produces a wide variety of clinical manifestations. Its most severe form attacks part of the central nervous system. After an incubation period of 3 to 35 days, the poliovirus infection may assume one of four forms: 1) Inapparent infection. 2) Minor illness, such as a transient respiratory or gastrointestinal disturbance. 3) Nonparalytic Poliomyelitis, which usually produces temporary stiffness of the neck and other symptoms of spinal meningitis. 4) Paralytic poliomyelitis.

In the latter, most serious form, the virus attacks specialized cells in the spinal cord and brain stem, producing paralysis in the face or extremities. This varies from mild affliction to respiratory paralysis. Some of the most heroic medical treatments have been developed to save the lives of these respiratory polio cases, often maintaining the patient for years in an "iron lung." Some of the most dramatic uses of hydrotherapy have also been effective in the treatment of advanced polio cases, especially the Kenny packs, used for severe muscle spasm. Rehabilitation in a specialized setting offers maximal potential for complete recovery. Prevention, however, is the best approach. With several vaccines available for each type of polio, childhood immunization offers an inexpensive and relatively safe medical practice to avoid this dreaded disease.

Rabies

All mammals are affected by this serious viral disease of the central nervous system. Usually, it is transmitted by accidental or traumatic inoculation with infected saliva. The bite of an animal may transfer this to humans. The **urban** type is propagated chiefly by unimmunized domestic dogs. Sylvatic rabies is propagated in skunks, foxes, raccoons, wolves, and bats. When the live rabies virus is introduced through an animal bite, there will be an early infection in 1-4 days, marked by fever, headache, fatigue, nausea, vomiting, or cough. Later, encephalitis develops with excitation, confusion, hallucination, combativeness, muscle spasm, and seizures. The latter dysfunction of brain stem centers brings the traditional picture of foaming at the mouth, followed by frank paralysis, coma, and death. Unless artificial supportive measures are instituted, the survival is seldom longer than four days!

Approximately 30,000 persons in the United States and 1,000,000 in the world are treated preventively for rabies each year. The local wound should be generously scrubbed with soap, then flushed with water or alcohol. Lacerations should not be sewed shut. Active immunization is then given with either nerve tissue derived vaccine (NTV) or duck embryo derived vaccine (DEV). When the vaccine is given alone, fourteen daily doses are sufficient. When rabies vaccine is given with antirabies antiserum, twenty-one daily injections, followed by boosters, ten and twenty days after the initial series is required. The antirabies antiserum from human origin is best, to avoid serum sickness so common when equine (horse) serums are used. Until recently, rabies in a human being was regarded as 100% fatal. With the advent of specific vaccines, as well as intensive cardiorespiratory assistance, for the first time in history there is hope of survival in this dreaded disease.

Gastrointestinal Viruses

Although tropical diseases and food poisoning may cause sudden vomiting, nausea, and diarrhea, viral infections are very commonly the cause of these symptoms. These are usually transmitted through stool-to-mouth contact. Personal hygiene, particularly hand washing eliminates the infectious cycle. Toddlers often bring intestinal viruses into a household. Insects, including flies and mosquitoes may act as carriers (vectors). Their incubation period lasts 2-5 days. Symptoms may be limited to the throat with soreness or tonsillar enlargement, but skin rash, and serious illness— hepatitis, viral meningitis, or pericarditis (inflammation of the pericardium)— is also seen. *Pleurodynia* (pain in the pleura or coverings of the lungs) also occurs in these viral infections, as well as malaise, sore throat, anorexia, fever and severe muscle and abdominal pain. Cardiac disease brings symptoms of heart murmurs, electrocardiographic changes, and even heart failure.

By far more common, though, is the illness we term *viral gastroenteritis*, also called "winter vomiting" or "intestinal flu". This disease is highly contagious; many cases are often seen in one family. Onset usually occurs within 48 hours, and recovery is rapid. Less commonly, mild diarrhea may persist for several weeks. General measures for the treatment of any infection, including adequate fluid intake, rest, and hydrotherapy (hot packs) to relieve abdominal pain, constitute the general measures most effective in these self-limited conditions.

Hantavirus

Carried by the deer mouse (*Peromyscus maniculatus*) this strain of virus caused in 1993 a serious outbreak of respiratory illness. Fever, muscular aching, and cough--all resembling flu symptoms--are followed by abrupt onset of severe respiratory distress. Patients had seemed otherwise healthy. Many (56%) of the victims died in our initial outbreak, located in the southwestern United States. Treatment was primarily supportive, with stabilization of serious cases in hospital intensive care.

To prevent **hantavirus** exposure, avoid occupational or leisure activities that bring individuals into contact with infected rodents, their excreta or bites. This requires caution in harvesting field crops, sleeping in vacant cabins, cleaning barns, or living in dwellings with indoor rodent populations. Prevention is the best approach to cure.

CHILDHOOD INFECTIONS

Measles

Measles *(Rubeola)* has increased its epidemic potential with the development of large city schools. Measles occurs naturally only in human beings. Usually after exposure, a child develops his first symptoms in 9-11 days. Malaise, high fever, and irritability is associated with inflammation of the eyes, tearing, a hacking cough, and nasal discharge. One to eight days later a rash develops, with small spots on the mucous membrane of the mouth and a red rash, at times slightly elevated, breaking out over the forehead, spreading downward over the face, neck, and trunk. Each spot (lesion) persists for about three days and disappears in the same order; total duration of the rash is about six days. Rarely complications of fluid retention or pneumonia develop; but most measles cases are self-limited, with a complete recovery conferring lifetime immunity. A vaccine is available to protect very young children, patients with tuberculosis, and others whose immune mechanisms are likely to be impaired.

Rubella *(German measles)* is a much more benign disease, often called the "three days measles". After 14-21 days from exposure, there will be a mild illness for 1-7 days consisting of malaise, headache, and fever. The non-blistering rash then develops on the forehead and face, spreading downward to the trunk and extremities. Recovery is usually complete. However, serious complications may be seen when a pregnant mother becomes infected. Within the first three months of pregnancy, the developing child is susceptible to *congenital rubella.* Fetal infection at such a vulnerable period may lead to severe handicaps—heart malformation, mental retardation, or deafness. For this reason it is important that the mother should avoid contact with anyone who might have measles during early pregnancy. She should **never** receive a vaccination if there is a possibility of pregnancy within the following two months.

Smallpox

The pox viruses are a disease producing family, including the severe contagious febrile illness *(variola)* commonly called **smallpox**. The disease involves a rash, characterized by small blisters and pustules, with an incubation period of about 12 days. There is no specific therapy for smallpox. Primarily one attempts to prevent bacterial infection and maintain a fluid balance. The *vaccinia* (cowpox) virus was purified and developed for inoculation to specifically prevent smallpox. Currently, these vaccinations are no longer used, for no smallpox cases have been found in the world in at least a decade. It is one of the few contagious diseases that science may have eradicated with strictly preventive measures. For this we thank the Lord! Individuals with immune deficiency, leukemia, or with a widespread skin rash, of course, should **never** be given the smallpox vaccination.

Chicken Pox and Shingles

Chicken Pox *(varicella)* is a contagious disease, usually seen in children. It is characterized by fever and a small blistering eruption. The same pox virus also produces *herpes zoster* or "shingles", characterized by a one-sided segmental inflammation of one spinal or cranial nerve. Painful localized blisters erupt on the skin over the distribution of the small nerve. Although chicken pox is more highly contagious, shingles is more distressing. Severe pain often lasts for weeks to months, particularly in older individuals. Acute shingles as well as post-herpetic *neuralgia* may respond to fever therapy, given early in the course of the disease. Given in the form of steam bath or at home in a bathtub, specific fever treatments can thwart the infection early and prevent many complications.

Cold Sores

Herpes simplex virus, a "second cousin" of the shingles virus, is the usual cause of cold sores. These painful lesions often erupt during a fever or other illness. They may also occur during times of stress. Except for drying agents, such as camphor or the use of topical steroids, no specific treatment is available.

37

Other viral diseases of the skin include the *foot and mouth disease* of children (Coxsackie virus), *warts, milker's nodule,* contracted from infected cows, and *molluscum contagiosum,* an infectious disease of the skin caused by the largest known viruses.

Cat scratch disease is a viral infection characterized by swelling of the regional lymph nodes, secondary to an animal scratch, usually a cat. The diagnosis is usually made from the history, with confirmation by a skin test or lymph node biopsy. The recovery is usually complete.

Infectious mononucleosis is a viral illness, and usually seen in young adults. A severe sore throat associated with a rash on the palate, enlargement of the lymph nodes and spleen, general weakness, muscle aching, and at times central nervous system symptoms are a result. Confirmatory blood tests (the Mono spot) can pinpoint the disease with accuracy in its early stages. Specific fever therapy associated with rest, a spare diet, and other symptomatic measures can usually provide a rapid recovery.

Chronic fatigue syndrome (CFS) is a more serious and lasting complication of viral illness. Unresolved infections with the Mono virus can sometimes result in a complex syndrome of recurrent sore throat, muscle aching, swollen lymph nodes, joint pain, and profound fatigue. Psychological disturbance results, with memory loss, difficulty concentrating, anxiety and depression. The *Epstein-Barr virus* is one of many organisms that can produce this syndrome. Specific serum antibody tests can evaluate this possibility. Some patients remain incapacitated for years. Crossover sensitivity to environmental toxins, fumes, industrial chemicals, and inhalant or food allergies are often seen.

At the **Poland Spring Health Institute** I have seen many patients with CFS recover their strength and energies. The combination of a simple, low-fat diet, and gradually increasing exercise helps to boost immune defenses. Chronic viral disease yields to the benefits of fever therapy, given over a two to three week period. Depression lifts, while new energy comes into the nearly disabled invalid. There is hope for most infections, especially the chronic viral ones producing fatigue.

Mumps is an acute communicable disease, characterized by painful enlargement of the salivary glands, and more specifically of the parotid glands, just in front of the ears. Sometimes the infection involves the testicles; rarely it produces meningitis. At times testicular involvement *(orchitis)* will result in lifetime sterility. There is no specific treatment, though swollen painful organs can be relieved with cold compresses while the disease runs its course and is treated at home with general measures.

Many tropical diseases, spread by mosquitoes, can be seen around the world. *Eastern* and *western equine encephalitis, dengue, yellow fever,* and *hemorrhagic fevers* are the more common of these. Treatment is generally symptomatic and supportive.

BACTERIAL INFECTIONS

Bacteria are one-celled living creatures, usually classified with the plant family. There are two general types of bacteria, one being spherical and the other rod shaped. These are called *cocci* and *bacilli*, respectively. We will first consider some specific infectious agents and subsequently general diseases caused by bacteria and their rational treatment.

Staphylococci

Staphylococcal infections commonly produce **boils** on the skin. They can also cause serious infections in the lungs, long bones, kidneys, and surgical wounds. Many of these are among the diseases of "medical progress,"**iatrogenic** (doctor caused) disorders seen in hospitals, complicating surgical treatment or the use of drugs. Staphylococcal infections may enter a newborn nursery, for example, and cause serious infection in premature or weakened babies. A number of enzymes are produced by small "*Staph*" germs that enable them the multiply in a walled off cavity, while pus develops as your body's defense.

The tendency of *Staphylococci* to change their reproductive needs (mutate) has caused them to develop frequent resistance to the older standard antibiotics. Pustules may occur in many locations— hair follicles on the face, under the arm, in the groin, and wherever the skin is broken. More extensive infection may appear among diabetics— carbuncles or deep infection of the bone (osteomyelitis). Any child who develops fever, limb pain, or joint pain should be suspected to have *osteomyelitis*. A physician, in such cases, should be contacted to obtain appropriate blood tests and cultures. Staphylococcal *pneumonia* may develop in children or hospitalized patients. Whenever the germs are present in the skin, they may enter the blood stream causing *bacteremia*.

Another type of infection with the Staphylococcal organism is *food poisoning*. A toxin is produced in contaminated food, which is frequently of animal origin, such as cream-filled pastries, cottage cheese, milk products, or meat. With improper refrigeration, the toxin is liberated. After about one to six hours, a sufferer will develop nausea, vomiting, cramps, diarrhea, and prostration. Rest and supportive treatment are needed during the acute phase, which is normally followed by a rapid recovery. Vegetarian foods are much less likely to be involved with toxins such as we see in food-borne epidemics.

Streptococcal Infection

These cocci appear under the microscope in the form of chains. Several types can be distinguished by culture. Those considered the most virulent are called *beta-hemolytic Strep.* These germs produce the typical **Strep. throat** and most cases of acute tonsillitis. In some people a rash will follow the acutely sore throat, in which case a diagnosis of *scarlet fever* is made.

Most of these Strep. infections need to be eradicated quite promptly to prevent serious potential complications of *rheumatic fever* and *glomerulonephritis.* Both can produce chronic disability and damage vital organs.

In throat infection, fortunately, alternating hot and cold gargles and heating compresses can be applied with considerable effectiveness. Complete avoidance of sugar during the acute illness is important to help white blood cell defenses and ensure rapid recovery. When skin or wound infections with the Streptococcal organism results, hot and cold compresses again will prove very beneficial. The fine red streaks that one sees in an infected finger or toe are caused by *lymphangitis*, usually related to this organism. I have used charcoal poultices with rapid benefit also.

Erysipelas is another Strep. infection of the skin. Aggressive hydro-therapy in the early stage must be used to prevent complications; for occasional deaths have been seen in this infection, particularly in young children.

Bacterial Meningitis

The organism most commonly responsible for meningitis is the *menin-gococcus* germ, also called *Neisseria meningitis.* This organism is seen in military recruits, and sporadically throughout the general population. The sudden onset of high fever, a hemorrhagic skin rash, low blood pressure, rapid heart rate and respiration, stiffness of the neck, and severe headache, should warn the family of the potential onset of meningitis and alert them to seek a physician immediately! Emergency medical treatment is needed to prevent serious complications—a tragic aftermath of arthritis, adrenal failure, blindness, deafness, seizures, or even death!

Gonococcal Infections

The most common "reportable" communicable disease in the United States today is *gonorrhea.* The genital organs are most commonly involved in this disease, considered sexually transmitted, especially through high-risk encounters with multiple partners. Currently this *venereal disease* (V.D.) is a formidable epidemic.

Usually in the male there is a discharge of pus from the urethra, associated with painful and frequent urination. Without immediate treatment, lymph node enlargement, pain in the scrotal sac (*epididymis*), and urinary outlet obstruction (*urethral stricture*) will result. Female patients frequently develop an increased vaginal discharge, with severe pain in the deeper pelvic organs. Abscesses may form. Prompt treatment is necessary to prevent the development of stricture in the Fallopian tubes, which could produce sterility.

Although in prior decades, fever therapy was used with success in the treatment of gonorrhea, current public health recommendations should be followed to prevent the spread of this disease associated with promiscuity and immoral behavior. Condoms are **not** the whole answer to V.D. We need to lift society to the higher moral standards of God's Word again.

Intestinal Bacilli

A number of germs are normally found in the intestinal tract. These include *Escherichia coli, Bacteroides,* and many other germs. Some of these are our friends in producing important substances for nutrition, such as **Vitamin K** and **inositol**. Invading the body outside the intestinal tract, however, *E. coli* (the most common intestinal germ, *Escherichia coli*) is definitely harmful. Infections of the blood stream may occur as a complication of urinary tract infection. These organisms can cause abscesses anywhere in the body tissues.

Children under two years of age sometimes develop an intestinal infection typified by nausea, vomiting, and diarrhea. Many similar outbreaks occurring in nurseries have been associated with a specific strain of *E. coli*. As with other infections, drainage of pus and the removal of foreign bodies are essential. Often the outcome of these infections depends upon the status of the associated disease, rather than the mere eradication of bacteria.

Next to *E. coli*, strains of *Klebsiella* and *Enterobacter* are the species of intestinal organisms most apt to infect man. *Klebsiella* is a well recognized pulmonary invader, causing serious bacterial pneumonia. Often the sputum will contain blood, and cyanosis or shortness of breath may develop rapidly. Chronic infections of the lungs are sometimes seen.

Proteus is another similar organism, which has whip-like projections called flagella to enable it to "swim". These bacteria may infect the urinary tract, also invading eyes, ears, mastoid sinuses, or blood stream.

Salmonella infections are common in the U.S. They occur frequently in travelers to underdeveloped nations. Various types of disease can result; usually they are intestinal in nature and result in diarrhea.

Typhoid fever is a systemic disease caused by *Salmonella typhi*. The disease is unique to man and characterized by malaise, fever, abdominal discomfort, rash, and enlargement of the spleen. The most prominent complications are intestinal hemorrhage and perforation. In a typical patient not treated with antimicrobials the illness lasts about four weeks. With supportive care, barring complications, the recovery is good, although some "carriers" are known. About 3% of infected patients will continue to excrete organisms in the feces for years. They have been known to infect others where careful screening for food handlers has been lacking.

Other *Salmonella* infections involve gastroenteritis, usually seen in large epidemics among individuals eating contaminated food. After incubating for 8–48 hours the organisms cause a sudden onset of abdominal pain and watery diarrhea, usually with mucus or blood. Low grade fever is common, and symptoms usually subside within 2–5 days. Public health organizations often attempt to isolate the germ carrier, in order to prevent the spread of this epidemic. The most important preventive, besides food surveillance, is personal hygiene, including hand washing. Minimizing the time that foods are allowed to sit at room temperature reduce the chances of growth of these infectious organisms.

The **rule-of-thumb** to prevent bacterial food poisoning is known as the two-forty-one hundred forty (2–40–140) rule. Simply explained, it means that any susceptible food—meat, milk, mayonnaise, poultry, custard, etc.—must **never** be left longer than two hours at a temperature either above 40 degrees F. or below 140 degrees F. Both refrigerated and hot foods are able to inhibit the multiplication of bacteria, thus avoiding toxin formation that would otherwise cause food borne disease.

Shigellosis is an acute self-limited infection of the intestinal tract, characterized by diarrhea, fever, and abdominal pain. This is frequently called *bacillary dysentery*. Severe dehydration may result in some patients who are not given adequate fluids during the diarrhea stage. As in *Salmonella* infections, the treatment of Shigellosis is primarily supportive, with the correction of salt or fluid abnormalities, followed by an uneventful convalescence. Proper sanitation and adequate sewage disposal will prevent most of these infections.

Hemophilus Infections

These bacteria, called *Hemophilus*, cause a variety of diseases. Pharyngitis (sore throat) is commonly seen in children. At times the throat may become severely inflamed, producing inflammation of the valve behind the tongue, the epiglottis *(epiglotitis)*. Shortness of breath, with a reddened, swollen, stiff epiglottis may constitute a medical emergency. *Croup* also develops in children with a raspy cough, and profound fluid accumulation in the larynx and trachea. If not treated promptly with cool mist and supportive measures it can prove fatal. Pneumonia caused by the *Hemophilus* organism is usually seen in children, as is also **otitis media**, a middle ear infection, and **meningitis**. In these complications prompt bacterial isolation with the appropriate medical treatment will usually prove effective.

Brucellosis

Brucellosis or *undulant fever* is caused by microorganisms transmitted from domestic animals. The acute illness is characterized by fever, while weakness and vague complaints may persist for months to years, when the disease becomes chronic. Three species are found in goats, hogs, and cattle. The infection is usually spread by cow's milk or skin contact (udder) with the *Brucella* organism. When the disease is suspected, appropriate blood tests are needed to confirm the diagnosis. Then specific medical therapy can be instituted. With the appropriate inspection of animals and the avoidance of contaminated milk and milk products, this occupational disease can be well controlled.

Plague

Various bacteria of the *Pasteurella* family have been associated with epidemics of plague around the world. About 200 species of rodents may harbor this organism. After an incubation period of 1-12 days a patient develops an acute severe illness. The more common **bubonic plague** develops abruptly with chills, headache, vomiting, rapid heart rate, prostration, and delirium. A flea bite at the portal of entry rarely can be seen. The "bubo" consists of a matted group of lymph glands, which usually develops pus and drains after 1-2 weeks. Plague may also take the form of pneumonia. Infection may localize in other regions of the body.

Although often misdiagnosed, plague should initially be treated with hot, moist applications. Specific therapy should await a bacteriologic diagnosis. A similar type of illness seen in animal bites with local cellulitis should be treated as most bacterial infections are. If plague is suspected, see a doctor immediately; this illness is extremely infectious.

Diphtheria

The *Diphtheria* bacteria that cause this acute infectious disease usually enter through the upper respiratory tract. During the incubation of one to seven days the germs make a toxin that is absorbed and carried through the blood stream to all parts of the body. Then a fever begins, associated with a membrane on the throat, listlessness, pallor, weakness, and finally vascular collapse. Although occasionally restricted to the nose, diphtheria usually involves the throat (the *pharynx* and *larynx*), and in tropical areas it is responsible for some cases of "jungle sore". Complications may involve the extension of the membrane, which obstructs the respiratory tract or equally serious a toxic *myocarditis*, a vascular collapse, or neuritis.

Patients with diphtheria should be isolated and kept on strict bed rest. Antitoxins should be obtained and given to the patient, while general supportive measures are carried out. Preventive immunization in infancy should be routine. The standard protocol of three initial **DPT** inoculations (or in the case of *Pertussis* sensitivity, a **DT** immunization is available) followed by booster doses at one and six years will usually confer lifelong protection.

Cholera

Cholera is an acute illness of the small intestine. Occurring in epidemic forms, a generally painless diarrhea follows the entrance of the germs by 6 - 48 hours. Several liters of fluid may be lost within hours, leading to profound shock. With prompt fluid and electrolyte replacement, dehydration can be combated, bringing a prompt physiologic recovery. Inadequately treated patients may die from shock, acidosis, or kidney failure (*uremia*). Therefore, prompt and massive fluid replacement is vital.

A satisfactory solution can be prepared by adding five grams of sodium chloride, four grams of sodium bicarbonate, one gram of potassium chloride to one liter of distilled water. Hydration must be maintained until the diarrhea subsides. Cholera prevention, for travelers, is available with a standard vaccination. In countries where cholera is epidemic, a single inoculation prior to departure is recommended.

Tetanus

This acute, often fatal disease is caused by a germ toxin (exotoxin) produced in any closed wound by the organism *Clostridium tetani*. Tetanus is characterized by sudden rigidity and convulsive spasms of the skeletal muscles. The tetanus bacillus grows *anaerobically*, that is, in a wound where oxygen is excluded. For this reason puncture wounds are often a source of tetanus infection. Gun shot wounds and animal bites also have been suspect, as well as lacerations that are sutured without adequate cleansing.

Supportive measures, usually in a hospital, are important to effect recovery from tetanus. Hot packs to relax the muscle spasm, adequate care of wounds, and the simple but effective toxoid vaccination can give protection. Vaccinations should be boosted every 10 years. In cases of an acute open wound, which appears contaminated, the human tetanus antitoxin should be given along with a tetanus toxoid vaccination to passively protect the individual from illness during early convalescence.

Botulism

This acute form of poisoning results from the ingestion of a toxin produced by *Clostridium botulinum*. Progressive paralysis descends from the brain stem to the skeletal muscles and is often fatal. This germ grows in improperly sealed non-acid canned foods, such as fish or beans, which have been cooked insufficiently to destroy all germs.

Outbreaks have been seen from commercially processed fish, tuna, peppers, and soups. It is impossible to tell that a food is infected by the taste. However, boiling a home-canned food for ten minutes will destroy the toxin completely. Because of the threat of respiratory failure, a person suspected of having botulism should be hospitalized. Artificial respiratory support may be required for a long time. Because of the current mortality rate of 25%, the primary prevention through proper canning procedures and food preservation is vital.

Gas Gangrene

Gas gangrene is another *clostridial* infection produced by the introduction of anaerobic organisms into a wound. Within a few days, severe pain develops in the injured part. Below this point the tissue becomes cold and swollen and eventually develops into gangrene. The wound drains a watery brown material, which may have a sweet odor.

Immediately opening the wound to permit adequate oxygen entrance is important, associated with hydrogen peroxide irrigation and therapies that draw fluid from the wound. This may include the use of dry sucrose (table sugar or honey), increased oxygen, and rarely in more serious cases amputation to prevent death from this severe complication. The most reliable protection against gas gangrene is **thorough cleansing** of the wound. Avoiding unsterile surgical procedures (septic abortion), prolonged labor, or operative interference with pregnancy can also help prevent these infections.

Tuberculosis

Once a prime cause of death around the world, **tuberculosis** is seen today mainly in underdeveloped societies. Fear of recurrence in the Western world is surfacing, especially in military barracks, prisons, inner city ghettos, and communities of immune suppressed men (AIDS). Pasteurization of milk has reduced greatly the incidence of *bovine* tuberculosis, which a generation ago commonly affected the intestinal tract. The lungs are now most often afflicted with development of characteristic abnormalities detectable by X-ray.

Symptoms of tuberculosis include fatigue, night sweats, cough, sputum production, shortness of breath, and rarely the coughing up of blood. During all of these activities droplets are sprayed from the lungs, which may contain tubercle bacilli. Using a tissue to trap the aerosolized particles, and disposing of it immediately will prevent most of the contagion due to tuberculosis.

In chronic pulmonary tuberculosis, chest x-rays show scars with scattered calcium deposits. These, however, during a time of lowered resistance may reactivate, producing illness and contagion once again. The **TB skin test**, when positive, indicates a person has previously contacted tuberculosis germs and that his immune system recognizes and sets up a battle against them. **PPD** (purified protein derivative) or **Tine** tests for tuberculosis are helpful screening procedures to detect active infection in the community. Public health laboratories then will perform sputum cultures and other needed follow-up measures in the detection and treatment of this illness.

Avoidance of contact with other people, particularly in the spread of the respiratory form, and hygienic healing measures, especially sunshine, adequate rest and proper diet, may produce a natural cure of most cases. Extrapulmonary tuberculosis involving bones and kidneys has responded to prolonged exposure to sunlight in some European health centers.

Leprosy

Knowledge of this widespread affliction of mankind has its root in Biblical history. Called "Hansen's disease" today, this organism is closely akin to the tubercle bacillus and belongs to the *Mycobacterium* family. Ten to twenty million persons in the world are affected with leprosy. It is more common in tropical countries; in many third world nations 1-2% or more of the population are affected. Leprosy is frequently a family infection. Several different types of the disease are known.

Early leprosy is usually seen on the skin with pigmented plaques and patches demonstrating anesthesia. The **tuberculoid leprosy** develops later with larger raised lesions having no sensation (*anesthesia*), associated with large painful nerves. These may occur behind the elbow or knee and are associated with anesthesia in the affected limb. Contractures of the hands and foot drop (*paralysis*) are frequent. Trauma, especially from burns and splinters, and excessive pressure lead to the secondary infection, ulcers, and the loss of fingers and toes.

Lepromatous leprosy creates an unusual appearance of the face, often making the hapless victim appear like a lion. The skin is primarily involved and early symptoms are those of nasal stuffiness or nose bleeds. Saddle nose, due to perforation of the septum (the wall between the two nostrils) may occur while lymph nodes may enlarge painlessly.

Although neurological involvement is less common, this type is actually more contagious. Other types of leprosy are seen with variations of the above. Although a specific drug (Dapsone) is widely used today, in reality there is no complete cure. It is suspected on the basis of animal studies that some form of fever induction may prove the therapy of the future, with public health control measures and quarantine limiting the spread. For further information you may wish to contact the following: *Leprosy Research Foundation, 11588 Lawton Court, Loma Linda, California 92354.*

Venereal Diseases

Venereal diseases are increasing in frequency today, due to the lack of moral restraint in society. **Gonorrhea** has been discussed above, but several other types are commonly seen. **Syphilis** is a chronic infection of the entire body, caused by *Treponema pallidum* and is usually sexually transmitted. After an incubation period of about three weeks, a primary sore develops with enlargement of the nearby lymph nodes.

Generalized rash on the skin develops in the secondary stage and after a latent period of many years, the tertiary stage can develop with progressive destructive lesions in the muscle, bone, aorta, or central nervous system. Although primary treatment with fever therapy was formerly effective in cases of syphilis, any current outbreak should be confirmed with appropriate blood (*serologic*) tests, a dark–field microscopic examination, and specific therapy as recommended by public health departments.

Other venereal infections include **chancroid** and **lymphogranuloma venereum**. These less common venereal disorders also must be treated definitively to prevent contagion.

AIDS

The preceding decade brought a new life-threatening disease into the vocabulary of every nation. **AIDS** (the *acquired immune deficiency syndrome*) is primarily transmitted as a venereal disease. First discovered in homosexual males, the syndrome quickly spread, soon encircling the world. Millions of women acquired the infection from their bisexual partners. Growing exponentially around our globe, this disease is caused by a virus called **HIV** (*human immunodeficiency virus*). A similar virus is now found in cows (the *bovine immunodeficiency virus*).

Drug abusing men and women pick up the virus from contaminated needles. Many *hemophiliacs* have acquired the infection from blood product transfusions. Sporadic case reports of hospital workers and physicians have raised the spectrum of risky needle sticks, surgery, and invasive medical procedures. Gloves are mandated for medical contact with all body fluids (called *universal precautions*). Latex is not adequate protection, however. It frequently contains microscopic pores, and the virus can pass through easily.

From their first knowledge of AIDS, physicians in hospitals began to practice isolation precautions. Lobbying tactics from homosexual advocates quickly pushed legislators into enacting laws preserving the confidentiality of AIDS carriers. This has increased the risks to dentists, paramedics, physicians, and all health care providers, who may not even know their patient is carrying a lethal virus. Most hospitals today refuse to isolate HIV carriers, ignoring its contagiousness and the scientific research provided.

There is no known cure for HIV infections. Most of the victims eventually develop full blown AIDS. This may develop in several ways. Sudden infection, with drug-resistant tuberculosis or pneumonia caused by an *opportunistic* germ such as *Pneumocystis carini*, may befall. This directly reveals the devastation of the patient's immune system. Lymphocyte counts are dangerously low; and the hapless patient must be supported with powerful and expensive drugs, usually for the rest of his life.

Unusual forms of cancer, such as *Kaposi's sarcoma*, may appear. One dentist, carrying several of these lesions in his mouth, continued to treat patients. Several of them eventually developed AIDS and died. This disease, as mentioned above, has run rampant in the militant homosexual population. Could there be any better warning to modern man? The Creator's plan for marriage, one man and one woman, mated and committed for life, is the only safe course for pure sexual harmony as well as disease prevention.

FUNGUS INFECTIONS

Except for the causative agent, infections caused by fungi differ little from bacterial disorders. Botanically, the fungi present peculiarities of life cycle that challenge the investigator.

Actinomycosis is a noncontagious infection produced by an organism normally resident in the mouth. This fungus also causes the so called "lumpy jaw" of cattle. A painful hard swelling results in humans, and can appear in the lower jaw, resembling the pain of a tooth extraction or fracture. The afflicted patient will then notice fever, cough, and eventually drainage. "Sulfur granules" appear in the pus draining from the lesion; these are especially evident if the pus is diluted with saline solution and filtered through gauze. Surgical drainage is helpful as an adjunct to specific therapy.

Cryptococcosis is a pulmonary infection caused by a yeast organism. It is occurring with increased frequency in patients with leukemia. At times it progresses to meningitis with visual disturbance, severe headache, vomiting, and even convulsions. Scientists are looking for safer treatments in this serious illness, which is fatal in many cases and difficult to diagnose.

Blastomycosis is a fungus infection of the skin and internal organs. It occurs in both North and South America and appears to enter the body via the lung. Dissemination to skin and bones may occur. The regional lymph glands and spleen are often enlarged. Although at times resembling tuberculosis of the lung, a skin test is available to aid in diagnosis. This condition can be cured if treatment is begun promptly.

Coccidioidomycosis is an infection acquired by the inhalation of a fungus. Most infections occur during the dry seasons, particularly after exposure to dust storms. The semi-arid region of the southwestern United States is a common location for this disease, often termed "desert" or "valley fever." The most frequent complaint is chest pain aggravated by breathing or coughing. Fluid accumulation in the lungs with x-ray changes are usually seen. A skin test is available for diagnosis, as well as confirmatory blood tests. Relief of stress, with increased rest, and in serious cases, specific antifungal agents may be needed to effect a cure.

Histoplasmosis is the eastern counterpart of "Cocci" found in the Mississippi River valley and the eastern United States. This fungus occurs in soil where bats, birds, and chickens are inhabiting the area. At times this illness is called "cave fever." City dwellers are also exposed, where starlings' or black bird's droppings collect. Signs and symptoms range from slight, self-limited infections to fatal disseminated disease. The skin test is very helpful in confirming the diagnosis. Lesions in the lung resemble tuberculosis in most respects. Cough is common. At times ulcers in the mouth, tongue, pharynx, or larynx can be seen. For the more serious cases, specific therapy is important as the disease can be fatal.

Sporotrichosis, another chronic infection is characterized by the formation of nodules, which drain a material resembling pus. These occur along the lymphatic vessel of the skin and underlying tissues. The first contact usually develops from the prick of a thorn, while the victim is working with plants. Rarely dissemination to the lungs, bones, or joints may be seen. The organism can be cultured. Treatment with potassium iodide drops is usually curative, except in the most disseminated forms.

Moniliasis is a common infection of the mucous membrane and skin, due to *Candida albicans*. At times in debilitated patients the fungus can cause widespread infection in the blood and internal organs. More commonly, it occurs as a diaper rash in babies, in the mouth as "thrush," and in diabetics usually in the skin or female organs. Vaginitis is very common, particularly with the increased wearing of nylon undergarments, panty hose, and the more widespread use of oral contraceptives. Oral suspensions or tablets of **nystatin** can be used in the mouth and antifungal tablets or vinegar douches for vaginal involvement. Control of blood sugar, diet, and adequate availability of fresh air and sunshine helps to increase resistance to this problem.

Skin involvement with fungi and yeast is quite common. Usually these organism cause **ringworm**, **athlete's foot, and jock itch**—an itching rash in the groin. Topical treatments, drying agents, and frequent changes of clothes, particularly dry socks on the feet are important to decrease the incidence of this summertime nuisance. Scalp involvement is more difficult to eradicate. Fortunately, the superficial fungi are quite sensitive to sunlight.

RICKETTSIAL DISEASES

A variety of afflictions are caused by this family of microorganisms. Rickettsia are smaller than bacteria. Most of these illnesses are transmitted by ticks, fleas, or lice. Serologic tests aid in the diagnosis.

Rocky mountain spotted fever is an acute febrile illness caused by a *Rickettsial* germ. It is transmitted to humans by ticks. The disease is characterized by sudden onset with headache and chill, with fever that persists for 2 - 3 weeks. A characteristic rash appears on the extremities and migrates to the trunk after about four days of illness. Those who become severely ill develop pain in the bones, delirium, shock, and kidney failure.

Many species of ticks are found infected with this organism. The **wood tick** is the most common vector in the west and the **dog tick** in the east. It is important to avoid crushing the tick when removing it from a person or animal. Carefully pull them off or apply heat, as with the head of a match which has just quit burning; or apply kerosene to their body. This will usually allow a tick to release itself and prevent leaving the head in the wound. Anyone suspected of having Rocky Mountain Spotted Fever should seek medical care for appropriate diagnosis and therapy. Prevention is attained primarily by the avoidance of tick infested areas.

Lyme disease is another tick borne illness, first described in the New York and Connecticut regions. It is carried by a deer tick, though other vectors have now been confirmed. Lyme disease begins with a mild fever, aching muscles and joints, and a "bull's eye" rash. Red in the center with an outer red ring, this rash begins on the trunk, then spreads and eventually fades. Blood tests are available to confirm the diagnosis. Long term complica-

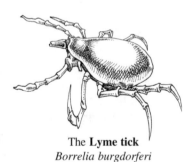

The **Lyme tick**
Borrelia burgdorferi

tions with arthritis, chronic fatigue, and vague internal complaints may result when the acute illness was not treated promptly.

I have found fever therapy to be helpful in both acute and chronic cases. The earlier the diagnosis, the better, since response from any therapy is more sure and rapid.

Lyme tick
top view

Other illnesses caused by Rickettsial organisms are as follows: **rickettsialpox** is a mild, nonfatal, self-limited illness transmitted from mites to humans. It is characterized by a skin lesion at the site of the mite bite, a one-week course of high fevers, and a rash resembling chicken pox. **Typhus fever** or **Murine typhus** is an acute illness with fever transmitted to humans by fleas. A headache and skin rash, together with muscle aching also develops, though serious complications are uncommon. The elimination of rodents and appropriate flea control measures in rat infested areas are the best for prevention of this disease. **Epidemic louse-borne typhus fever** is caused by another Rickettsial organism. Headache, fever, and a skin rash are sometimes complicated by vascular and neurologic disturbances. Specific therapeutic agents are available.

Scrub typhus, Q fever, and **trench fever** are other Rickettsial infections, the latter transmitted by the human body louse. Since these are uncommon, you may refer to a standard textbook of infectious diseases for clinical description and specific treatment.

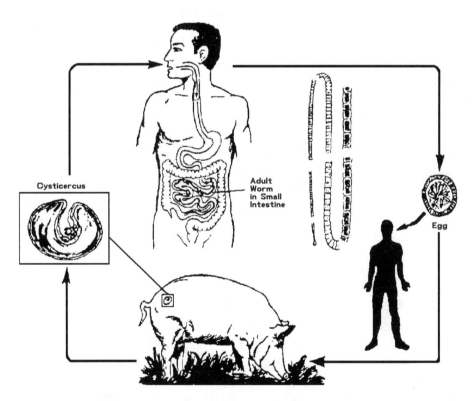

Life cycle of the Pork Tapeworm. The eggs of this parasite, *Taenia solium*, are first ingested by the hog. The embryo is then released from the egg. When an individual eats pork (especially undercooked) the egg penetrates his intestinal wall, is carried by vascular channels to all parts of the body, then encysts as a larvae (called *bladder worms*) and lives in the muscles causing pain or weakness. With brain involvment the patient may even develop seizures, symptoms of meningoencephalitis, and other neurologic disorders. The pig is a scavenger. **Do not eat it!**

PARASITIC INFECTIONS

There are a number of worms that parasitize humans. These can be divided into three major groups: roundworm *(nematodes)*, tapeworm *(cestodes)*, and flukes *(trematodes)*. Only the most common infections that are likely to be seen in North and Central America will be discussed.

Roundworms

Pinworms are intestinal parasites transmitted by the ingestion of the egg form. This roundworm is called *Enterobius vermiculari* and is a small white worm about one-half inch in length. An estimated 200 million people in the world are infested with parasites, 18 million in the United States and Canada. Children are particularly affected. Rectal itching is present, due to the unique nocturnal habits of the female parasite, that nightly leave the anus to lay eggs on the skin surrounding it. Scratching leads to reinfection by ingestion. Usually all members of the family should be treated simultaneously.

The **whipworm** or *Trichuris* infection is more serious with invasion of the colon mucosa by the adult parasite. This is found more commonly in the tropics, especially in children. At times abdominal pain, diarrhea, and dysentery results with a chronic blood loss that may produce significant anemia.

The **roundworm** or *Ascaris lumbricoides* migrates first to the lungs and later lives in the intestinal tract. It is estimated that 25% of the world's population is infected with this nematode. Ascaris worms are quite large and cylindric in size. Muscular activity maintains them in within the small intestine. Amazingly, the daily egg output of the female is estimated to be 200,000 per worm! Their larva are liberated into the small intestine, migrate through the wall, and are thus carried by the blood stream to the lungs. Thus, without specific treatment, the condition is quite chronic and debilitating.

Ascaris is primarily a household infection of rural areas. Adequate toilet facilities, hand washing, and strict personal hygiene are good preventives.

Hookworm disease is a symptomatic infection caused by two parasite living in the Americas. Hookworm infestation causes significant suffering; an estimated loss of seven million liters of blood occurs daily in the 700 million people infected throughout the entire world. Abundant rainfall, shade, and well-drained, sandy soil are conditions conducive to the development of the hookworm egg into an infective larval form. Walking barefoot in the area allows the larvae to migrate through the sole of the victim's foot into his blood stream. There it enters the lungs, is coughed up, and later is swallowed, thus reaching the intestines.

The major manifestation of hookworm disease is iron deficiency anemia, due to chronic blood loss. Specific treatment must be followed by adequate iron and protein intake in the diet in order for an individual to completely recover.

Common eggs of the *roundworm* types as seen under the microscope. Their proper identification aids in treatment, as pictured below.

HUMAN ROUNDWORM EGGS

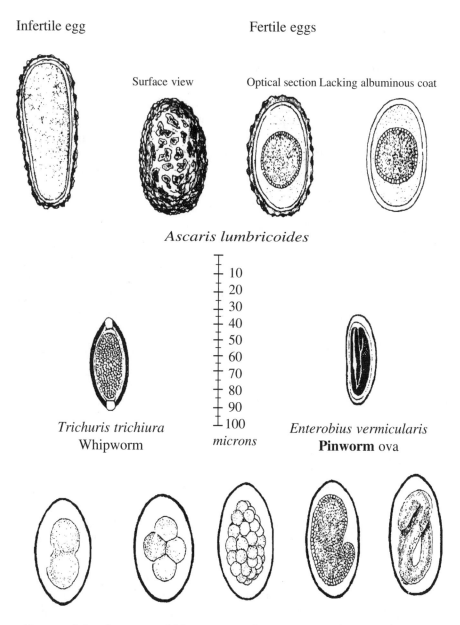

Infertile egg

Fertile eggs

Surface view

Optical section   Lacking albuminous coat

Ascaris lumbricoides

10
20
30
40
50
60
70
80
90
100
microns

Trichuris trichiura
Whipworm

Enterobius vermicularis
Pinworm ova

Stages of development of *Necator americanus* or *Ancylostoma duodenale*. These are the eggs of the common **hookworms** that infect humans.

Several intestinal worms, including *Toxicara* (the dog and cat hookworms), produce **visceral larva migrans**, and a disease called **creeping eruption** or **cutaneous larva migrans**. In this situation the parasite migrates in the skin causing intense itching. *Strongyloides stercoralis,* another roundworm, causes a serious intestinal infection. The preventive measures are similar for all of these: wear shoes, wash hands, cook vegetables.

Flatworms

Trichinosis is one of the most common flatworm infections in North America. This intestinal and tissue infection of man is caused by the nematode *Trichinella spiralis*. The disease is characterized by diarrhea during the development of the adult worm in the intestine. Later there is a syndrome of muscle pain, fever, prostration, edema of the eyelids, and occasionally by myocarditis or encephalitis during the stage of larval migration in the tissues. Trichinosis in humans is contacted by ingesting meat containing larvae in its dormant stage called a cyst.

The meat has almost always been pork, but about 10% of cases reported in recent years have been attributed to bear meat. Butcher shops often use the same knife or cutting board for different kinds of meat, so cross contamination may occur. Humans are particularly susceptible to this infection. Cooking the meat thoroughly usually kills the larva and reduces the risk of infection. Specific treatment has not always been available and the prevention of Trichinosis lies mainly in the observance of an ancient Biblical injunction to shun swine's flesh as food.

Schistosomiasis or **Bilharziasis** can be produced by three closely related flatworms of the Schistosoma family. These parasites live in the blood vessels of humans who dwell in tropical countries. The organs most frequently affected are the colon, urinary bladder, liver, lungs, and central nervous system. The best attack on this disease is preventive. Public health measures, including proper disposal of human excrement, provision of pure water supply, and snail control methods in the epidemic areas can be helpful. The parasite, which is harbored by snails, enters the body through the skin of people wading, planting rice, or working in gardens. Specific treatment is difficult and relapses are frequent.

Tapeworm infections are usually acquired through the mouth. Eating raw or undercooked beef will allow introduction of embryos of the cestode *Taenia saginata*. There is also a **pork** tapeworm, *Taenia solium*, and the dwarf tapeworm *Hymenolepsis nana*. A broad fish tapeworm, *Diphyllobothrium latum*, is also parasitic in humans and can rob the body of Vitamin B_{12}. Anemia and other symptoms of B_{12} deficiency can then result. The most practical control measure of the tapeworm is to avoid disposing of untreated sewage in fresh water lakes. Personal hygiene should be stressed. The contamination of food by rats and mice should be prevented.

PROTOZOAL INFECTIONS

Protozoa are one-cell animals. They infect man usually when introduced by mosquitoes or other insects. These infections remain among the major causes of human sickness and death in the world today. Over 500 million people still live in malaria areas. It is estimated that 100 million of these are infected at any given time. Of those infected one million die of malaria annually.

One of the most lethal of all human diseases, **sleeping sickness**, is carried by the *Tsetse* fly. In South America, another related organism infects several million people leaving many with severe heart and gastrointestinal lesions (**Chagas' disease**). It is carried by the kissing bug, found in many homes of underprivileged people living in South America.

Ten percent of the world's population, including 2-5% in the United States are infected with the intestinal protozoa *(Entamoeba histolytica)*. **Toxoplasmosis, giardiasis**, and **trichomoniasis** are three cosmopolitan protozoan infections well known to American physicians. Some of the most common of these will be discussed briefly.

Amebiasis is an infection of the large intestine, produced by *Entamoeba histolytica*. It produces a disease ranging from chronic mild diarrhea to life–threatening dysentery. Liver abscesses may result, at times rupturing into the abdominal or chest cavities. These diseases are diagnosed primarily by an examination of the stool. Careful microscopic investigation can disclose the presence of the cyst or adult form, a *trophozoite*. Treatment should be aimed at relief of symptoms, replacement of fluids, elec-

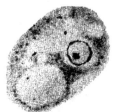

Entamoeba histolytica causes **amebic dysentery.**

trolytes, and blood loss, and eradication of the organism. The prevention of amebiasis is even more important. For example, the avoidance of contaminated food and water, scalding of vegetables, and the use of iodine release tablets in drinking water are important measures. Improvement in the general sanitation, detection of "cyst passers", and their removal from food-handling duties, are general measures in prevention.

Malaria is a protozoal disease transmitted to humans by the bite of the *Anopheles* mosquito. It remains the major infectious disease problem in the world. Malaria is characterized by enlargement of the spleen, fever, anemia, and a chronic relapsing course. Today malaria survives best in areas of South and Central America, Africa, and Asia, where the mosquito and the infected human population co-exist. The incidence of the disease has decreased since 1945, due to an active international cooperative program aimed at its eradication.

Several types of the organism, *Plasmodium vivax*, *P. malaria*, and *P. falciparum* exist. The cycles between the muscle aching, headache, and fever vary from 48–72 hour periods. "Cerebral malaria" can lead to paralysis, convulsions, delirium, coma, and rapid death. "Black water fever" is a type of malaria associated with *P. falciparum*. Massive destruction (*hemolysis*) of red blood cells is followed by jaundice, kidney failure, and vascular collapse. The most important diagnostic test in the search for malaria parasites is the examination of a stained blood drop under the microscope.

Final cure of malaria is difficult, but mild cases often respond to the timely use of fever therapy. This is given as a rapid sweating steam or tub bath, bringing the body temperature up just as the chills begin, and before fever crests. The treatment should finish as usual with a *cold mitten friction* or a cool shower (see Chapter 17). Repeat this treatment on successive days if the chills return. Performed faithfully in conjunction with a simple diet, extra rest, and other hygienic measures, control can usually be obtained.

The prevention of malaria involves primarily mosquito control, using netting, repellents, and the draining of swampy areas to reduce their breeding potential. Travelers or missionaries to countries where resistant malaria is endemic may want to take preventive medication for added protection.

Leishmaniasis is seen in various forms in the new and old world. **Trypanosomiasis** or "sleeping sickness" is primarily a disease seen in Africa. **Toxoplasmosis** is a protozoa infection widely distributed among mammals and birds. In humans it can produce both congenital and acquired brain infections. Specific diagnosis is important before determining the appropriate therapy.

Minor protozoal diseases are a common nuisance, and at times are resistant to therapy. **Trichomoniasis** is a venereal infection caused by the protozoan *Trichomonas vaginalis*. This organism may survive in the bladder and the genital tract. Itching, burning, and a profuse, malodorous creamy-yellow discharge may persist for weeks. Usually the symptoms subside after the passage of time. Medicated douches as well as careful hygiene are important in the control.

Giardiasis is an unusual appearing organism. This protozoa infection is a significant cause of "traveler's diarrhea". It comes from drinking contaminated lake or river water, often while camping. Although the symptoms may persist for several weeks, most infections are asymptomatic and the symptoms are self-limited.

Giardia lamblia, the culprit in many diarrhea cases.

* * * * * * *

There are a number of other diseases resembling infectious processes where no organism has been identified. **Sarcoidosis** is one of these, often affecting the lungs and lymph nodes. Diagnosis is obtained by a skin test in association with chest x-ray or biopsies. We have found fever therapy to be helpful in these cases, like many other infectious diseases of uncertain origin. Many other diseases can mimic the above described processes. With new organisms being discovered each year and new diseases being described, only a cursory review of the latest research is possible in the scope of this book.

Some **general principles** can be helpful in the treatment of infections, however. **Fever** is one of the most common symptoms. It is usually thought to be a body defense against infection, since viruses do not multiply well at temperatures over 102 degrees F. Other germs are actually destroyed when the temperature reaches 104-105 degrees. Unless the symptoms caused by the fever are severe, it should not be totally obliterated, but rather modified by such treatments as moist sponges, cool baths, or the *wet sheet pack* (Chapter 17).

Hydrotherapy is an extremely valuable treatment for infections of the lungs and the gastrointestinal tract. Hot and cold moist towels are used freely on the extremities and with the exception of tuberculosis, the same contrasting temperatures are useful in helping the lungs to increase their resistance and throw off the invaders.

Many other diseases are self–limited if supportive measures, such as adequate fluids, rest, proper nutrition, sunlight, and judicious balance of all hygienic remedies are combined. In spite of the many so-called "miracle drugs," the increase of infectious diseases of uncertain origin and the emergence of resistant organisms continue to challenge patients, as well as physicians in the pursuit of simple remedies.

I have been increasingly impressed with the potential of simple home remedies. As the future ravages of infectious diseases will be more common, more virulent, and people increasingly susceptible to their invasion, everyone must find better ways to treat illness. Even more vital, perhaps, we must learn how to protect ourselves from the diseases of civilization.

CHAPTER FOUR

DISEASES

OF THE

HEART

AND

CIRCULATION

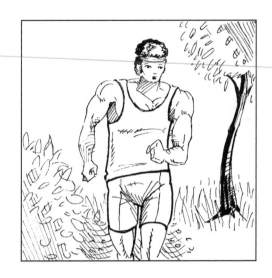

Interest in improving our heart and circulation has never been greater than in our world today. **Coronary heart disease** leads all other causes of death. Circulatory conditions (including stroke) take even more lives, and force millions into premature retirement, disability, or nursing home care. Thus the prevention and treatment of cardiovascular disease deserves our utmost attention. The fact is that about 750,000 die annually in the United States from heart disease and over 260,000 by stroke. These are prime reasons why the United States today is nowhere near the top of the list (actually 19th) for life expectancy in *men* compared to other world nations. For *women* we are 10th from the top of lifespan leaders. Heading the list of degenerative diseases, these fearsome afflictions of the circulation clamor for attention.

The human heart is without doubt the world's most amazing pump. About the size of a fist in the average man and weighing less than one pound, it pumps every day the equivalent of 7,000 quarts of blood! This precious fluid, weighing about seven tons, distributes itself through more than 60,000 miles of blood vessels in an average person. During our lifetime, the heart beats two and one half billion times, resting only between beats, and moves some 75,000,000 gallons of blood with all its life-sustaining oxygen and various nutrients!

In actuality, the four chambers of your heart constitute four pumps, with two pairs working in series. From the vascular circulation of your body — head, arms, legs, internal organs —blood is brought to the right*atrium*. Here is located the pacemaker, which begins an electrical impulse every second and initiates the beat of your entire heart. Blood is then pumped into the right *ventricle* and distributed to both lungs through the pulmonary arteries. Here your blood receives oxygen and gives off carbon dioxide, the two principle gases exchanged in respiration.

The fresh, oxygenated blood then returns to the heart, this time through pulmonary veins to the left atrium. Blood is thoroughly mixed in this chamber, since some of the blood cells received more oxygen than from other parts of the lungs, depending upon the posture and depth of respiration. Blood then passes through the mitral valve, into the left ventricle, the strongest portion of the heart muscle. Your heartbeat then contracts and propels blood through the aortic semi-lunar valve into the aorta, whence it is distributed to the extremities, brain, and all internal organs. Oxygen in the blood is delivered to cells, aiding the body in respiration, while the waste products carried by the same fluids and blood cells return through the veins to complete the cycle.

A number of diseases can occur, affecting this marvelously designed circulatory system. The heart can be affected by inherited or congenital disease. The aftermath of infection with Streptococcal organism can produce a condition known as **rheumatic fever** with its feared complication, **carditis**. This may damage heart valves, producing lifelong disability. Infections, as well as malignancies (cancer), can involve the heart. By far the most common affliction is **arteriosclerosis**, a degenerative disorder affecting the arteries.

Since the heart muscle receives blood through its own special system of coronary arteries, it is certainly true for this organ, as for the whole body that "The life of the flesh is in the blood."

HOW TO EVALUATE THE HEART

Many signs can reveal the existence of impaired circulation. The **color** of the body is extremely important. Since skin color is partially due to blood circulating just beneath it, it is important to compare skin hues in areas where your skin is particularly thin. The conjunctiva of the lower eyelid, the lips, the fingernail beds, and the palm are often valuable indicators of the state of your oxygen supply. A dusky color or bluish cast *(cyanosis)* indicates an inadequate supply of oxygen in the blood. Cyanosis may be seen in congenital heart afflictions, as is the case with "blue babies." Sometimes cyanosis develops when the blood is too thick *(hemoconcentration)* and the flow is sluggish.

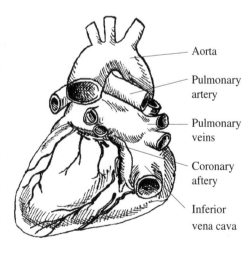

Aorta

Pulmonary artery

Pulmonary veins

Coronary aftery

Inferior vena cava

59

Frequently in advanced heart failure, cyanosis will be seen. Deep breathing, sitting upright, or administering oxygen may correct this problem.

The **pulse** should be examined; remember my description in Chapter One. It is normally regular and equal from side to side in the respective wrist arteries. Your **blood pressure** can also indicate the general state of the circulation, as well as the force of contraction in your heart itself. The veins along side your neck also are indicators of cardiac function. Normally little pulse waves are seen, but unusual distention usually means that the right side of the heart is unable to keep up with the demand. Examine the jugular veins particularly when a patient is sitting upright.

Finally, your heart itself is evaluated by first looking at the chest to see if there are unusual pulsations, then feeling with the hand to detect unusual vibrations or heaves, and finally listening with a stethoscope. The presence of turbulence, as the blood flows through the valves is reflected in sounds called *murmurs*. These can occur during either phase of the heart cycle. Considerable practice is needed to hear these specific sounds and understand their meaning.

Diagnostic tests are frequently performed to evaluate the efficiency of the heart. A **chest x-ray** can determine enlargement of one or more chambers. The **electrocardiogram** provides an excellent look at your electrical activity during each cardiac contraction. During exercise your heart rate should increase. An evaluation of the pulse and blood pressure during mild exercise on a motorized treadmill or bicycle (called a **stress test**) can be extremely helpful in assessing the dynamic function of this marvelous organ. More specialized tests are done in hospitals today, using x-rays, flow studies involving radioactive isotopes, **Thallium scanning** procedures, and the **coronary angiogram** which x-rays the heart in rapid sequence while a radiopaque dye is simultaneously injected into a coronary artery or blood vessel. This helps to visualize the heart chambers and vessels, and may indicate the need for surgery.

Arteriosclerosis

Hardening of the arteries, or arteriosclerosis, is the most common cause of serious heart disease today. This condition primarily affects your coronary arteries and large vessels. It is a disease intimately related to our fast-paced lifestyle, and principally involves the type of food eaten and other unhealthful habits formed. Arteriosclerosis actually begins in early childhood. Thus our preventive efforts must be directed toward infants and children to truly prevent the relentless progression of this degenerative condition.

Arteriosclerosis develops as our dietary fat intake increases. The modern unhealthful, refined diet uses large amounts of grease, oil, sugar, soft drinks, and desserts producing a state in the blood known as *hyperlipidemia*. The sluggish circulation of this excess fat promotes deposits in the walls of the arteries. Normal arteries have three layers, the middle one being muscular and the inner and outer layers being thin, delicate linings. Cholesterol enters the inner cells and deposits throughout the first two layers of the artery. This frequently occurs where there is a division or bend in the vessel.

The habit of smoking is especially harmful, as **carbon monoxide** in mainstream cigarette smoke tends to open these tiny lining *(endothelial)* cells and actually creates openings in the vessel wall, enabling cholesterol to penetrate more easily. As the years go by, this cholesterol plaque builds up, becoming thicker and eventually obstructing the vessel. Roughness in the lining cell creates more turbulence, which adds to the danger of *thrombosis*, or sudden clot formation in the vessel. That is the event which is known as a heart attack, or *myocardial infarction*.

It is not known why some individuals tend to form these deposits in the heart more readily, while others select out the brain, the aorta, or other vascular structures. Nevertheless, arteriosclerosis is affecting nearly every American and was even significant in 70% of the American youth killed in action during the Korean War. For reasons of lifestyle, mostly lower animal fat intake, few Koreans or Japanese get coronary heart disease. The picture changes rapidly, though, when they move to Hawaii or the continental USA.

A number of risk factors are directly associated with the development of arteriosclerosis and the inherent risk of coronary heart disease. **Obesity**, afflicting over one third of all adults, is directly associated with heart risk. Every five pounds of extra body fat requires four extra miles of blood vessels just to keep the cells nourished . Not only consult height and weight charts, but also measure skin folds to evaluate a person's obese potential. If the fold of pinched abdominal skin is an inch or more thick, men are definitely obese; for women the skin fold measure allowed is 1½ inches.

Insurance statistics show the obese individual to be at high risk, not only for cardiac disease, but also for several types of cancer, diabetes, gall stones, and numerous other health problems. America's overweight now number over 50 million people, still growing both in population and total accumulated pounds. Excess calories in the diet are either burned up or stored, but all calories must be accounted for. Our appetite problem is right in the center of a major preventive health program today,

Smoking directly causes an increased risk for coronary heart disease. **Nicotine**, the addictive alkaloid in tobacco, abnormally speeds the heart rate and raises the blood pressure. Carbon monoxide, as mentioned above, "shoots holes" in the artery walls for cholesterol to enter. An average tobacco smoker, according to the Framingham study has three times the risk for a heart attack and more than a 75% increased chance of dying from one! With increasing non-smoking years, these risks fall gradually to normal for the ex-smoker.

Hypertension or high blood pressure is a major risk factor in both heart attacks and strokes. The extra load imposed upon the heart as it pumps against increased resistance is a major factor in congestive heart failure, which may occur either gradually or in association with a sudden heart attack. This problem will be considered below, as it frequently is preventable.

The sedentary habits of Americans have also come under scrutiny. Inactivity is another major risk for the development of heart disease. Exercise is protective in many ways. It not only improves the peripheral circulation elsewhere in the body, but lowers the resting pulse rate, improves the volume of blood delivered with each heartbeat, and dilates the coronary arteries, both large and small. Many research studies comparing active with sedentary workers have demonstrated numerous protective benefits of moderate exercise in avoiding a fatal heart attack. Walking is especially beneficial. Nearly everyone can do it, too.

Other factors, such as the excessive intake of sugar, a positive family history for heart disease, longstanding presence of diabetes, advanced age, and male gender are related to a higher risk. Some of these can be modified in a healthful way.

Because dietary prevention is so important concerning the risk of coronary heart disease, we wish to spend more time on this vital yet controversial factor. Several simple principles must be understood and applied by anyone desiring to have a healthy heart. First of all, our dietary fat intake must be reduced. The average American takes in daily over 40% of his or her calories as fat. Half this much fat (10 to 20%) would definitely be more optimal. This would of necessity involve the elimination of many unnecessary fats, such as butter, fried greasy foods, flesh meats, rich pastries, oily salad dressings, and the excessive use of cheese, all having increased in Western dietaries over the past two decades.

An intelligent return to natural foods, such as whole grain cereals, and the increased use of fruits and vegetables, will aid you greatly in reducing fat intake. One fringe benefit of this adjustment will be the increased intake of **fiber**. Bran, found abundantly in whole grains and legumes, is an excellent source of dietary fiber. Increasing your fiber intake has been shown to help with elimination of **cholesterol** from arteries via your liver and the intestinal tract. Plant *sterols* present in whole grains and some vegetables will inhibit in a competitive fashion the absorption of cholesterol from the intestines. All these changes will make your food more interesting and grant much improved health for heart, brain, and longevity.

Most shoppers are aware that cholesterol is *always* of animal origin. With increased meat being used, the intake of fruits and vegetables as dietary staples have fallen off conspicuously for the average household. The richest source of food cholesterol is the yoke of an egg, over 230 mg. in one of medium size. The butterfat portion of milk and all derived milk products—such as cheese, butter, ice cream and cottage cheese—contain cholesterol. Meats, especially those rich in fat, are exceptionally abundant in cholesterol. Even poultry and fish are not excepted. The more cholesterol you take into your body, the higher the level blood cholesterol is likely to be. This accelerates the development of arteriosclerosis. I advise that as much as possible all dietary sources of cholesterol be eliminated. Then comes the good news; for most people coronary heart disease can begin to regress.

Actually, contemporary and very encouraging data is available to show that the cholesterol problem is in fact reversible. First you should begin with a change in diet and curtailment in the type of fat eaten. By lowering the total fat intake and eliminating cholesterol, your special protein-fat carriers, called lipoproteins, are mustered to mobilize cholesterol for transportation to the liver and eventual excretion in the bile. Modern measurements of blood **HDL** *(high density lipoprotein)* cholesterol have enabled even more accurate prediction of the state of this efficient cleansing mechanism.

Second, the avoidance of excess calories and refined sugars also helps combat the problem of fat deposition in the vascular structures. Combining a natural diet with adequate exercise will increase the preventive dividends.

With your general decrease in the use of fat, it is time next to take a look at oil. Biochemists agree that some fat is needed in the diet. For most people this can be obtained entirely from non-animal sources, such as nuts, olives, or avocados. In areas where these are scarce, in colder climates, or for extremely active occupations where more calories are needed, some vegetable fats could be taken in their refined form. Usually these are combined in the cooking process, as in making bread.

Certain fats, however, are clearly better from the standpoint of cholesterol control. Measuring the ratio of *polyunsaturated* to *saturated* fat (**P:S Ratio**) will help to establish the relative risk or benefits of certain seed oils. Corn, safflower, and soy oils are the best from the standpoint of polyunsaturated fats. The *monounsaturated* fats found in olives and olive oil convey a protective benefit on the heart and arteries. Peanut and cottonseed oil are of lesser value. It is crucial to avoid entirely the consumption of shortening, lard, and butter, for these hardened fats will always tend to increase the cholesterol content of the blood. Recipe books are available, which enable the average cook to lower greatly total fat consumption as well as choose the most healthful sources.

Signs and symptoms of heart disease challenge medical experts as well as laymen to find an accurate diagnosis. Chest pain is usually one of two principal qualities in heart disease. One type, called *angina pectoris*, is a transient pain, usually described as a pressure, aching, or squeezing in the area behind the left breast and associated with exercise. It may come on gradually as in walking up a hill or while mowing the lawn, or the pain may be triggered by stress, as in watching violent sports on television or by getting into an argument. Sometimes angina may arise after a heavy meal, because of the increased work load that digestion imposes on the heart. When exercise is a triggering factor, rest will within minutes relieve the pain. Sometimes an improvement of circulation results in the hands or feet by immersion in warm water to accelerate this relief process. In fact, it is important to keep the extremities warm when exercising on a cold day, to avoid chilling and thus reduce congestion around the heart.

The **heart attack**, or *acute myocardial infarction*, presents suddenly with chest pain of a much different character. Although in the elderly this serious event may occur silently, for most younger individuals a sudden heart attack produces definite symptoms. Occasionally, however, it may resemble heart-burn, a digestive problem, or may be thought to be related to indigestion. Classically the pain of a heart attack is located beneath the breast bone or left portion of the chest. Patients describe their chest pain as vise-like, squeezing, a tense, aching pain that at times radiates into the left shoulder or arm, or up into the neck or jaw. This pain persists, sometimes for hours, and may be associated with collapse or a catastrophic sudden death. About two out of seven individuals having an acute heart attack will die before reaching the emergency room.

Your physician's advice can be reassuring, and is particularly beneficial in establishing a prompt and accurate diagnosis. Electrocardiograms and blood tests for heart enzymes can aid in establishing the diagnosis. Temporary monitoring of the heart rhythm may be essential to observe for threatening signs of rhythm abnormality *(arrhythmia).*

With our modern technologic emphasis on cardiopulmonary resuscitation and emergency care, many lives have been spared. Nevertheless, it remains questionable whether our state-of-the-art coronary care units considered so essential in the United States do significantly reduce **mortality** from these attacks. In Great Britain, many heart attacks are treated at home, and with careful observation, rest and home nursing care, survival is about the same.

Usually the sufferer of a heart attack is well advised to stay in bed, With frequent movement of arms and legs to prevent blood clots (thrombosis) and deep breathing exercises to keep the lungs ventilated (preventing *atelectasis—* collapsed air sacs in the lungs), bed rest provides the safest treatment for each acute episode. Oxygen is usually administered and vital signs carefully monitored to detect any rhythm disturbances or signs of heart failure. Serve the patient a liquids only diet for a day or two, then a gradual progression to healthful solid foods at regular intervals (5 or 6 hours between each meal).

Recommended exercise consists of steady, progressive activity in the room, then inside the home, and finally carefully supervised cardiac reconditioning through prescribed outdoor exercises such as walking. These methods will enable most of afflicted heart patients to return to their desired level of function, eventually enjoying as good if not better health than before the heart attack. We have seen this happen in reconditioning centers around the country, including at Poland Spring.

Cardiac preventive exercises today are taking many forms. Although some doctors recommend no specific program, most physicians believe in exercise. Many are enthusiastic about fitness, some even joggers. Because of the orthopedic disadvantages, the risks, and the lack of objective data that running really saves lives, I believe that our main emphasis should be on **walking**. After a brief warm-up period, the fitness walker can begin at his most comfortable leisurely pace, then gradually increase the time, distance, and speed of this activity. Dr. Kenneth Cooper's "Aerobics" program, Dr. Dean Ornish's books, and many other popular books on heart disease prevention contain guidelines for the prudent approach to heart reconditioning.

Years of experience at both the **Wildwood Lifestyle Center & Hospital** and the **Poland Spring Health Institute** have convinced me that walking is your best overall protective exercise for the heart, the nerves, healthy blood vessels, optimum weight control, and normalizing the blood pressure for optimum prevention of arteriosclerosis. Any physical activity must be pursued regularly with enthusiasm and consistency in order to be effective, however. Noncompetitive sports, swimming, bicycle riding, and cross-country skiing, wood chopping, and gardening make excellent seasonal variations to the daily walk.

HIGH BLOOD PRESSURE

Medical authorities estimate that from 15-25% of Americans suffer from high blood pressure or **hypertension**. Our most conservative figure in this country is already over 25 million persons with hypertension. No single cause for this is proven. It appears that there are numerous types of hypertension, some related to chronic diseases and other patients with causes potentially reversible.

Salt ingestion is well known to be a risk factor in causing high blood pressure. More then four thousand years ago a Chinese by the name of Ch'i Po noted the "If too much salt is used in the food, the pulse hardens." The average American consumes from 6-13 grams of salt daily. Some in Western countries and many in the Orient use as much as 18-24 grams of salt a day! The incidence of high blood pressure in a population is increased in proportion to the sodium intake of the diet. The Japanese illustrate this, with increasing strokes as their major cause of death.

Sodium chloride, or table salt, is hidden in many foods—soups, canned vegetables, crackers, dried meats. It consists of about 40% sodium and 60% chloride. A teaspoon of salt contains about 2.3 grams of sodium. Your body needs only 220 milligrams (about a 10th of a teaspoon) of sodium a day. Most experts recommend that you consume no more than a teaspoon of salt a day in your diet.

Too much salt gets sprinkled on our food, often before even tasting it. Another portion appears in particularly salty types of foods, such as potato chips, salted nuts, and other snack foods. Prepared foods usually have their ingredients listed on the label in order of their proportion. Read the labels carefully; they may even have an analysis of sodium content printed with other nutrient values.

Not only is salt a problem, but other substances, such as baking soda, monosodium glutamate, and other sodium containing food additives will supply hidden forms of dietary salt. First, eliminate all added salt at the table—just remove the salt shaker. Next, cut back on excessively salty foods. These can easily bring down your sodium intake to approximately two grams per day. When you do buy processed foods, read the labels. Choose those foods that are lower in sodium. Further restrict sodium by avoiding milk and milk products, even salty vegetables, such as celery, beets, and leafy greens.

If you plan carefully, and use only salt-free breads and cereals, it will be possible to lower the sodium intake to one gram. Periodically, for patients in congestive heart failure, even a stricter regulation of salt intake is necessary to prevent fluid retention and to lower the blood pressure. Fruit and most natural vegetables are very low in sodium. More and more dietetic foods are supplying the needs for convenience in packaging without the danger of a hidden sodium content.

Symptoms of hypertension are variable. Most patients with high blood pressure have no symptoms at all. In actuality, well over half of the cases of high blood pressure in the Unites States are presently undetected. Physical symptoms such as headache, nosebleeds, visual disturbance, and signs of heart failure or kidney disease coexist in conjunction with high blood pressure. Home measurement of blood pressure is simple and becoming more convenient. Nearly all pharmacies carry blood pressure cuffs (the *sphygmomanometer*) for home use, together with detailed directions. And coin operated blood pressure machines are available in many shopping centers.

Numerous less common types of hypertension are surgically curable. Tumors of the adrenal gland, such as the adrenalin producing *pheochromocytoma* and cortisone producing *adenomas* can cause hypertension, among other symptoms. A third type of adrenal tumor produces the hormone *aldosterone*, which increases sodium retention, thereby elevating the blood pressure. Chronic diseases of the kidneys, due whether to infection, nephritis, or congenital cysts can cause hypertension. Arteriosclerosis, which narrows the arteries to one or both kidneys can also trigger a renin-angiotensin hormonal cycle that results in high blood pressure. Specialized tests are needed to diagnose these "curable" hypertensive diseases. Nevertheless, all of these together comprise only 5% of the total hypertensive patients.

In addition to a salt restricted diet, the individual with hypertension must learn to control **stress**. Our emotions are profoundly related to the incidence of hypertension. Furthermore, these tendencies are aggravated by excessive noise, a harried schedule, lack of sleep, and lack of exercise. Most of the time,

SODIUM AVERAGES FOR COMMON FOODS			
Food Group	Household Measure	Weight (g.)	Sodium (mg.)
Milk Exchanges	8 oz. (1/2 pt.)	240	120
Eggs	one	50	70
Vegetable Exchanges	1/2 cup	100	9
Fruit Exchanges	1 serving	varies	2
Bread Exchanges	1 serving	varies	5
Fat Exchanges	1 tsp.	5	0

fortunately, adherence to these simple preventives can help a person regain good control of his blood pressure.

STROKE

In the United States more than 200,000 people die annually from stroke. Many more are handicapped for life, and spend months to years in nursing homes. Stroke, formerly called *apoplexy*, now goes by the more modern term *cerebrovascular accident*. It is the culmination or combination of several health problems. **Thrombosis**, blood clotting, involving one of the major arteries to the brain, or a smaller artery within the brain can affect neurologic function and produce serious symptoms.

Blood clots may form elsewhere in the body and break off, forming an *embolus*. Going to the brain as a "cerebral embolism" initiates another type of stroke. In younger people a sudden *hemorrhage* in the brain may produce a stroke; it may be associated either with congenital defects in the artery wall (aneurysm) or some episode of trauma.

The symptoms of a stroke can vary widely. The most mild ones involve temporary slurring of speech, dizziness, weakness in a hand or arm, numbness. They may occur suddenly, then clearing within minutes to hours. This is called a **transient ischemic attack** (T.I.A.) and indicates the risk of more serious and more permanent damage, as well as the definite presence of arteriosclerosis.

The first major stroke usually occurs in the midportion to one hemi-sphere of the patient's brain. Usually one side is affected, with paralysis or weakness in an arm or leg. Sometimes both the arm and leg are involved, producing one-sided paralysis called *hemiplegia*. Occasionally some facial muscles will be involved as well. If the brain damage is on the dominant side — usually the left in a right-handed person — the speech will be impaired also.

Recovery from a stroke represents a triumph of determination on the part of the patient, and wisdom and skill by the rehabilitative medical team. Rehabilitation is often a costly and prolonged procedure, with hospitalization in the acute stage, and long-term physical therapy for vocational re-education in most activities, including the use of wheelchairs, walkers, braces, canes, and a gradual return to normal activities. Local heart associations have informative literature concerning the treatment in a home-like setting for a person who has had a stroke. Continued effort for many months is frequently rewarded by the recovery of a loved one to productivity and self respect.

The prevention of stroke primarily falls into the dimensions of diet and other lifestyle changes. Control of stress, adequate daily exercise, and a balance between mental and physical labor are extremely important. Some time each day should be spent outdoors, especially if your work is basically sedentary. The diet should be limited in sodium to a maximum of 2 to 3 grams of salt intake daily. Your low fat vegetarian diet helps maintain the blood cholesterol as low as possible. These measures will prevent a gradual buildup of cholesterol plaques, leading to arteriosclerosis in your brain arteries. Home treatment of stroke is an outstanding ministry for nurses, well worth your thought and study.

ANEMIAS

Because of television advertising of vitamins and the contemporary dependence on supplements, *anemia* has almost become a household word. Lowering of hemoglobin and/or scarcity of red blood cells in the circulation manifests this condition. The delivery of oxygen to the cells is impaired, and predictable symptoms will result. Most causes of anemia are still nutritional.

The nutrients necessary for the formation of red blood cells by our bone marrow are usually available in a varied vegetarian diet. Adequate quantities of iron, folic acid, vitamin B_{12}, and protein are especially necessary. Each one of these nutrients can become the limiting factor in blood production and, when deficient for a period of time, can produce anemia.

The symptoms of anemia are frequently profound **fatigue, dizziness**, particularly on arising suddenly, limited exercise tolerance, and **pallor** or paleness to the skin. Many physicians can estimate the degree of anemia by looking within the individual's lower eyelid (*conjunctiva*). Hemoglobin determination involves the laboratory; measuring the red blood cell count and hematocrit (the per cent ratio of blood cells to whole blood) are useful to evaluate the extent of anemia. Microscopic view of the red blood cells may give some hint concerning the cause. The iron level in your blood, serum vitamin B_{12}, and other similar factors can be measured in most laboratories.

Iron deficiency is the most common cause of anemia. This is seen most commonly in lower socioeconomic classes of society. A diet that is low in greens and whole grain cereals will be more likely to lack iron and produce anemia. Babies are normally born with a high hemoglobin, but receive some iron from their mother's milk. Those on cow's milk without supplemental iron will develop progressive anemia. Some of this may be "physiologic", but most of it can be prevented with appropriate baby formula. Iron-rich foods include dark green vegetables such as spinach, kale, broccoli, and chard.

Whole wheat and other unrefined grains contain iron, and in "enriched" flour most of the lost iron is replaced. Certain fruits, such as grapes, raisins, strawberries, and blackberries contain liberal amounts of iron. These are the best food sources and can adequately nourish a growing child, adult, or even mothers during pregnancy. The use of iron kettles in cooking will also add iron, particularly when boiling acid fruits or sauces. Some iron may be available in community water supplies.

The adequate intake of Vitamin B_{12} has stirred many controversies among vegetarians. It is well established that some vegetables fresh from the ground many contain trace amounts of vitamin B_{12} or *cobalamin*. However, the

B_{12} availability is no where near adequate for normal nutrition. Some B_{12} is made by bacteria in the colon, but it is not known that this will be adequately absorbed. Most dietary Vitamin B_{12} is obtained from foods of animal origin, particularly milk and eggs. This is made available to our bodies for absorption by *intrinsic factor*, supplied in the stomach.

The vitamin B_{12} is then absorbed in the small intestine and stored for long periods in the liver. In actuality, most individuals can thrive without B_{12} for many years before developing symptoms of the deficiency. Unfortunately for the few, **neurologic problems** can develop with tingling, numbness, weakness in the extremities, due to degenerative breakdown in the posterior portion of the spinal cord. Some functional deficit may remain permanently, even though the anemia is reversed.

Folic acid deficiency can produce a similar anemia, but without the neurologic problems. This B vitamin is seldom deficient, though, except in certain disease states involving malabsorption. The individual who is eating a total vegetarian diet, without milk, eggs, or other animal foods would do well to obtain some source of vitamin B_{12} as a tablet, an injection, or in various fortified foods at least every month. Thorough chewing of any B_{12} vitamin supplement assists absorption. There appears to be a second hormone in the saliva to assist this process.

Other causes of anemia include *chronic blood loss* from heavy menstruation or hidden (*occult*) bleeding in the intestinal tract. Older individuals should definitely have a complete examination if anemia is discovered, to exclude the possibility of undetected cancer. During the menstrual years, a woman may lose excessive blood in the monthly period and, not obtaining adequate replacement, could develop anemia. Iron is occasionally needed in supplemental form during pregnancy to correct a developing anemia that results in dizzy spells or weakness.

Any persistent anemia not related to blood loss or nutritional deficiency, and refractive to simple therapy, should be investigated by a physician. Chronic disease of the kidneys, acute or chronic leukemia, or abnormal destruction of the blood cells (*hemolysis*) may require examination of the bone marrow and a careful medical investigation to discover and remove their causes. Most anemias can be treated and cured, the detective work involved providing a challenge to every medical diagnostician.

VARICOSE VEINS

Abnormal dilation of leg veins may occur from many causes. **Varicose veins** usually appear on the surface of the skin. Most common in the legs, they may also occur in the entire lower extremity, the perineum, the pelvis, or the abdomen. Dilation of rectal veins are usually called *hemorrhoids*, while in the scrotum, they are termed a *varicocele*.

The late Dr. Dennis Burkett of England taught for decades that varicose veins result from a deficient intake of fiber in the diet. This creates, he said, the necessity for increased straining, thus elevating the abdominal pressure, and stretching the veins. While this may constitute one cause, I believe that there are many causes of varicose veins. Some of these follow episodes of *thrombophlebitis*, an inflamed blood clot in the same involved veins. Unwisely wearing tight constricting garments around the upper thigh or waist, as well as prolonged sitting or standing, can promote the development of unwelcome varicosities. They are usually aggravated by pregnancy or any other condition that raises the pressure within the abdomen.

Although some writers think that vitamin E is curative, scientific evidence is presently inconclusive. We know that exercise and the use of whirlpool baths are beneficial in chronic disease involving the veins. An increase of fiber in the diet will provide better elimination, decreasing the need for straining with unnatural elevation of the abdominal pressure.

Symptoms of aching in the legs or unsightly deformities of the skin can be treated with the wearing of elastic support hose. These should be of a surgical quality and appropriately fitted to the patient's size. **Jobst** company will custom design your hose after careful measurement, if you want the best, most expensive product. Many people with varicose veins below the knee should wear support stockings up to the knee, while others require a full length hose to appropriately compress the veins and prevent them from dilating further. Occasionally, surgery is indicated, called a vein *stripping and ligation,* to remove the offenders. Most varicose veins, nonetheless, can be treated at home.

One dreadful complication that patients fear is the varicose ulcer, usually developing on the inner side of the ankle, below a varicose vein. This needs urgent treatment to reduce the hazard of infection and promote rapid healing. Bed rest is combined with elevation of the affected limb, together with hot and cold soaks, and careful antiseptic cleansing of the ulcer. This method, even at home, will usually promote rapid healing. Swelling in the ankles needs to be reduced by the combined influence of gravity (elevate the legs) and salt restriction. At times a topical application of vitamin E, aloe vera, or the healing effect of oxygen administered with a plastic bag around the foot can help to promote more rapid healing.

THROMBOPHLEBITIS

Clots may form at any time in stagnant or injured veins. The smallest veins on the skin surface become red and tender. Inflammation of the veins, with clotted blood inside obstructing flow, is called *thrombophlebitis*. This condition does not constitute a great threat to health, however, and responds to a few days of bed rest with elevation of the extremity and frequent application of moist, hot compresses. *Deep vein thrombosis* is more serious. As the clot extends into a deeper vein, it may break off or fragment, migrating through the larger veins to the lungs. A sudden clot in the lungs, *pulmonary embolism*, may tragically be fatal. Usually an embolism produces chest pain, cough, and some transient shortness of breath.

Hot packs and bed rest are helpful in the management of this type of acute thrombosis. The diet must be very low in fat, particularly eliminating any meat or swine's flesh, since the chemicals derived from these toxic foods tend to promote clot formation. Platelets in the blood, which normally being protective and serve to prevent bleeding, will become sticky and adhere to one another, increasing the tendency for thrombosis to occur. The use of estrogen supplements and oral contraceptives significantly increases the risk of thrombosis. Tobacco also produces spasm of the vessels, compromising the circulation, and may trigger development of an abnormal clot within a blood vessel.

CONGESTIVE HEART FAILURE

When one side of the heart pumps less than the other side, congestion results. Usually the left portion of the heart first becomes weak, forcing the blood to back up into the lungs, with resulting congestion. Shortness of breath associated with cough, the coughing of blood *(hemoptysis)*, or inability to lie flat in bed will result from this type of *passive congestion*.

When the right heart chambers are unable to keep up with the pumping load, congestion develops in the general circulation. Distention of the neck veins ensues, with swelling of the liver and retention of fluid in the abdomen *(ascites)*, the legs, and the ankles. Sometimes an unusually ruddy complexion will result, with *cyanosis* in more serious cases.

Symptoms of shortness of breath on exertion will be followed by nocturnal episodes of air hunger. The patient may be unable to sleep lying down, and require a recliner lounge chair, or he may sleep in bed propped on several pillows. His weight increases rapidly, due to fluid retention. If treatment is not received promptly, *acute pulmonary edema* may develop, requiring emergency hospitalization.

Common causes of congestive heart failure include hypertension, with its frequent problem of excessive salt intake, and arteriosclerosis. Less common causes are thiamine (B_1) deficiency, hyperthyroid conditions, heart muscle inflammation (*myocarditis*, usually viral), or tumors involving the heart.

Bed rest in the acute stage requires a limitation of exercise, associated with strict control of dietary salt intake and, for serious complications, even fluid restriction. These remedies will bring relief for most cases of heart failure. A careful investigation into the causes will generally provide a basis for more specific therapy. Warmth to the extremities, a calm peaceful mind, and the avoidance of drugs which adversely affect the cardiac rhythm will likewise prove beneficial.

Kidney function can be enhanced with hot packs across the low back. Ice packs over the heart can slow its rate in most cases, except the rhythm disorder called atrial fibrillation. Unusual irregular pulses and very rapid heart rates should be evaluated by a physician.

Of great importance in congestive heart failure, as in treatment of hypertension, is a strict limitation of sodium intake. I have seen in my institution many heart patients recover from congestive failure on a salt restricted diet. Sometimes they improve only to indulge in salt again through ignorance or habit when returning home. Then, promptly, their fluid retention and heart failure return. Appetite control, a knowledge of nutrition, and carefulness in exercise are fundamental to properly maintain a healthful circulation.

THE FOLLOWING PAGES WILL HELP YOU PREPARE A DIET LOW IN SODIUM, SATURATED FATTY ACID, AND CHOLESTEROL. THERAPEUTIC USE OF THESE GUIDE-LINES WILL REDUCE YOUR RISK OF HEART ATTACKS AND IMPROVE RESISTANCE TO ARTERIOSCLEROSIS.

LOW SODIUM DIET

500 Milligram Sodium Diet (with adaption for 250 and 1000 mg.)

INCLUDE IN EACH DAY'S DIET

Milk, skim or soy	2 cups
Milk, low-sodium	1 cup
Soups, unsalted	1 serving
Bread, unsalted	3 slices
Cereal, unsalted	1 serving

Fruit and Juices

Citrus	1 serving
Other fruits	3 servings

Vegetables and Entrees

Potato or substitute	1 serving
Other (one should be green, leafy, or yellow)	2 servings
Legumes - beans, peas	1 serving
Meat Alternates (see List)	2 servings

Miscellaneous

Desserts (see List)	1 serving
Sweets (jelly, honey)	as desired
Margarine, unsalted	4-5 servings

HELPFUL SUGGESTIONS:

1. Do not use salt, baking powder, baking soda, MSG (*monosodium glutamate*) or anything with added sodium in cooking or seasoning food.

2. Use distilled water for drinking and cooking.

3. Read all labels and avoid foods that contain salt or sodium (*Na*) preservatives.

4. Do not use foods that have been cured, smoked, pickled, corned, or processed in any way with salt or sodium.

5. Since salt is restricted, it is important to plan flavor combinations from the seasonings suggested to enhance the flavor of foods used. See Lemon, Butter, Sweet-Sour Sauce, Unsalted Mayonnaise, and Hot Low-Sodium Salad Dressing.

MENU PATTERN

Here are some simple meals for a starter.

BREAKFAST

Fresh fruit or juice or both
Unsalted whole-grain cereal with milk
Peanut butter or nuts
Unsalted toast with unsalted margarine
Low-sodium milk
Honey or jelly

BREAKFAST

Orange Juice
Unsalted oatmeal with milk
Scrambled tofu
Unsalted toast with unsalted margarine
Fresh fruit or applesauce
Jelly, jam, or honey

LUNCHEON OR SUPPER

Unsalted tomato soup, if desired
Unsalted meat alternate (see list)
Unsalted vegetable
Fruit as salad or dessert
Unsalted bread
Unsalted margarine

LUNCHEON OR SUPPER

Unsalted vegetable soup
Unsalted cottage cheese
Unsalted broccoli with soy cheese
Tossed fresh salad
Unsalted bread
Unsalted margarine
Skim milk

DINNER

Unsalted meat alternate (see list)
Unsalted potato or substitute
Unsalted vegetable
Vegetable salad (unsalted)
Fruit or allowed dessert
Unsalted bread
Unsalted margarine
Skim or soy milk

DINNER

Unsalted soy beans
Baked potato with unsalted margarine
Sliced tomatoes with unsalted soy mayonnaise
Banana orange fruit cup
Unsalted cookies
Unsalted bread
Unsalted margarine
Skim or soy milk

For a 250 mg. sodium diet, you may substitute dialyzed or low-sodium milk for skim milk at dinner and supper.

For a 1000 mg. sodium diet, try to substitute skim or soy milk for low-sodium milk at breakfast, tap water for distilled water. Use beets, celery, chard, and other "greens" as desired.

Try this tasty **LOW-SODIUM SALAD DRESSING**

> Canned tomato, tomato juice, or puree (no sodium added), flavored with lemon, sugar, onion, garlic, and herbs as desired.

YOU MAY USE THE FOLLOWING SEASONINGS:

Almond extract
Anise seed
Bakon yeast
Basil, sweet
Bay leaf
Caraway seed
Cassia
Chives
Cumin seed
Dill
Fennel seed
Garlic
Lemon juice
Lemon extract
Maple extract
Marjoram
Mint
Onion
Oregano
Paprika
Parsley, fresh only
Peppermint extract
Rosemary
Sage
Sesame seed
Vanilla

HERB BUTTER FOR VEGETABLES, etc.

Basic Mix for **Lemon Butter**:

> Water, boiling   1 1/2 teaspoons
> Margarine, unsalted 2 tablespoons
> Lemon juice   1 tablespoon
> To the Basic Mix add
> 1 teaspoon to 1 tablespoon herbs, such as minced parsley, scraped onion, minced garlic, paprika.

SWEET-SOUR SAUCE FOR VEGETABLES

> Lemon juice and sugar seasoned with grated onion, and herbs as desired.

You May Also Use:

Beverages and Soups

> Cereal beverages (Pero, Postum, Roma, etc.) with distilled water. Hot carob beverage made with skim or soy milk allowed.
> Unsalted broth or soup made from low-sodium milk and allowed vegetable.

Breads and Cereals

> Breads made WITHOUT salt, baking powder, baking soda, eggs, or preservatives containing sodium.
> Unsalted bread, unsalted Pita bread.

Fruits and Juices

> Use any fresh, canned, or frozen fruit or juices except limited amounts of raisins and dried figs. Include one citrus fruit or other food high in vitamin C daily.

Vegetables

> White or sweet potato, macaroni, noodles, rice, spaghetti, all prepared without salt.
> Fresh, canned, or frozen WITHOUT SALT asparagus, eggplant, string beans, peas, pumpkin, squash, lettuce, tomatoes, kale, mustard greens.
> The strong-flavored vegetables - broccoli, Brussels sprouts, cabbage,

cauliflower, cucumber, onions, radishes, turnips - should be limited if they cause distention.

Use ONLY ONCE A WEEK: beets, beet greens, celery, Swiss chard, spinach, carrots.
Use one green or yellow vegetable daily.

Meat Alternates

Unsalted cottage cheese, soy beans, tofu (soy cheese), dried legumes (beans, garbanzos and lentils); unsalted nut butters; unsalted prepared meat alternates (vegetable protein products).

Desserts

Vegetable gelatin desserts made with canned or frozen fruits allowed; ice dream (homemade), using fruit whiz.

Fats

Unsalted salad dressing without eggs; vegetable oils, soy cream.

Miscellaneous

Seasonings (except those listed under *You may not use*), unsalted nuts, unsalted popcorn.

YOU SHOULD NOT USE the following:

Beverages and Soups

Buttermilk, regular milk in excess of 2 cups
Instant cocoa mixes, "Dutch process" cocoa.
Salted tomato juice, coffee, tea.
Water which has been run through water softening equipment.

Breads and Cereals

Commercial bread, biscuits, pancake or waffle mixes. Salted bread, self-rising flours; pretzels; white and graham crackers.
Quick-cooking cereals containing salt. Roman meal, oven cooked wheat, dry prepared cereals except allowed unsalted ones.

Fruits

Those containing sodium benzoate as a preservative as *Maraschino* cherries. Raw apples and melons should be avoided only if they cause discomfort.

Vegetables

Vegetables prepared with salt.
Frozen corn, frozen lima beans, frozen peas and mixtures of these vegetables. Sauerkraut, white turnips.

Limit these to ONCE A WEEK since they are higher in natural sodium: beets, beet greens, carrots, celery, spinach, Swiss chard.

Desserts

Any prepared with salt, baking powder, baking soda, eggs, regular milk; commercial gelatin dessert; commercial ice cream; rennet desserts.

Fats

Salted butter, salted margarine, salad dressings made with salt and egg white.

Miscellaneous

Catsup, chili sauce, salted gravy, salted nuts, salted popcorn, salt, seasonings such as celery salt and celery seeds, garlic salts, onion salt, monosodium glutamate (*Accent*), Bakon yeast, meat tenderizers, chemically softened water.

STRICT DIET for LOWERING CHOLESTEROL and BLOOD FATS

This diet is formulated to be cholesterol free, very low in fat, and high in complex carbohydrates, with no refined sugar. Foods should be chosen from unrefined sources, eating the food in as natural a state as practical. Animal products are omitted, except for a limited use of skim milk and egg whites.

This diet meets the daily requirements for vitamins, minerals, protein, and fat. **Calories** are restricted to aid in weight reduction (special 1200, 1500, and 1800 calorie plans are included).

If sodium restriction is also desired, this diet will meet your requirement by simply following the procedure of not adding any salt, and not buying foods with salt added in processing (be sure to read labels).

This diet provides the following approximate composition:

Fat - 10-12% of the calories, all from vegetable fat sources.

Protein - 15-18% of calories (55 to 68 gms. of protein).

Carbohydrate - 73% of calories, composed primarily of complex carbohydrates in as unrefined a state as practical.

INSTRUCTIONS

Foods are listed under two main categories: Foods Permitted, and Foods Omitted. The various types of foods are then broken down into six basic food groups, vegetables, fruits, grains, milk, fats, and protein rich foods. Specific foods are listed with serving sizes. Follow the recommended number of servings per food group as specified for the 1200, 1500, or 1800 calorie diet listed below. Suggested daily menus and some recipes are provided in the following pages to assist you in meal planning.

FOODS PERMITTED

VEGETABLE GROUP

One serving provides approximately 2 gms. of protein, 8 gms. of complex carbohydrates, a trace of polyunsaturated fats, and 40 calories.

Asparagus, 7-8 spears
Beans, Green snap, 1 cup
Bean Sprouts, 1 1/2 cups
Beets, 2 beets, 2" dia.
Broccoli, 1 1/2 stalks, or 1 cup
Brussels sprouts, 7-8 medium
Cabbage 1 1/2 cups raw shredded, 1 cup cooked
Carrots, 1 large, 2 small raw, 3/4 cup cooked
Cauliflower, 1 cup, raw or cooked
Celery, no restriction
Chard, 1 cup, cooked
Collards, 1/2 cooked
Cucumbers, no restriction
Egg plant, 3 slices
Kale, 3/4 cup cooked

Lettuce and other salad greens, no restriction
Mushrooms, 12-14 small, 6 large
Mustard green, 3/4 cup cooked
Onions, 1 small
Onions, green, 4 small, including tops
Parsnips, 1/2 of a small parsnip, 1/3 cup cooked
Peas, 1/2 cup
Peppers, green, no restriction
Potatoes, 1/2 of a small potato, 2/5 cooked
Pumpkin, 1/2 cup cooked
Radishes, no restriction
Rutabagas, 3 oz. raw, 1/2 cup cooked
Spinach, 1 cup cooked
Squash, summer 1 cup cooked
Squash, winter 2/5 cup cooked
Sweet potatoes 1/3 small
Tomatoes, 1 medium
Tomato juice, 1 cup
Turnip greens, 1 cup cooked
Vegetable juice cocktail, 1 cup
Yams, 1/4 cup cooked

FRUIT GROUP

One serving of fruit provides approximately 20 grams of carbohydrates, a trace of protein and fats, and 80 calories.

Fruit should be fresh or preserved without added sugar.

Apple, 1 medium
Apricots, 4-5 medium
Banana, 1 small
Blackberries, 1 cup raw
Blueberries, 1 cup raw
Boysenberries, 1 cup raw
Cantaloupe, 1/2 medium melon
Cherries, sweet - raw, 18 large
Dates, 3 medium
Figs, fresh, 2 large
Grapefruit, one medium
Grapes, fresh, 3/4 cup
Guavas, 1 medium
Lemons, 2 medium

Mangoes, 1/2 medium
Nectarines, 2 medium
Orange, 1 medium
Papaya, 2/3 medium
Peaches, 2 medium, 1 cup sliced raw
Pear, 1 small
Persimmon, 1 medium
Pineapple, raw, 1 cup
Plums, 2 medium
Prunes, 3 medium
Pomegranate, 1 large
Raisin, 2 1/2 t.
Raspberries, fresh, 1 cup
Strawberries, fresh, 1 1/3 cups
Tangerine, 2 large
Watermelon, 1 slice, 6 inch diameter, 3/4" thick

CEREAL-GRAIN GROUP

One serving of cereal-grains provides approximately 3 grams of protein, 18 grams of complex carbohydrates, and 100 calories.

Bread, whole grain, 1 1/2 slices
Roll, 1 average
Tortilla, corn, 1 1/1 6" diameter
Pancake (made with egg white and whole grains), 1
Rice, brown, 3/4 cup cooked
Sweet corn, 1 medium ear
Corn, canned, 3/4 cup
Cornmeal, whole grain, 1/4 cup
Oatmeal, dry, 1/4 cup
Oatmeal, cooked, 2/3 cup
Wheat, cracked, 2/3 cup cooked
Wheat flour, whole grain, 1/4 cup
Rye flour, 1/3 cup

Breakfast cereals, prepared
All Bran, 1/2 cup
Bran Flakes, 40% 3/4 cup
Grape nuts, 1/4 cup
Shredded wheat, 1 1/4 biscuits
Wheat chex, 1/2 cup
Rye crisp 4-5 small wafers.

MILK GROUP

One serving of milk provides 9 grams of protein, 12 grams of carbohydrate, and 90 calories.

Skim (non-fat) milk, 1 cup
Butter milk, 1 cup
Soy milk, 2/3 cup

FAT GROUP

One serving of fat provides 5 gms. of fat and 45 calories.

Vegetable oil, 1 teaspoon
Margarine, soft tub, 1 1/2 teaspoons
Peanut butter, 1 1/2 teaspoons

PROTEIN GROUP

One serving of protein rich foods provides approximately 15 gms. of protein, 40 grams of complex carbohydrates, 2.5 gms. of fats (polyunsaturated), and 240 calories.

Legumes:
Brown beans, 1 cup
Chickpeas (garbanzos), 1 cup
Cuban black beans, 1 cup
Kidney beans, 1 cup
Lentils, 1 cup
Lima beans, 1 cup
Pinto beans, 1 cup
Soy beans, 4/5 cup (higher fat content, 9 gms.)
Split peas, soup (made with skim milk), 1 1/2 cups
White navy beans, 1 cup

Entrees (Legume, Grain, Vegetable combinations)

Bean-oat patties, 2 patties
Bulgur Chick patties, 2 patties
Chili beans, (made with TVP), 1 cup

Garbanzo roast, 4/5 cup
Garbanzo-rice patties, 2 patties
Lentil roast, 4/5 cup
Lentil-millet roast, 4/5 cup
Savory patties, 2 patties
Soy-oat patties, 2 patties
Soybean casserole, 4/5 cup
Vegeburgers, (made with TVP and/or egg whites), 2

Meat Alternates

Cottage cheese, 1/2 cup
Egg white, one (5.5 gm. protein, but only 16 cal.)
Use egg whites in food preparation, count as part of the entree instead of separately.
TVP (textured vegetable protein), dry, 2 oz.
Tofu

FOODS OMITTED

If on a sodium restriction, **omit** pickles, sauerkraut, and processed foods with salt added.
Read the labels carefully!

Canned and frozen fruits that have added sugar:

Refined cereal products, such as: White flour, white bread, noodles, macaroni, white rice, pastry, cookies, cake, crackers.

Omit whole milk, ice cream, non-dairy creamer substitutes.

All solid fats, and animal fats, especially lard.

Meat, fish, poultry, cheese, shellfish, and foods containing these animal products.

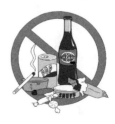

MEAL PLAN

FOR 1200 CALORIES, 1500 CALORIES, AND 1800 CALORIES

FOOD GROUPS	NUMBER OF SERVINGS FOR:		
	1200 calories	1500 calories	1800 calories
Vegetables	3	4	6
Fruits	2	3	3
Cereals–Grains	3	4	6
Milk-skim & soy	1	1	1
Fats	1	2	3
Protein rich foods	2	2	2

Sample Meal Plan for One Day
(1200 calorie plan)

Breakfast	**Lunch**	**Supper**
Fruits — 2 serv.	Vegetables — 1 or 2	Vegetables — 1 or 2
Cereal-Grains — 1	Cereal-Grains — 1	*(Depending on lunch)*
Milk group — 1	Protein food — 1	Cereal-Grains — 1
Protein food — 1		

Fat serving may be used in preparing entree or wherever desired.

TYPES OF FATTY ACIDS IN COMMON FOOD OILS

Vegetable Oil	Saturated Fatty Acids *	Monoun-saturated Fatty Acids *	Polyun-saturated Fatty Acids *
Coconut	86	7	. .
Cocoa butter	56	37	2
Olive	11	76	7
Peanut	22	43	29
Cottonseed	25	21	50
Soy	15	20	59
Corn	10	28	54
Safflower	8	15	72

* Grams per 100 g. of ether extracted or crude fat.

From **USDA Home Economics Report No. 7**, and Brown, H.B., and Farrand, M.G.: *Journal of the American Dietetic Association*, 49:303, 1966

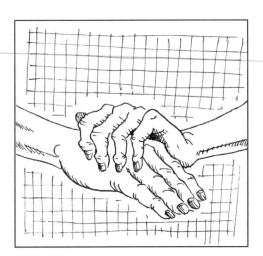

CHAPTER FIVE

ARTHRITIS

There are many degenerative diseases which involve our joints and their connective tissues. The causes of these afflictions are varied and include accidents, injuries, infections, hormone disorders, cancer, and aberrations of the immune system. Most of these conditions involving the joints can generate pain, stiffness, swelling, redness, increased warmth, or progressive limitation of motion. The involvement of a single joint or of several joints may actually be a manifestation of systemic illness or caused by a disorder confined to the particular joint. It is crucial to consider **all** of the above possibilities in ascertaining the precise cause. Some disorders are self-limited and leave no residual handicap, whereas other illnesses become chronic and may lead to progressive joint destruction.

An initial step in evaluating painful diseases of our joints is to confirm whether the symptoms involve the joint itself or the structures around the joint. **Bursitis, tendonitis**, and **cellulitis** can usually be distinguished from actual joint disease, through the withdrawal of joint fluid with a sterile needle and syringe, and its examination under the microscope. Accurately taken x-rays are necessary to provide the most accurate diagnosis.

Depression or anxiety often exists in conjunction with joint symptoms. Most of the time *"psychogenic rheumatism"* coexists without obvious signs of abnormalities in the muscles or bones. Articular (joint) involvement manifests itself, however, by joint tenderness, increased warmth, redness, the collection of fluid in the joint, and restriction of motion. Sometimes in the knees, one feels a click or grating sensation with rapid movement. Be sure to look the body over in its entirety for other signs of disease. The eyes, the skin, any presence of fever, the blood pressure are all valuable indexes to a general state of health.

RHEUMATOID ARTHRITIS

Of all forms of joint inflammation, rheumatoid arthritis is the most disastrous, destructive, and disabling. It may strike suddenly, then progress rapidly to an acute and seriously damaging stage. Although seven out of ten cases of rheumatoid arthritis occur between the age of 20 and 60, its onset could come at any time during life. Frequently, it advances subtly and deceptively. The initial symptoms appear for a few days and go away, then come back later slightly worse. There may be weeks or months between goings and comings. Gradually the disease reappears at shorter intervals, until it is a daily problem, which cannot be ignored. No two patients are quite the same. No one can say how any given instance is going to heal, except there will for certain be ups and downs.

Physicians use the term *remission* to describe times when a disease seems to go away by itself. The pain, stiffness, and swelling of rheumatoid arthritis even in severe cases may suddenly subside and disappear for months or even years. For about 25% of these fortunate individuals, it never comes back. Damage already done, though, does not miraculously disappear, even if the victim cannot tell by pain or other symptoms that the disease is still there. Moreover, his or her arthritis is likely to flair up again in the same insidious way that it first appeared.

People with rheumatoid arthritis can feel sick all over. The main targets of rheumatic disease are the joints of both hands, the arms, the hips, the knees, and the feet. People may be affected generally with fever, fatigue, and poor appetite. They may lose weight and develop anemia. Occasionally the lymph glands or spleen may become enlarged. It is quite common for the arthritis patient to be troubled by coldness, trembling of the hands and feet, or excessive sweating.

Rheumatoid arthritis usually affects more than one joint. The joint first stiffens, then swells and becomes tender, eventually making its entire motion difficult and painful. These symptoms are typically at their worst when the patient first arises in the morning. Pain and stiffness tend to get better after he or she has been up and moving for a while. Some patients develop small lumps under the skin, called *rheumatoid nodules*. These are usually at the elbows, knees, or ankles, and may be quite tender.

Progressive damage may occur inside the joint. Here is what happens. The area where two bones meet is enclosed, usually in a capsule that contains fluid. This joint capsule has an inner lining called the *synovial membrane*. The inflammation of rheumatoid arthritis starts here, swelling this membrane and spreading to other parts of the joint. An outgrowth of inflamed tissue invades the cartilage surrounding the bone ends, eventually eating it away. Finally scar tissue forms between the bones. Sometimes a scar transforms itself into actual bone, permanently fusing and rendering it immovable.

While a joint is undergoing this destruction, muscle contraction can cause contracture and severe deformity. This is most apparent when the disease attacks the hands; the fingers can become so distorted that they are virtually useless.

Even though the *cause* of rheumatoid arthritis is not completely known, scientists believe it is due to some type of a germ, possibly a bacterium or virus. The immune system is involved also, and harmful antibodies frequently form, attacking our own body tissues, in this case the joints. The key to success in combating the long term complications of rheumatoid arthritis is a treatment program begun **early** and carried out **faithfully** for a life time.

The diet of the patient with rheumatoid arthritis is exceptionally important. Refined sugars, all sweets and excessive fats in the diet should studiously be avoided. Meat intake should be curtailed and ultimately eliminated, as well as spices, condiments, and unnecessary food additives. It is worth trying to eliminate nightshade plants from the menu. These include tomatoes, potatoes, eggplant, and peppers. At least 20% of our patients have benefited from this restriction, especially with relief of joint pain. The diet should be simple, of good quality, with a variety of natural foods, eaten at regular intervals. Adequate water intake is important to insure good hydration of joint tissues, as well as maintaining a vigorous circulation.

As part of the treatment program, one should also find the ideal personal balance between **rest** and **exercise**. This may vary from person to person depending upon how severely the disease process is raging. The acute stages of arthritis require more rest, while with improvement, exercise is most essential. Inflammation usually subsides with bed rest, but prolonged immobility can rapidly lead to stiffening and contracture of diseased joints.

Incorrect **posture** in standing, walking, sitting, or lying down puts unnecessary strain on inflamed joints. This is why guidelines for correct posture are part of the treatment. Rarely, an inflamed joint might be splinted to protect it from the abnormal pull of muscle spasm, yielding contractures which cause painful deformities. Particularly is this important in the hands and fingers, to keep them functioning smoothly.

Much of the crippling of rheumatoid arthritis develops because the painful joints are kept for long periods in what *feels* like a comfortable position. They then become frozen or stiffened, while muscles around the joint are weak from inactivity. The way to keep your joints mobile is to move them. In rheumatoid arthritis an exercise prescription does not mean athletics, lifting heavy things, jogging, or any strenuous activity. Quiet exercises tailor-made for the problem must be performed every day, putting the joints through their full range of motion.

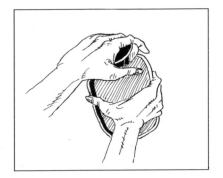

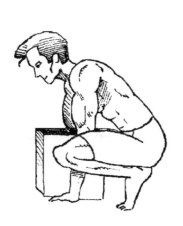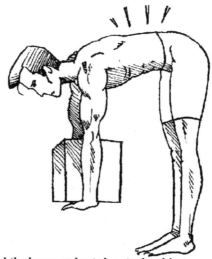

Healthful method of lifting. Bend the knees and get close to the object. Grasp it firmly and hold it close to you. Rise from the squatting position, using the leg muscles and keeping the back erect. When carrying large parcels, always look where you are going; maintain an erect posture at all times.

The muscles must be kept strong, so that the joints can function as they are meant to. The key word is **balance**. Too much rest can result in stiff joints and muscles. Too much exercise may damage joints. Physical therapists, as well as physicians may be helpful in outlining a program for rehabilitation.

Moist heat is relaxing and soothing to the inflamed joints. Various types and forms of heat are used to treat rheumatoid arthritis. They all help joints to move better with less pain. Hot baths are useful for the larger joints, such as the hips, knees, or elbows. They may be given in the bathtub or kitchen sink, and usually will last 15-30 minutes at a time. **Hydrotherapy** is the science of treating disease with water. Many clinics and hospitals have departments devoted to this medical specialty. Some physicians specialize in it. (See chapter 17.) Hot packs, fomentations, heat lamps, and paraffin wax applications can all be used with success to treat specific joints for the relief of pain, spasm, and inflammation.

Also important is our **disposition** in preventing flare-ups of rheumatoid arthritis. Emotional upsets, tension states, depression, and sudden traumatic shock frequently aggravate the symptoms. Patients who already have this disease may actually get worse during periods of upset, then better when such stresses are relieved.

This is not to say that these psychological factors cause rheumatoid arthritis, but only that they may *contribute* to the problem in some way. Achieving peace of mind through trust in our all wise Creator, helps remove all causes for bitterness and grief. Cultivating a life of prayer and Bible study will greatly help the arthritis sufferer to regain health right at home. (See chapter 27.)

DEGENERATIVE JOINT DISEASE

Of the 17 million arthritis sufferers in the United States, over 10 million have degenerative types of arthritis. Sometimes called **osteoarthritis**, the degenerative joint disease occurs twice as often as rheumatoid arthritis and usually begins later in life. In fact, almost everyone will get "a touch of rheumatism" sooner or later, if he lives long enough.

Usually osteoarthritis is mild. It seldom cripples, but often produces pain. Weather changes, storms, and cold may aggravate the symptoms, making the sufferer somewhat of a weather prophet. This type of arthritis confines its attack locally to individual joints and rarely spreads to distant joints or affects the whole body. Primarily osteoarthritis is a matter of "wear and tear" of the mechanical parts of the joint, the cartilage cushions wearing out as the patient becomes older. Most often affected are weight-bearing joints, such as the knees, hips, or spine. One variety of this disease, which does not seem to have anything to do with strain on the joints, affects younger women. The joints of the fingers are the chief point of attack, often showing bony enlargement on the hands, called *Heberden's nodes.* These can be quite painful.

In the normal joint where two bones meet, their ends are covered with layers of smooth elastic material called cartilage. These surfaces are designed to slide smoothly across each other, lubricated by the joint fluid. In osteoarthritis the bone ends become thicker, then bony spurs develop. The surrounding ligaments and membranes may also become thickened, changing the whole shape of the joint.

Muscles in the region of the arthritic joint tend to become tense and contract unnaturally as a reflex reaction to pain. They may likewise become weak. Obviously when the mechanical system breaks down in this way, the joint is not going to work properly.

A number of **causes** can progress into osteoarthritis. Joints which take unusual punishment or abuse, such as the hips and knees of obese or overweight patients are likely to develop these changes. Joints injured in an accident or an athletic injury may also deteriorate early. Sometimes a hip defect is present at birth. Inherited tendencies can predispose people to osteoarthritis. Fundamentally for most of us, this degeneration of tissue in the body is a normal process of aging. There is much we can do to protect these important structures and continue living free from pain.

Although many people have x-ray changes characteristic of osteoarthritis without symptoms, most patients develop pain in or around the joint. This may be mild aching and soreness, or a nagging constant pain. The pain of joint disease is caused by pressure on nerve endings, and by tense muscles and their rapid fatigue. Sometimes pain is felt at a distance from the joint where the trouble is. Second, one experiences the loss of ability to move his or her joints easily and comfortably. Usually part of the problem is an advancing muscular weakness. Obvious distortion of the joints will develop later. X-rays often aid doctors to make a correct diagnosis.

Early treatment is helpful to limit the troublesome symptoms. I place great importance on healthful mental influences. Recommended nutritional measures with a natural vegetarian diet are nearly identical to principles mentioned above for rheumatoid patients. Chili-containing creams such as *Zostrix* are valued to quell the ache of chronic joint pain. Containing the ingredient, **capsaicin**, the cream appears to affect a chemical "pain messenger," *substance P*, responsible for transmitting pain signals along nerve pathways to the brain. The capsaicin cream, which burns slightly on the skin, triggers the release of substance P from the nerves in the area where it's applied.

Hot packs, special baths and other forms of external heat, combined with rest, and exercises to protect the joints from stress and strain, may all be helpful. Most important for any overweight or obese patient, though, is a **weight reduction** program. Remember that osteoarthritis is a chronic disease and may last for life. This makes obvious the conclusion, for treatment must continue for a long time. Disability can nearly be prevented by early attention to the above simple measures.

GOUT

Gout is an acutely painful form of arthritis, attacking at least one million victims in the United States. This disease usually results from an inherited defect in body chemistry. **Uric acid**, a normal body substance is either overproduced or delivered faster than the kidneys can get rid of it. Great excesses of uric acid form needle-like crystals in joints, leading to severe inflammation. The affected joints become hot, swollen, and exquisitely tender.

Although gouty arthritis can settle in almost any part of the body, the large joint of the big toe is attacked most commonly. Your diet must be regulated to lower the *uric acid* intake. This can be done most naturally by eliminating meat and cola beverages, then substituting unrefined whole grain cereal foods, fruits and vegetables. The use of hot packs, or in the case of extremely acute inflammation ice packs, may reduce the inflammation and bring rapid resolution.

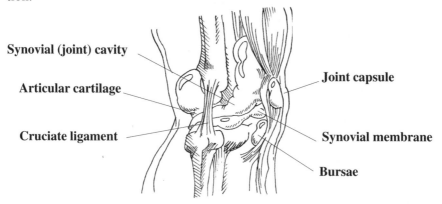

Synovial (joint) cavity

Articular cartilage

Cruciate ligament

Joint capsule

Synovial membrane

Bursae

91

Also dangerous for patients with gout is the crystallization of uric acid in the kidneys. Actual stone formation can occur with the typical symptoms of colic in the ureter. Occasional deposits of uric acid, called *tophi*, can occur in the skin around the ears, the hands, and the elbows. Strict control of dietary uric acid, elimination of alcohol and caffeine, and adequate fluid intake are good preventive measures. A physician should be consulted when difficulty arises.

Other types of joint pains may be related to **bursitis**, **tendinitis**, and the other painful afflictions of musculoskeletal tissues discussed in chapter two.

Finally, it is important to emphasize a few major misconceptions about arthritis. First of all, arthritis **can** be a serious disease. It is very important to make an accurate diagnosis, particularly of the rheumatoid type. Many people are under the impression that nothing much can be done for arthritis. This is definitely untrue. With early, proper, and continued treatment, a great deal can be done.

A short stay in a lifestyle or wellness center for nutritional education, hydrotherapy, and diagnostic evaluation is well worth the time and money. Sometimes all progressive crippling can be prevented. Distortion of the joints which has already occurred may be greatly reduced if not corrected. It is likewise *not* true that arthritis affects only old people. Some of the elderly were struck with arthritis when they were relatively young. Juvenile forms of rheumatoid arthritis are also known and rarely may be seen from infancy. Find out what kind of arthritis it is, then go to work in removing the cause, aiding nature in her valiant effort to combat this problem.

WARNING SIGNS of CANCER

1. Unusual bleeding or discharge.
2. A lump or thickening in the breast,
   or elsewhere in the body, especially if new.
3. Discovering a sore that does not heal.
4. Any changes in bowel or bladder habits.
5. Indigestion, or difficulty in swallowing.
6. Hoarseness or cough, chronic & persisting.
7. Any decided change in a wart or mole.

This brings us to the next chapter. Study it carefully, not only to learn about the subject of cancer, but for means of prevention. That will be even better than cure!

CHAPTER SIX

CANCER

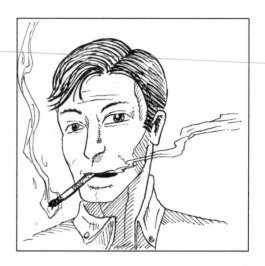

The magnitude of the cancer problem may be appreciated by these few statistics. One in four Americans will develop cancer during his or her lifetime. More than 400,000 Americans died of cancer in 1990. Not only is cancer a momentous health problem, but the management and care of these patients is frequently quite complex and heartrending.

The much-feared word, **cancer**, is a term used to characterize an aberrant growth of cells, which ultimately results either in the invasion of normal tissues, or the spread to other organs, called **metastasis**. The degree of threat or malignancy (from the Latin roots *malignus*, and *genus*, meaning "engendering harm") of a particular cancer is based upon the propensity of its abnormal cells to invade surrounding tissues or spread to other organs.

Cancer is not one disease. There are more than one hundred distinct forms of cancer with differing biological behavior and clinical manifestations. The natural course of some kinds progresses rapidly, and takes the life of the victim within weeks to months. Others are very slow growing and may metastasize to distant areas, spread rapidly, or extend the tumor locally and invade the surrounding tissues.

Some types of cancer are quite predictable in their behavior, while others are just the opposite. The factors that allow aberrant cancer cells to invade tissues are not well understood. Some individuals appear to be resistant to the invasion of cancer. Not only do they resist the disease, but if they have a malignant growth they may undergo spontaneous remission leading to a complete cure.

Some of the basic types of cancer have general features that characterize their behavior. **Carcinomas** are cancers involving glandular or covering tissues, such as the intestinal tract, lungs, or skin. These are more apt to spread by invasion of the lymph vessels, initially involving the nearest lymph node. This is why the lymph nodes are carefully examined in the diagnosis and treatment of breast cancer, for example. **Sarcomas**, on the other hand, are cancers of connective tissue, such as muscle, cartilage, or bone. These characteristically spread via the blood stream, and distant metastases to the lungs or brain are common.

Two properties of tumor cells probably contribute to their spread to distant sites. One is decreased "adhesiveness" of tumor cells to each other with the resulting ability of these clumps of cells to break off and enter the lymphatics of blood stream and to lodge in other tissues. The second is the elaboration of a *"tissue angiogenesis factor,"* which results in rapid development of local blood vessels, thereby feeding the growing tumor cell mass and hastening its development.

Common symptoms that are seen with most malignancies are those of weight loss, loss of appetite, and unexplained bleeding. The *American Cancer Society* has popularized the seven danger signals, which although helpful in early detection, at times show up too late for an actual cure by surgical removal. The change in a wart or mole, unexplained bleeding, difficulty swallowing, loss of appetite, a persistent cough, particularly with the production of blood, a lump developing in some part of the body, and a change in bowel habits - these are the signs that should alert one to seek comprehensive investigation for the possibility of cancer.

Many *causes* of cancer have been suggested. A great deal of evidence has accumulated in recent years. For a long time, it was known that certain hereditary disorders may increase the risk of cancer. For example, if a relative of a patient has breast cancer, the risk increases 3-5 times in females. Individuals with multiple polyps in the colon, or other hereditary disorders, such as Down's syndrome, have increased risk of developing certain cancers.

Viruses can cause development of cancer in almost every mammal, as well as fish, frogs, and other species. Some may be transmitted to humans through meat eating, milk, or eggs. These tumor viruses transform cells, but occasionally may lie dormant for many years without producing disease. It is felt today that many cases of breast cancer, leukemia, and other cancers of the lymph organs (*lymphomas*) are caused by viruses. One of these is the *Epstein-Barr virus* known to cause **infectious mononucleosis**.

Carcinogens are chemicals that can produce cancer. Most of these are present in the environment. They were first demonstrated by Dr. Potts in England, who linked the increased incidence of scrotal cancer in chimney sweeps with exposure to soot. We now know that it was creosote and tars which adhered to the skin, that eventually caused skin cancer.

Lung cancer is much more common today, caused by one or more of the dozens of cancer-producing chemicals present in main-stream tobacco smoke. People working in occupations where dusts are inhaled, as asbestos workers and coal miners, and some who in painting the luminous dials of watches exposed themselves to radium,—all can develop cancer from these environmental agents.

95

In fact, **radiation** in any form, as well as numerous **drugs** have been unequivocally shown to be associated with the induction of cancer. The survivors of the atomic bombing of Hiroshima and Nagasaki showed an increased incidence of acute and chronic leukemia that reached a peak approximately seven years after their exposure to radiation. As this research points up, it is right to minimize ones exposure to radiation and x-rays.

Drugs are also capable of interacting with cells to form various types of cancer. Radioactive isotopes and immune suppressive agents, as well as some hormones have been known to cause cancer. Exposure to **estrogens** has increased the incidence of cancer of the womb. **Arsenic** exposure has been associated with skin cancer. Many other common drugs, such as **coal tar** ointments are being related to skin cancer. Amphetamines, male hormones, and in fact, practically all of the anticancer chemotherapy drugs can in susceptible individuals produce malignancy.

More recent research has focused on the role of **diet** in possibly causing (called the *etiology*) certain cancers. We know, for example, that in undeveloped nations where the fiber intake is high the incidence of cancer of the colon is exceptionally low. Cancer of the stomach, as well as the colon has been related to certain Oriental food patterns. **Meat** intake is being implicated more and more as a possible cause of cancer. Evidence supporting this assertion indicates a higher rate of cancer in the northern United States and New Zealand where beef consumption is high. In fact, colon cancer risk seems directly proportional to the amount of meat taken by a given population.

Nursing a baby appears to protect a mother against developing breast cancer later in life. Some additives in foods, such as the artificial sweeteners, *saccharine* and *cyclamate*, have been related to cancer of the bladder in experimental animals. So you can see that our environment may contain many agents with malignant potential. This makes it mandatory to guard your personal health and fortify your body's resistance to disease with the purest air and water, and the most natural sources of food that you can find.

Certain **examinations** should always be carried out in high risk patients for early detection of possible cancer. Probably the most valuable screening test is the **chest x-ray**, a must in smokers. Preferably, in tobacco users a chest x-ray should be taken every three to six months. For the general population, an annual chest x-ray can determine the earliest presence of most lung cancers, as well as tuberculosis and several other pulmonary diseases.

Routine annual x-rays of the breasts (called a **mammogram**) should be performed especially in ladies with unusually large breasts, fibrocystic disease, or with a strong family history of breast disorders or cancer. The cumulative radiation exposure makes mammography's routine use unadvisable for women without any risk factors or symptoms.

The complete blood count is the best screening procedure for leukemia and many other diseases involving the blood. Urine tests can be done to evaluate the kidneys, bladder, and urinary tract for bleeding or other suspicious abnormalities. Many other blood tests and x-ray procedures, as well as the actual obtaining of tissues through a biopsy can diagnose with certainty most specific types of cancer. Brief clinical descriptions and some principles of tumor management will be discussed below.

BENIGN TUMORS

Benign tumor growths, although not true cancers, share some of their same characteristics, such as viral causation, transformation of cells, and autonomous growth. A number of specific viruses are known to cause benign tumors. They are by far the most common of any new growths a person might have.

Warts are benign tumors that occur in almost any location. They are very common on the hands. However, in spite of folklore rumors, they are not caused by handling frogs! A wart virus penetrates the skin and transforms dermal cells causing this unusual growth. When it occurs on the sole of the foot, around the nail beds, or in the genital organs, it may be difficult to eradicate, even quite painful.

Warts can usually be frozen with liquid nitrogen, or may be removed chemically, such as with strong acids. Many physicians prefer to destroy the wart with an electric current (*cautery*) after appropriately anesthetizing the skin. Many of these can be successfully frozen or removed at home, if appropriate antiseptic precautions are observed.

Skin tags and **papillomas** are growths that protrude from the skin or mucous membrane. Some of these can be tied off with a strong silk string, while others with a larger base require local excision, freezing technique, or chemical cautery. Soft lumps of varying sizes under the skin are often **lipomas**, fatty tumors that usually develop autonomously in the fatty tissue beneath the skin. Sometimes for cosmetic reasons these are removed by a simple surgical procedure done under local anesthesia. Fibrous tumors (**fibromas**) and various types of moles also can be removed to prevent cosmetic blemish, irritation, or the avoidance of further growth.

LUNG CANCER

Cancer of the lung is the most common cancer in men and increasing rapidly among women in the United States. There are a number of types of lung cancer, but the most common is called *bronchogenic*, since it originates in the bronchial tubes. By far, the most common cause of lung cancer is tobacco smoking with the risk directly proportionate to the number of cigarettes smoked and the amount of inhaling. It appears that in the tobacco tar, we find not only *benz-0-pyrene*, but dozens of other cancer-producing chemicals, as well as other substances that sensitize the tissues to the destructive action of these agents. Over a period of years the hapless smoker accumulates an increasing amount of tar, until some of the lining cells, which at first increase in number as a protective measure, finally become transformed into malignant cells, which invade local tissues and eventually metastasize.

Extensive research on tobacco was sponsored by the **American Cancer Society**. Also, momentous publications by the recent **Surgeon General** of the United States, especially his dynamic governmental *Report on Smoking and Health*, underscore clearly the detrimental effects of tobacco use and its potential for producing malignancy in vital organs. In spite of many medical and surgical advances in the treatment of advanced cancer, lung cancer still takes the lives of about 95% of its victims. Tragically, most cases are discovered too late for any hope of cure, although this disease is almost entirely preventable.

An individual developing cancer of the lung may have no **symptoms** at all until the cancer is far advanced. Others develop a cough that may be confused with the smoker's cough of chronic bronchitis. At times the expectorated mucous may contain blood, a rather late sign in the development of this cancer. Some unfortunate cases have spread to involve vital blood vessels, the brain, or bones before adequate diagnosis has been made. Occasionally, the removal of the lung or part of a lobe may eradicate the tumor early enough to effect a cure.

BREAST CANCER

Cancer of the breast is the leading cancer among women in Western countries. It appears that this cancer is caused by one of several viruses and is increased in certain population groups. As mentioned before women who breast-feed their babies seem to be protected. Those with fibrocystic disease, a condition where the mammary glands enlarge and become engorged with sacs of fluid have an increased risk of breast malignancy.

Recent evidence points to the intake of caffeinated beverages, such as coffee, tea, and colas as factors in the production of this fibrocystic change. Beverage alcohol is believed to be one major risk factor in breast cancer. Men may also have breast cancer, but it is about 1/125th as common. Periodic self-examination is an excellent aid to early detection of breast cancer, especially if it remains the same throughout the menstrual cycle.

A great deal of controversy is raging in the medical world concerning the best treatment for breast cancer. Some types seem to be adequately treated by locally excising the tumor. The removal of a portion of the breast obviously preserves normal anatomy and is far less mutilating than the more traditional radical mastectomy.

Many types of breast cancer are quite adequately treated and often cured by a modified approach removing the breast only, while preserving the muscles in the chest and dissecting the lymph glands in the arm pit only when the risk of metastasis is high. This to me seems like a much more "middle-of-the-road" approach, avoiding the extensive mutilation and more serious complications of the radical surgery commonly performed.

CANCER of the GASTROINTESTINAL TRACT

For the last three decades, cancer of the **stomach** has been decreasing in frequency in the United States. It remains high in Japan and certain other Oriental nations, and is probably related to the intake of certain foods, some highly seasoned, others extremely hot. The second most common type of cancer in our country is cancer of the **colon** and **rectum**. This often produces a change in bowel habits, the stools becoming more constipated or of small caliber. Bleeding from the rectum is occasionally seen. This is usually red when the tumor growth is low in the colon and darker, brown to black (called *melena*) when the lesion is high in the colon or coming from the small intestine or stomach. This color change is due to the partial digestion of blood products by bacteria and enzymes in the bowel.

The rectal examination is helpful in detection of many cancers in their early stages. A ten-inch tube with attached light, called a *sigmoidoscope* can be used to look into the lower bowel, where nearly three-fourths of the cancers are seen. This should be done in conjunction with a complete annual exam for individuals over the age of 40. A new technology in fiberoptic viewing, called *endoscopy*, has developed instruments that can examine the stomach and duodenum (*gastroscopy*), and the entire colon (*colonoscopy*). These procedures are often done on an outpatient basis, and provide even more adequate confir- mation than the traditional barium x-rays.

The **cause** of these colon cancers is still somewhat uncertain. It is felt that a high fiber diet, which increases the rapidity of transit through the bowel, will decrease the incidence of cancer. This is probably because the waste products contain many toxins. In contact with the mucous lining of the bowel these can cause irritation and eventual malignant change in the cells. A number of foods, most notably meat, contains toxins (*carcinogens*) that can be directly associated with cancer. The *benz-0-pyrene* in a charcoal broiled steak may be equivalent to that found in about 600 cigarettes. *Methylcholanthrene* is also a dangerous substance found in many types of meat. Recently discovered is the chemical *malonaldehyde*, which seems to be increased when the meat is cooked!

Certain vegetables are not exempt from association with cancer. **Moldy** corn, peanuts, soybeans, and other seeds contain a factor called *aflatoxin*, which has been associated with liver cancer in several countries. It is interesting to note that the incidence of cancer is increasing in many fish that inhabit polluted streams and rivers. Problems with meat inspection also contribute to risk of cancer, in that certain portions of an animal carcass may be preserved for food, while another part of the animal may have actual malignancy.

All of these danger signals are turning more food buyers to a vegetarian diet. In fact the numbers are growing rapidly in the United Kingdom, where a disease called *bovine spongiform encephalopathy* was discovered in 1985. It will undoubtedly spread to other nations. Often called the "**mad cow disease**," this condition results from using animal products such as a bone meal in cattle feed. The cows after a few years go crazy, and become violent. A virus-like particle called a *PRION* is found in the animals brain. Currently it is resistant to most germ killing procedures, including boiling, radiation, and disinfectants. Modern cancer virus research points out the "ounce of prevention" at your supermarket being worth much more than "pounds of cure" in the hospital.

Another bit of good news in the treatment of cancer of the colon is that some types can be removed without radical resection of the organ. Many snares, cauteries, and forceps have been devised to remove these cancers from the rectum through the sigmoidoscope. Sometimes when the malignancy is present only as a growth on a stalk, the area involved can be followed with periodic examinations. Other times the removal of a portion of the colon is necessary to effect the cure. The possibility of metastasis to the lymph nodes or liver makes it important to achieve early diagnosis and therapy, if life is to be maximally prolonged.

CANCER of the UTERUS and CERVIX

Routine screening has decreases the incidence of cervical cancer in recent years. Called the "**Pap smear**", this screening tool developed by Dr. Papanicoleau has allowed for the early detection of change in the cells of the cervix. Being less common in nuns, in Jewish women, and in those with less sexual activity, this type of cancer merits great interest from a preventive standpoint. A virus similar to the *Herpes virus* that causes cold sores has been implicated in the development of some of these cancers.

More and more nurses, as well as many midwives are learning how to take these smears, thus increasing the acceptance of the pap smear to many women as well as making the procedure more available. It certainly should be part of an annual examination from the time of marriage on through life. Early diagnosis with surgical removal of the uterus and cervix can well be curative.

Cancer of the lining of the womb *(endometrium)* is less common, but is still taking many lives. This has definitely been related to the use of estrogens, the female hormone used traditionally to lighten symptoms of the menopause. Avoidance of these hormone preparations, as well as prompt medical treatment in the event of unusual menstrual flow can provide the early diagnosis needed.

An outpatient procedure, using techniques similar to the pap smear (e.g. *Vabra aspiration*, or the *Pipelle*) can with less expense and discomfort provide the reassurance needed to evaluate this bleeding.

LEUKEMIA

Cancer involving the blood and bone marrow is most often seen in children. Several types of leukemia are described, based upon the type of blood cells involved and their appearance under the microscope. Samples from the blood and bone marrow are usually compared.

Ionizing radiation, whether from nuclear sources or x-ray therapy, is clearly associated with an increased incidence of these leukemias. Chemical agents, such as the anticancer drugs and occupational exposure to *benzal* have been associated with increased leukemia. Some hereditary factors have also been linked with this disease.

Most interesting is the firmly established viral theory in relation to acute leukemia. In rodents, fowls, cats, and monkeys certain viruses are known to cause leukemia when experimentally inoculated. These animals can pass viruses to their offspring through the ovum or shed it in their milk or other secretions, thereby transmitting it to unaffected animals. Again it makes one wonder how much leukemia may actually be transmitted to human beings through the use of animal foods, such as meat, eggs or milk. Milk is increasingly suspect for cancer viruses, especially the *bovine leukemia virus* (BLV) and the *bovine immunodeficiency virus* (BIV, a relative of HIV).

A disease in chickens *(fowl leukosis)* is estimated to affect up to 15% of the birds used for food, and many cases escape the casual inspection at the mass production slaughterhouse. The virus definitely passes into the egg, and can infect a baby chick even before hatching. It would take very high or prolonged cooking temperatures to be sure the virus was inactivated in eggs used for food.

In spite of the fact that the common treatment of leukemia today is with cellular poisons (*cytotoxic* drugs), it is my hope that a much more physiologic treatment will soon become available, and, in the right setting be demonstrated as superior. Combining a proper diet with the judicious use of fever therapy should induce the appropriate antibodies to aid in virus destruction and the maintenance of health, as well as a decrease in complications. This type of therapy has been used with increasing success in the treatment of related tumors, such as Hodgkin's disease, chronic lymphocytic leukemia, and some other lymphomas. These closely related malignancies all seem to have a common viral origin. Thus, they should respond to the intermittent induction of high fever. However, it must be given in a controlled setting for safety.

SKIN CANCER

Although more skin cancers are seen than malignancies involving any other organ, this is least commonly a cause of cancer death. Inasmuch as the lesion can be seen with the naked eye in an early stage, the potential for cure is well over 90%. It is thought that the single most important factor in the cause of skin cancer is chronic exposure to ultraviolet light of the sunburn wave length **(UV-B)**. Individuals who are intensely pigmented are quite well protected from these rays. Fair-complexioned individuals and albinos should especially use sun screen preparations. All should avoid unnecessary exposure to x-rays, coal tar products, and arsenic preparations known to be carcinogens.

Seventy-five percent of all skin cancers are of the *basal cell carcinoma* type. These rarely metastasize, but are locally invasive. The cancer typically begins as a noninflammed, smooth, waxy nodule. Usually a number of small blood vessels are visible near the surface. These nodules often ulcerate and form a crust. Biopsy and excision will confirm the diagnosis, as well as treat the lesion. Simple excision gives the best cosmetic results. Liquid nitrogen may be used for local freezing, called **cryosurgery**. In combination with curettage or **electrocautery**, a cure rate of more than 95% may be expected.

Squamous cell carcinoma is the second most common type, developing also from the surface layer of the skin, but having more propensity to metasta-size. Most of these lesions are painless. They show up with firm, red plaques, displaying visible scales on the surface. They may arise from pre-existing *solar keratoses*, premalignant lesions developing from repeated sunburn. Treatment is similar to that of basal cell lesions described above, namely removal.

Malignant melanoma is the most deadly type of skin cancer. They also are related to excessive sunburn and exposure. Pigmented moles are among the most common growths on the skin of humans. Some of these ultimately may change in their color, size, or hair pattern, which is often an early sign of their malignancy. Irregularities in surface pattern and varying colors are character-istic of the melanoma. Shades of red, white, or blue (no patriotism here) and other mixtures of brown and black, may indicate the development of this cancer.

Melanomas should always be removed with wide excision, since their propensity to spread to other organs, such as the liver, eye, and other areas of the skin is great. Therapy utilizing the immune mechanism (immunotherapy) has been used widely in the treatment of metastatic melanoma. Although still experimental these approaches offer an exciting alternative with less cost in toxicity to the individual. BCG vaccine, used for years to prevent tuberculosis, has found its place in the treatment of these melanomas with encouraging results in many cases.

The PREVENTION of MALIGNANCY

Based upon the evidence currently available, it is my conviction that a rational plan can be designed to prevent most types of cancer. Summed up in one word, **moderation**, the preventive approach involves several factors:

Your **diet** should be simple, utilizing natural foods as much as possible. Adequate amounts of fruit, fresh vegetables, and whole grain cereals should be included together with some nuts and natural sources of dietary fats, such as olives, avocados, and a most sparing use of vegetable oil. Any **excess** of oil, sugar, salt, or any single food, especially refined ones, in the diet should be shunned.

The low-fat **vegetarian** diet has been associated clearly with an increased resistance to many types of cancer. When individuals abstain from milk and eggs, as well as meat, the cancer risk becomes even lower. Naturally these total vegetarians must have a considerable knowledge of nutrition in order to maintain balanced nutrition, and provide optimum vitamin and mineral intake to maintain excellent health. Thousands of discriminating consumers, however, are rapidly adopting a vegetarian lifestyle as fast as they are able to learn how to select and prepare the foods. In this change is found the key to preventing not only many cancers, but also atherosclerosis and numerous other diseases.

Reasonable amounts of **exercise** should be obtained daily for a lifestyle that is low in occupational stress, while satisfying and productive. A moderate exposure to **sunlight** prevents detrimental premalignant skin changes that many acquire as their skin ages. The use of a broad-brimmed hat, sun screen lotions, and avoidance of excessive sun bathing can bring about vibrant health, without wearing out or prematurely aging the dwelling of skin we live in.

Temperance advocates for many years have proclaimed the key to prevent one most common cancer. Those who abstain completely from tobacco smoke, and even avoid settings where the involuntary inhalation of stale second-hand smoke is required, will reduce their risk of lung cancer dramatically. Even ex-smokers who quit before a cancer develops, have a much lower rate than the devotee who continues to use cigarettes. Although pipes and cigars may produce less lung cancer, their stronger forms of tobacco still show malignant potential in cancer of the lip, tongue, throat, and larynx far too often.

Chronic use of **alcohol** increases the risk of cancer in the breast and liver, as well as seriously irritating the stomach and several other organs. Exposure to **drugs** of all kinds, including sex hormones, antibiotics, anticancer agents, and coal tar preparations can increase the incidence of malignancies in many organs. True temperance requires us to dispense entirely with all things hurtful, and use in moderation those things healthful. This principle of moderation can help to prevent many cancers.

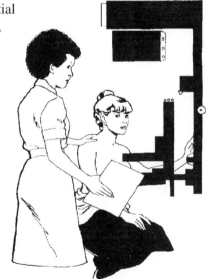

Early detection of breast cancer is best accomplished with a screening mammogram, combined with periodic examinations.

103

Routine physical examinations and **periodic self-examination** of the breasts and skin, with careful observation for the symptoms of cancer described above can detect abnormal lesions in the earliest possible stage, when surgical removal is a possibility. A regular annual physical should usually include the annual **Pap smear**, a biennial sigmoidoscopic examination, together with the appropriate laboratory testing for additional aid in early diagnosis. On the other hand, it may just give satisfying reassurance concerning one's state of health.

Rational **treatment of cancer** falls into several areas. Whenever possible the malignancy should be removed. Some natural "healers" have spread the erroneous message that surgery spreads cancer. This is only true if the disease is widespread and unresectable with any treatment. Early surgery in breast cancer can be curative in about three-fourths of patients. The treatment of colon cancer by surgery is well accepted to be not only curative in many, but helpful in avoiding obstruction of the bowel or profound chronic loss of blood that can complicate these cases.

The **diet** for any cancer victim should be such that will maintain health and function of all body organs, particularly those systems of elimination. Eating a high fiber, low fat diet as described above is extremely helpful. But extremes should be avoided, such as prolonged fasts, the use of a single fruit juice, or a total reliance on certain vitamin preparations thought to be curative.

Certain types of **hydrotherapy** include the judicious use of cleansing enemas, fever therapy, or local heating of the tumor may prove therapeutic, particularly in those tumors of viral origin. Cytotoxic drugs should be avoided. Their complications, numerous high-risk symptoms, usually makes the side-effects worse than the "cure." Radiation therapy, in general, should be reserved only for those cases where metastasis has produced intractable pain, or a "pathologic" fracture is imminent from bone destruction.

Although this conservative approach to cancer treatment could well be challenged, it is my conviction that clinical trials of natural therapies will produce resulting longevity and survival statistics equaling the best experimental programs, and with great savings in patient cost and safety. Our principal fear in such a natural therapeutic approach to cancer is founded upon the failure to follow the simple preventive approaches or seek adequate care early if such disease strikes. Widespread promotion and the practice of these "simple remedies" could in time bring populations, as well as individuals, into a state of health promised by the One who offered *"none of these diseases"* (see *Exodus 15:26)* only on condition of obedience.

CHAPTER SEVEN

DISEASES

OF THE

KIDNEY

AND

URINARY TRACT

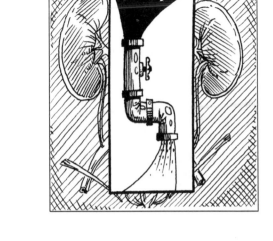

The production, transport, storage, and discharge of most liquid wastes by the human body is accomplished by the marvelously engineered, highly complex and integrated urinary system which includes several vital organs. The kidneys and ureters operate together, with delicately controlled cellular mechanisms in each kidney, giving finesse to the passage of urine through a muscular contraction called *peristalsis,* ending finally with the act of urination. Each kidney weighs less than a pound, yet contains over two million microscopic filtration units. These*nephrons*, if stretched out end-to-end, would be fifty miles long!

Every day our kidney tubules perform the amazing feat of removing about 300 pints of water from the blood. All but around three to six pints of this filtered water is returned (98-99%), purified of waste and mineral-balanced to perfect accuracy. Proper treatment of urinary problems requires an understanding of the physiology of this process, making possible most methodical analysis, then guiding medical practitioners to an accurate diagnosis. This in actuality, is usually derived from the history of the illness, together with certain physical findings; and most simply the examination of the urine.

A patient may develop a life-threatening disease in the genitourinary tract with few, if any symptoms. However, the following symptoms at least suggest urinary tract disease. *Nocturia* is the awakening at night to void, usually unnecessary for the ordinary person. Nighttime urination may be caused by bladder dysfunction, infection, or the presence of stones. Metabolic disorders, such as diabetes, congestive heart failure, or the intake of some drug can also produce these symptoms. Usually, though, it results from excessive water intake, drinking particularly late in the day.

Frequency: The normal person voids three to four times a day. Increased urinary frequency may be due to several causes. *Polyuria* means larger than normal total urine volume. This is characteristic of metabolic disorders such as diabetes, as well as inordinate fluid intake. Diminished urine volume is called *oliguria*. At times complete suppression of urine formation occurs. This is termed *anuria*.

The sudden desire to void, called *urgency*, makes control difficult, even impossible at times. Occasionally this is associated with pain or discomfort on urination, called *dysuria*. When it is severe, bladder spasm may follow voiding, and usually indicates the presence of an irritated or infected bladder.

Hesitancy denotes undue delay and difficulty in initiating the voiding process. With infection blood may be present in the urine *(hematuria)*, or pus may appear *(pyuria)*. A kidney or bladder stone may be passed occasionally. *Incontinence* is another distressing symptom, where involuntary loss of urine occurs. The stress of coughing or straining may cause this, or it may occur in association with urgency.

Pain from a kidney disorder may vary from dull aching discomfort in the flank to very sharp flank pain radiating into the lower abdomen or buttocks. Renal pain may be episodic or persistent. Often it is associated with loss of appetite, nausea, or vomiting. When a stone is passing through the ureter, pain is quite excruciating, causing the patient to move about restlessly, holding the area of discomfort, often by grasping the flank between his thumb and forefingers. Kidney pain tends to radiate into the lower abdomen and genitalia. A stone lodging in the junction between the ureter and bladder may also cause frequency, urgency, and pain on urination.

Individual cases may present with severe or mild symptoms, and the diagnosis may be immediately apparent or thoroughly obscure. A careful examination of the affected area and scrutiny of the urine, both with light illumination and, when possible the microscope, is of considerable help in establishing numerous causes.

URINARY STONES

Stones in the kidney or ureters may occur at any age, but are more common in the third and fourth decades. These *calculi* may be single or multiple, firmly lodged or free. Kidney stones often cause pain, produce blood in the urine, and symptoms of vague abdominal distress. Occasionally, even when large, stones may occur without symptoms, while causing serious and insidious kidney damage.

Characteristically, as mentioned above, renal calculi cause severe, sharp flank pain, which is often acute in onset and present intermittently. A small stone being passed in the ureter creates painful colic and the patient usually moves about restlessly, vainly seeking relief. Blood is frequently present in the urine, but at times requires the microscope for its detection. Physical findings may be entirely normal, although tenderness, muscle spasm, or even a lump may be felt in the location.

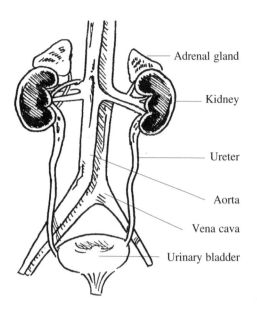

— Adrenal gland

— Kidney

— Ureter

— Aorta

— Vena cava

— Urinary bladder

It is important to search for the original cause of the stone, then attempt to correct it. Most stones after bladder passage can be analyzed to determine their composition. Some are composed of calcium salts, others of oxalate crystals, and less commonly uric acid or cystine may precipitate to form stones. Each of these causes needs to be ascertained in order to correct the diet, avoiding future recurrence.

One of the commonest situations that sets the environment for an attack of colic is inadequate fluid intake. Normally our kidneys require at least one and a half to two quarts of fluid a day! That will maintain urine volume at diluted concentrations, to avoid the precipitation of these salts. A high consumption of milk may result in calcium precipitation and the formation of a stone. Ice cream, cheese, and soft drinks such as cola beverages, and foods high in oxalic acid may provide the situation where stones begin to crystallize.

Uric acid stones usually result from a high intake of purines, found in meats, particularly sweetbreads, and other flesh foods obtained from animal organs. Uric acid calculi are usually seen in combination with other symptoms of **gout**, a metabolic disease traditionally associated with indulgence in rich foods and alcohol. A discriminating, well-balanced diet associated with adequate fluid will usually bring relief to patients who form uric acid stones frequently.

The treatment of colic in the urinary tract usually begins at home. Drink a high intake of water, at least one glass of liquid hourly, and begin immediately. Urinary acidifying agents are helpful to deter stones of calcium or oxalate composition, while for uric acid stones the urine should be alkalinized. Vitamin C and cranberry juice are both good acidifying agents for the urine, and are also helpful in treating urinary infections. Diuretic herbs, such as Buchu tea may also be helpful, when combined with a high volume of fluids.

Relief of acute urinary pain can be obtained in a hot tub bath, or with intensely hot fomentations applied to the flank and hip region. At times when flank pain is severe, the treatments will not only modify the pain, but through reflex pathways may help to relax the ureter and alleviate the spasm. Most often the smaller stones *(calculi)* will pass down into the bladder, where they are then excreted. Since obstruction in the urinary tract can progressively damage the kidney, as well as be painfully disabling, any urinary stones that do not resolve promptly should be evaluated be a competent physician. Newer diagnostic techniques using x-ray contrast, and *cystoscopic* basket stone retrieval, water immersion shock (sound) wave *lithotripsy*, and other types of surgery may be necessary to save the kidneys from permanent harm.

URINARY INFECTION

Bacterial infections of the urinary tract are extremely common. Some are also notoriously resistant to treatment and thus likely to reoccur. Yet the majority of persons with urinary tract infections are unaware of it. On other occasions, infections take the form of a acute disease usually with characteristic symptoms. The commonest symptoms are pain on urination, urinary frequency, and a strong urge to void. More serious infections may produce fever, pain in the bladder region, or over the kidneys.

Many different causes can produce infection. The commonest of these come from the group of gram negative bacteria (such as *E. coli*) inhabiting the digestive tract. Cultures of the urine can usually pinpoint the exact offender. Most of the time these *coliform bacteria* gain access to the bladder through the urethra. Under normal circumstances the urine in the bladder is sterile and large numbers of bacteria can be cleared rapidly in both humans and animals. Slight physiologic alterations, however, may permit survival of as few as ten microorganisms which multiply rapidly, then persist for prolonged periods.

Some associated conditions that may contribute to the formation of urinary infections are as follows: One to four percent of females from childhood to the childbearing age may harbor bacteria in the bladder or urethra, sometimes without the presence of symptoms. In men urinary infections are quite rare below the age 50. Four to eight percent of **pregnant** women may have infections, some of them without symptoms. **Diabetes** is another contributing factor, particularly when sugar is present in the urine. Any impediment to the free flow of urine—tumor, stricture, or stones—results in distention of the kidney and greatly increased frequency of urinary infection.

In fact, the reflux of urine in the bladder cavity up to the ureter occurring during voiding will contribute to more infections, particularly children. Infection of the lower urinary passages is sometimes initiated by bacteria carried on catheters or other instruments passed into the urethra and bladder. Sterile technique in catheter insertion can help to reduce this risk. Kidney diseases with resulting high blood pressure may also contribute at times to the lowered defense against infection.

Once the diagnosis has been established, treatment can be begun at home. The fluid intake should be increased, usually with water as well as **Vitamin C** or **cranberry juice** to render the urine more acid. A special protein found in cranberries and blueberries can combat most urinary tract infection by causing the causative germs to lose their grip on the bladder wall. Thus, the infective organisms become more amenable to bladder rinse-out with normal urination. One glass of liquid per hour up to 12-16 cups per day is recommended. In at least half such cases, the urinary infection will clear itself, with symptoms subsiding over 24-48 hours.

Hot and cold **sitz baths** (see Chapter 17) are helpful, as is the **half bath** in a hot tub of water followed by a cold spray. Increasing blood flow to the urinary organs, these hydrotherapy treatments aid the body in natural resistance to infection and the clearing of disease. Persistence of symptoms or the underlying presence of diabetes, high blood pressure, or chronic kidney disease should be evaluated with appropriate urine tests, cultures, and medical counsel.

INCONTINENCE

Involuntary loss of urine is a very troublesome symptom. This may occur in children and when associated with bed wetting is usually termed *enuresis*. Up to 4-5 years of age this may be quite common, and when persistent usually indicates some psychological distress. Congenital defects in the formation of the urinary organs may contribute to this disorder, and they can be evaluated with a specific x-ray study, the *intravenous pyelogram*.

Most cases of childhood incontinence subside with the passage of years. Women of childbearing age may have incontinence after the delivery of a large baby. Or with successive pregnancies, the support of the bladder and urethra may be weakened, producing a hernia or prolapse called a *cystocele*. Often this is associated with stress incontinence on sneezing, coughing, or straining. The **Kegel exercises** described in the chapter on gynecology are often helpful in alleviating these symptoms. If persistent anatomic defect is demonstrated, surgical repair may be indicated to restore continence and alleviate the anxiety that inhibits social interaction.

Men seldom have incontinence until advanced age. This may occur at times after operations such as a *prostatectomy*. If the incontinence does not improve during convalescence it should be evaluated by a urologist since research centers have developed a number of surgical approaches to this troublesome problem. Mechanical devices to preserve social acceptance and self-confidence are also available.

KIDNEY FAILURE

Failure of the kidneys to form urine properly can be either of an acute or chronic nature. The acute types are called *nephritis*, referring to the inflammation of the functional kidney complex. This may occur in conjunction with a Strep. throat or other bacterial infection. At times it develops suddenly, associated with protein loss, edema, and high blood pressure. These cases need to be evaluated with laboratory tests and medical expertise. But several simple approaches are helpful.

First of all it is important to recognize the influence of diet on kidney function. Many years ago it was discovered that a high protein diet predisposes to kidney complications. For this reason it is wise to avoid an excess of animal products, particularly flesh foods. Adequate fluid intake is also important. In treating these symptoms hot packs as well as hydration will be beneficial.

Chronic failure of the kidneys frequently produces metabolic disturbances in water, sodium, potassium, calcium, and acid-base balance. The onset of renal failure is usually insidious. Excessive formation of urine and passage of urine at night may be only signs at first. Later a patient complains of feeling weak, fatiguing easily, sleeping poorly, and becoming slightly breathless. The appetite is lost and there is a bad taste in the mouth. Nausea, especially in the morning or anemia may be present. With increasing kidney failure, a person becomes lethargic, may develop twitching of the limbs, hemorrhages, and eventually develops a breath with an odor of urine, dry skin, and if not treated may progress into a coma and die.

Therapy of kidney failure demands an early determination of the cause. The role of dietary protein is very important. To reduce the blood urea accumulation a good quality protein is used with restriction in quantity to around 20 gm. daily. Sweating treatments may help eliminate toxins through the pores. The most efficacious are usually the hot blanket pack or steam bath. However, the latter is not advised (*contraindicated*) in severe hypertension.

Scientific research has offered a number of artificial approaches to kidney disease, such as dialysis of the blood (*hemodialysis*) or abdominal (*peritoneal*) fluid, and even transplants from a healthy donor. All of these have hazards, however, and if approached early and controlled, many cases of chronic kidney failure can be arrested.

TRAUMA TO THE KIDNEY

Injury to the urinary tract may at times produce blood in the urine. This is particularly a problem in contact sports, since the kidneys are easily traumatized. Long distance runners also frequently show signs of kidney damage with elevated enzymes and blood in the urine. This may be related not only to the metabolic breakdown of muscle during severe exercise, but also to the dehydration that results from profound sweating. In most cases of urinary trauma where the urethra, bladder, or ureters have not been ruptured bed rest combined with hot packs and adequate fluid intake will produce a rapid cure.

URINARY RETENTION

Inability to void may develop abruptly, but is usually preceded by a history of diminished size and force of the urinary system, hesitancy, nocturnal urination, and dribbling. Many of these individuals are older men, having developed gradual prostate enlargement, but scarring and stricture from infection in the urinary tract can also produce these symptoms.

One of the most important ways of relieving these conditions, short of actual surgical cure, is the use of the urinary catheter. Unless the obstruction is severe this soft, flexible tube with a rounded end can be passed successfully into the bladder in most people. The catheter should be sterilized, the opening of the urethra (meatus) cleansed carefully with antiseptic solution, and with appropriate lubrication the catheter passed gently into the bladder. Usually relief is obtained and this technique is easily learned at home thus allowing either for the necessary time to seek medical care or a chronic relief in older patients deemed unsuitable for surgery.

The *Foley catheter*, which contains an inflatable balloon, can be used for indwelling drainage of the bladder. This, connected to a closed, sterile system of collection can provide comfort for a longer time. However, infection may result from the presence of this foreign substance after only two to three days. In association with gentle catheter placement techniques, bladder irrigation may be learned.

Different patients require varying intervals between catheter change and this can often be prolonged by the use of irrigating solutions. Some of these inhibit bacterial formation and others improve patency of the catheter by reducing bladder sludge. All instrumentation of the bladder may produce *hematuria* or the presence of blood. Persistence of this and other urinary symptoms should cause a patient to seek counsel from a competent physician.

Although the urinary tract is complex and mysterious it is usually amenable to simple home remedies. The early use of these preventive measures can frequently restore health before chronic illness or disability becomes a problem.

EXCHANGE SYSTEM FOR CALCULATING PROTEIN, SODIUM, AND POTASSIUM RESTRICTED DIETS

Food Exchanges	Household Measure	Grams	Protein (g.)	Sodium (mg.)	Potassium (mg.)*
Milk	½ cup	120	4	60	170
Egg	1	50	7	70	100
Vegetables					
Group A	½ cup	100	1	9	150
Group B	½ cup	100	2	9	240
Fruit					
Group A	varies	varies	1	2	100
Group B	varies	varies	1	2	145
Breads, unsalted					
Group A	varies	varies	2	5	25
Group B	varies	varies	3	5	50
Fat, salted	1 tsp.	5	0	50	0

Handbook No. 8, USDA, 1963

PROTEIN, SODIUM, AND POTASSIUM EXCHANGE LISTS

Milk Exchange

One serving contains 4 g. of protein, 60 mg. of sodium, 170 mg. of potassium.

Milk, whole	½ cup
Milk, skim	½ cup

Egg Exchange

One egg contains 7 g. of protein, 70 mg. of sodium, 120 mg. of potassium.

Vegetable Exchanges: Group A

One serving contains 1 g. of protein, 9 mg. of sodium, 150 mg. of potassium.

Beans, green or wax	½ cup
Beets*	½ cup
Cabbage	½ cup
Corn, whole kernel	½ cup
Eggplant	½ cup
Summer squash	½ cup
Zucchini	½ cup

All vegetables *cooked* or *canned* without salt and *well-drained.*

* Reduce to 1/3 cup if sodium restricted to less than 500 mg.

Vegetable Exchanges: Group B

One serving contains 2 g. of protein, 9 mg. of sodium, 240 mg. of potassium.

Asparagus	½ cup
Broccoli	½ cup
Brussels sprouts	½ cup
Carrots[1]	½ cup
Potatoes[2]	½ cup
Pumpkin	½ cup
Winter squash	½ cup
Tomatoes	½ cup
Tomato juice, low-sodium dietetic	½ cup
Turnips	1/3 cup

All vegetables *cooked* or *canned* without salt and *well-drained*

[1]Reduce to 1/3 cup if sodium restricted to less than 500 mg.

[2]Pare, soak in water ½ hour, discard water, cook in fresh water.

Fruit Exchanges: Group A

One serving contains 1 g. of protein, 2 mg. of sodium, 100 mg. of potassium.

Apple, raw	1 small
Apple juice	½ cup
Apple sauce	½ cup
Blueberries	5/8 cup
Peach nectar	½ cup
Pears, canned	1/3 cup
Pear nectar	½ cup
Pineapple, canned	1 slice

Fruit Exchanges: Group B

One serving contains 1 g. of protein, 2 mg. of sodium, 145 mg. of potassium.

Blackberries, fresh	½ cup
Fruit cocktail	1/3 cup
Grape juice, canned	½ cup
Grapefruit, raw	½ medium
Grapefruit, juice	1/3 cup
Grapefruit sections	½ cup
Pear, raw	½ medium
Pineapple juice	1/3 cup
Plums, purple, canned	3 medium
Raspberries, fresh	½ cup
Strawberries, fresh	½ cup
Tangerine	1 medium
Watermelon, cubed	¾ cup

Bread Exchanges: Group A

One serving contains 2 g. of protein, 5 mg. of sodium, and 25 mg. of potassium.

Low-sodium bread	1 slice
Unsalted cooked cereal	
Rice	½ cup
Farina	¾ cup
Corn grits	¾ cup

Use regular only. Do not use instant or quick cooking varieties.

Dry cereal	
Puffed rice	1 cup
Unsalted cornflakes	1 cup

Bread Exchanges: Group B

One serving contains 3 g. of protein, 5 mg. of sodium, 50 mg. of potassium.

Dry cereal	
Puffed wheat	½ cup
Unsalted, cooked	
Macaroni	½ cup
Noodles	½ cup
Spaghetti	½ cup

Fat Exchanges

One serving contains no protein, 50 mg. of sodium, no potassium.

Butter, salted	1 tsp.
Margarine, salted	1 tsp.
Mayonnaise, salted	1 tsp.

Unsalted butter and margarine and vegetable oil may be used as desired.

Beverages

Juices and milk are counted as part of total fluid allowance.

Miscellaneous

These items may be used as desired.

Flavorings

Caraway	Sage
Thyme	Garlic
Turmeric	Garlic powder
Vanilla extract	(not salt)
Peppermint extract	

Small amounts of the following may be used in food preparation:

Celery	Mushrooms
Onions	Green pepper
Mint leaves	

CHAPTER EIGHT

HORMONE

RELATED

DISEASES

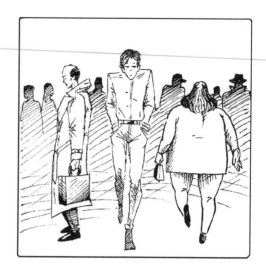

One of the rapidly growing areas of scientific research involving body processes is the specialty of **endocrinology**. This science deals with hormones and the related glands producing them. Interacting closely with all hormone mechanisms is the field of nutrition. Dealing primarily with the science of body chemicals, nutrition relates to foods and diseases produced by overabundance or lack of these specific nutrients. It is now generally agreed that hormones do not *initiate* new events in the complicated chemistry of metabolic processes, but rather produce their effect by regulating enzyme systems of the body. From this one may conclude that a true understanding of any disease and the factors regulating their production. Characteristically, abnormalities in the hormone or endocrine system arise from either an increased or decreased hormone secretion. This deviation from "normal" produces the characteristic syndromes of endocrine disease.

The suspicion that a hormone problem may play a role in the patient's illness often comes initially from the physical appearance of a patient. **Hypothyroidism** or *myxedema* often produces puffiness of the face and appearance of mental dullness, with drying of the skin, hair loss, and tendency to fluid retention. Overactivity of the thyroid gland, on the other hand produces just the opposite **hyperthyroid** state, with nervousness, tremor, weight loss, prominence of the eyes, and a continuous perspiration.

Dwarfs and giants are commonly produced from variation in pituitary glands secretions, particularly growth hormone. The adult form of **giantism** is called *acromegaly* and occurs after the normal body height has been reached.

This hormone excess often enlarges the hands and feet. Overactivity of the cortex of the adrenal gland, called **Cushing's syndrome** produces a characteristic obesity with thin arms and legs, increased tendency to bruising, a hump on the back of the shoulders, and roundness of the face like a full moon. Reduced function of the adrenal cortex is called **Addison's disease**. It is characterized by increase pigmentation of the skin, weakness, salt craving, weight loss, and low blood pressure.

A rapid step towards the accurate diagnosis of these hormone problems has come with new laboratory tests, such as the radioimmunoassay. Most of the body's endocrine hormones can be analyzed now. Although the tests are expensive they are available in most large cities. One single determination of the hormone level does not necessarily establish or exclude an endocrine abnormality. Wide fluctuations in hormone secretions are seen during a twenty-four hour period. Some disorders of the adrenal glands, particularly, may result from a loss of the normal cyclic 24-hour pattern. This is particularly seen in conjunction with disturbed sleep pattern, work schedules, and other tendencies toward irregularity.

SYMPTOMS RELATED TO THE ENDOCRINE SYSTEM

We now present a few common symptoms and the possible relationships to specific endocrine diseases. Clinical experience is certainly important in interpreting these relationships. Nevertheless, the suspicion that there is something wrong is often the first step toward an accurate diagnosis.

Weakness and increased fatigability are without doubt the most frequent symptom of adults seeking medical diagnosis. In the majority, these complaints derive primarily from emotional or psychological disturbances. When hormone abnormalities are suspected, one should inquire first whether the symptoms have been accompanied by weight loss. If so, insufficiency of the adrenal gland, overactivity of the thyroid, and diabetes mellitus should be considered.

Adrenal insufficiency is usually accompanied by increased pigmentation, low blood pressure, and perhaps salt craving. **Hyperthyroidism** is suggested by *goiter* (enlargement of the thyroid gland), bulging eye changes, tremor, and heat intolerance. **Sugar diabetes** is usually accompanied by excessive urination and increased thirst. Without weight loss, but with symptoms of weakness and fatigability one could consider underactive thyroid, underactive pituitary gland, overactive parathyroid gland with high calcium levels, and hypersecretions of aldosterone, another hormone from the adrenal gland regulating the salt balance. The first of these are associated with hypoactive reflexes, intolerance to cold, dry skin. **Hypopituitarism** is suggested by delayed or absent menstrual cycle, impotence, decreased tolerance to cold, hypoglycemia, and low blood pressure. **Hyperparathyroidism** is usually

115

associated with bone pain, kidney stones, and increased urination. Elevated aldosterone levels are accompanied by high blood pressure, muscle weakness, and signs of potassium depletion.

Menstrual irregularities are associated with four major hormone disturbances. Primary failure of the ovaries prior to a natural menopause is characterized by hot flushes, weight gain, emotional instability. Secondary ovarian failure, associated with reduced stimulating hormones from the pituitary gland is often related to diseases in the thyroid or adrenal. Underactive thyroid gland is often associated with excessive menstruation, as well as decreased flow. The final, but much more rare syndrome is seen in conjunction with adrenal gland dysfunction. The menstrual irregularities in this case are usually associated with increased muscle development, increased body hair (**hirsutism**) and other signs of masculinization. The use of birth control pills should always be investigated as a cause of menstrual irregularity.

Breast changes are also commonly associated with hormone disorders. Enlargement of the breast in males (**gynecomastia**) occurs normally at puberty and may persist through adolescence. Rarely, hormone-secreting tumors of the adrenal gland or testes may also produce these problems. Several varieties of drugs may cause breast changes as well. Abnormal lactation (**galactorrhea**) is sometimes observed in patients with tumors of the pituitary gland. A number of drugs, including some antihypertensive and tranquilizing preparations may also produce this problem.

Hypertension may also be associated with hormone disorders, although it is more commonly related to stress, salt intake, and obesity. **Cushing's syndrome** or adrenal gland excess can definitely cause high blood pressure and should be considered if unusual obesity, associated with a tendency to bruising, is present. An episodic hypertension is caused by secretion from the adrenal medullary tumor called *pheochromocytoma*. The picture of rapid heart rate, nervousness, sweating, although classic, is infrequent. Increased secretion of the parathyroid hormone or the adrenal hormone *aldosterone* can also cause hypertension, and should be excluded in complete diagnosis of the problem.

Obesity suggests the possibility of a hormone disturbance, but it is usually caused by habitually increased food intake or deep-seated emotional problems. Diabetes should definitely be investigated and excluded in the presence of obesity, particularly in adults. Thyroid disorders are commonly related and can be evaluated with simple blood measurements. One must also consider the possibility of problems induced by hormone administration, as we see the frequent prescribing of cortisone preparations, thyroid or sex hormone in nonspecific therapies for varying symptoms. These so-called *iatrogenic* (physician caused) problems can often be improved by the discontinuance of the offending drug.

DIABETES MELLITUS

We now turn to the common problems of metabolism that can often be treated, controlled, or prevented in a home setting. A knowledge of sugar diabetes is important, because of its high prevalence. This disease has been recognized from antiquity. Both Greek and Chinese writings have mentioned it; and in the sixteenth century Paracelsus initiated the study of the chemistry of diabetic urine. The word **mellitus**, introduced by Thomas Willis one hundred years later, describes the sweetness of the diabetic urine, "as if imbued with honey." This rapidly led to a dietary approach to this disease, until finally Langerhans, a medical student, in 1869 described the islets in the pancreas where the basic production of insulin occurs. Two Canadians, Banting and Best, finally prepared the extract from dog pancreas that was capable of reducing the elevated blood glucose level. A fascinating long history of discoveries marks the approaches to understanding and treating this common disorder.

It is estimated that there are about 200 million diabetics in the world and approximately 4.2 million in the United States. This disease is more frequent in older people. Hence, as the population grows and becomes older, diabetes will continue to increase. With treatment, the life expectancy of the diabetic is increasing, and since inheritance is an important factor, the more diabetics that have children, the greater will be the prevalence of this disease. Obesity is also on the rise and appears to precipitate diabetes among those predisposed to it.

Next to obesity and thyroid disorders, diabetes is the third most common problem in metabolism. Interrelated are the metabolic or hormone, and vascular or long-termed components of this disease. The latter consist of an accelerated arteriosclerosis, that leads to premature aging and particularly affects the eyes and the kidneys. Gangrene of the foot, arteriosclerotic heart disease, blindness, and kidney failure (*uremia*) are the most frequent manifestations of the vascular syndrome. Statistically, the diabetic is faced, not only with a decreased life expectancy, but also with the eventual possibility of disabling complications.

The early detection of diabetes first involves a high index of suspicion. This disease is two and half times more frequent in relatives of known diabetics. Furthermore, 85% of diabetic patients were or are overweight. Four out of five diabetics are over 45 years of age. Mothers who deliver large babies have a high potential for the development of diabetes.

The simplest screening test for this disorder is a urinalysis for sugar. Measurement of the blood sugar (glucose) level in the fasting patient should also be encouraged as a screening tool. The five-hour **Glucose Tolerance Test** is less commonly performed for diabetes, but is usually used to diagnose and evaluate hypoglycemia. Pathologic changes occur with the passage of time in diabetes, and seem accelerated by failure to control this disease. The *islets of Langerhans* in the pancreas typically deteriorate, resulting in the lack of insulin production.

Atherosclerosis occurs earlier in a diabetic patient, often leading to coronary artery disease and stroke as the most frequent cause of death. These

117

also occur from the lack of insulin production. The eyes show changes after 10 to 15 years of diabetes. Small retinal hemorrhages, dilated sacs in the weakened blood vessel (*aneurysms*), and waxy patches (*exudates*) develop. Later a dangerous type of new blood vessel forms, then further hemorrhages and gradual or sudden loss of vision. Although marvelous advances in the diagnosis and treatment of these visual complications have been made, diabetic eye disease remains the second most frequent cause of blindness in the United States. Increased tendencies toward cataract formation also occur.

In the kidney, characteristic damage to the filtering unit (*glomerulus*) progresses to destroy renal function. Infections of the kidney and urinary tract are common, and many patients go on to develop high blood pressure, serious loss of protein, and later kidney failure.

The symptoms of diabetes, as mentioned above, are multiple. Increased fatigability and weakness is common. The diagnosis is frequently suggested by history of increased thirst (*polydipsia*), increased urination (*polyuria*), and excessive hunger (*polyphagia*) in association with weight loss. Long standing disease is reflected in the pathologic changes mentioned above.

Two typical types of diabetes mellitus are seen. The **juvenile onset** type is characterized by a rapid onset, with instable diabetes, associated with loss of weight and strength, irritability, and the three "polys" mentioned above. Insulin therapy is mandatory in this type of patient and long-term medical counseling is needed. The second type of diabetes is termed **maturity onset**. Frequently symptoms are minimal or absent at first. Weight loss or weight gain may be present. These may be increased tendency to urinary infections or vaginitis. Blurred or decreased vision, anemia, loss of sensation, or other neurologic problems may send the patient to the physician. Since many patients are obese, the reduction of weight associated with a careful diet can bring a return of health to most people who will cooperate with simple health principles.

The **treatment** of diabetes involves several basic principles. Doctors aim to correct the underlying metabolic abnormalities and thereby reduce diabetic symptoms. This is associated first of all by the achieving and maintaining of an ideal body weight. Our third goal is the prevention or delay of the specific complications associated with diseases of the eye, kidney, and nerves. Finally, we try to stem the accelerating atherosclerosis to which the diabetic is particularly liable. Success in these therapies depends on how well the patient has been instructed and his conscientiousness in following directions. The avoidance of cigarette smoking, with regular daily exercise, the monitoring of the urine and blood sugar, cholesterol and triglycerides, blood pressure and body weight are all imperative. Basically, however, the treatment of diabetes revolves around an appropriate diet.

The **dietary** treatment must meet the basic nutritional requirements. These are usually the same as those of a nondiabetic patient and, of course, to be acceptable, taste, variety, economy, and other nutritional factors should be considered. The prevention of high blood sugar occurring after a meal is important to avoid aggravating the symptoms. On the other hand, if a person is taking insulin it is important to provide enough calories of the right type to prevent hypoglycemic reactions. Ideal body weight should be achieved as soon as possible. In order to delay the atherosclerotic complications, the diet should be low enough in fat and animal products to normalize the serum cholesterol and triglyceride levels.

The basic caloric requirement is dictated by age, ideal weight, physical activity, climate, and the patient's occupation. An approximate calculation can be obtained by multiplying the ideal weight in pounds by ten. Individuals who are less active or past middle-age should reduce their calories somewhat. Meals should be regular, usually spaced 5-6 hours apart. They are ideally limited to two or three meals a day, the latter especially for those taking insulin. I recommend taking the greater number of calories at breakfast, in order to provide energy during the active part of the day. Suppers should be light, eaten several hours before going to bed.

Careful regulation of the insulin level can usually avoid the necessity of a bedtime snack. The fat content of the diet should definitely be reduced from the 40% eaten by the average American. Protein should also be reduced slightly. The remaining calories should be obtained from complex carbohydrates. This can lower the insulin requirement dramatically, and in many maturity onset diabetics, make a need for the needle entirely unnecessary. Some dietary suggestions for diabetics, as used in my institution, are presented in the accompanying tables.

Insulin therapy is usually necessary for diabetes of juvenile onset. Several types are available, having fast, intermediate, and long duration of action. Most of the insulin used in the United States today contains 100 units per milliliter. This has helped considerably to standardize the syringes and simplify the self administration of this hormone. Regular or crystalline insulin is the shortest acting and is usually used for emergencies. Its duration of action is 6 to 8 hours. Intermediate acting insulins, such as NPH or Lente have a peak effect in 8-12 hours and usually last for 24. The longer-acting insulins are seldom used. At times, a second small dose of intermediate insulin before bedtime is preferable to increasing the daily dose.

It is preferable to have a small amount of sugar spill in the urine during the day than achieve such rigid glucose control as to render the patient hungry all the time or prone to *hypoglycemic reactions*. Be sure to rotate the sites of injections and use sterile techniques in the administration of all insulin hormones. Although many diabetic patients develop antibodies to the insulin used, only a few, about 0.1% will develop insulin resistance. A regular exercise program helps, in combination with the low fat diet, to lower daily insulin requirement. Using the more convenient but less physiologic oral diabetic pills should be discouraged, because of numerous side effects, particularly an increased acceleration of vascular complications. Hope is definitely on the way for patients with diabetes, who will eat properly, exercise regularly, and keep their weight under control.

HYPOGLYCEMIA

Low blood sugar, usually called *hypoglycemia*, has many causes. The most common one relates to our fast-paced lifestyle. Excessive sugar intake, frequent snacking, and caffeine or cola beverages contribute to this frequent malady. When the blood glucose level falls rapidly, emergency "fight-or-flight" stress responses take over. The individual feels weak, very hungry, and frequently becomes irrational. Emotional reactions to hypoglycemic episodes vary from agitated to angry, depressed to suicidal. Personalities change rapidly, but return to normal function with some form of food.

Rather than frequent feedings such as the "six meal a day" diet, I recommend the following regimen: First, begin the day with a wholesome, hearty breakfast. Some whole grain cereal, bread, nut butter, or fruit makes a great way to start the day. Avoid coffee and frequent snacks. They both aggravate any tendency to low blood sugar. Mealtimes should be at regular intervals, usually five or six hours apart. Stress factors can affect hypoglycemia. Exercise is a great way to reduce or relieve stress. Try for an hour or two of extra sleep at night. Or find a weekend for a refreshing mini-vacation.

Careful testing of your blood, including the five hour Glucose Tolerance Test (GTT), may help your medical advisor to "fine-tune" your dietary and lifestyle regimen. Most individuals can overcome this metabolic imbalance, particularly the so-called *reactive hypoglycemia*. This type comes several hours after a meal or sugar-rich snack. It responds very well to the remedies mentioned above. Rarely, tumors of the pancreas may produce abnormal secretions of *insulin*. In such case the symptoms of hypoglycemia occur during a fast, often early in the morning. Removal of the tumor is necessary to cure this uncommon condition.

Finally, diabetes mellitus may be associated with hypoglycemia. It occurs in the context of early diabetes, erroneously termed *borderline*. Overdoses of insulin will produce hypoglycemia. They occur during vigorous exercise or at night. Adjusting the insulin dosage along with dietary modification will level the blood glucose fluctuations in all but the most "brittle" diabetics.

WATER RETENTION

Adults who suddenly increase their body weight may have an increase in fatty (*adipose*) tissue, accumulation of fluid (*edema*) or both disorders. Weight gain in excess of two pounds per day usually implies excess fluid retention. It is easy to confirm this by comparing the body weight in the morning and then again in the evening. Weight gains of less than two pounds during one day usually will subside by the following morning. Fluid retention may disclose increased salt and water intake or decreased sodium and water secretion.

Checking weight changes from morning to evening often provides early evidence of disease. Dietary indiscretion, the use of diuretics, excessive intake of licorice root, or a cortisol-type drug preparation may also be responsible.

A special type of fluid retention called **cyclic edema** occurs predominantly in women. This is characterized by periodic episodes of fluid retention, frequently accompanied by distention of the abdomen. Patients may weigh several pounds more in the evening than in the morning. Although there is some relation to the menstrual cycle, evidence suggests also that psychologic and hormonal factors may be related. The treatment of cyclic edema includes restriction in salt intake, rest in the feet elevated (*supine*) position for several hours during the day, and the use of elastic stockings. Careful medical work-up is sometimes indicated to evaluate underlying causes.

OBESITY

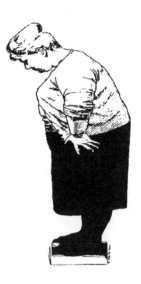

The single most prevalent metabolic disorder in countries where food supplies are abundant is **obesity**. A person is considered *over weight* if his weight exceeds the upper range of ideal weight for his body frame. He is considered *obese* if his weight exceeds by 15-20% his ideal weight. Obesity occurs when the caloric intake exceeds the energy requirement of the body for physical activity and growth, with resultant accumulation of fat. This excessive *adipose tissue* may be distributed generally over the body or may be localized. Hormones from the pituitary, thyroid, adrenal, and sex glands all play important roles in fat distribution.

For the most part, obesity is preventable. Unfortunately, however, the follow-through of treatment for prolonged periods is usually difficult. Relapse becomes extremely common.

The amount of body fat can be estimated from the measurement of skin fold thickness with calipers. Most commonly employed, however, are bathroom scales, and the commonly available tables for estimation of desirable weight with relative guidelines for determining obesity. Some physiologists claim that certain persons are more efficient than others in their ability to digest, absorb, and utilize food. Although this theory is not completely substantiated it has been observed many times that some obese patients lose weight much easier than others, on a given caloric intake.

Direct study of fat cell **size** by biopsy and the subsequent measurement of the isolated calls permits calculation of the total number of fat cells in the body. The average non-obese adult has approximately 40 trillion fat cells. Individuals who develop obesity in the middle years of life develop larger fat cells. Those who develop obesity during their growing years increase fat cell numbers, as well as size. This potential of forming new fat cells, with excessive food intake during growth, enhances our emphasis on prevention in childhood. Most studies demonstrate weight loss in both types of obesity to be associated with reduction in cell size, but seldom is there actual loss of fat cells.

Psychological and cultural factors influence our tendency toward obesity. Certain persons may have abnormal appetites, using food as a substitute for satisfaction that ordinarily would be supplied in other ways. In this respect, these persons resemble somewhat the alcoholic, hence are often termed "*foodaholics*."

Increased food intake may also result from depression or anxiety. The resulting obesity may increase a persons tendency toward isolation. Merely reducing food intake without understanding the underlying emotional problems is usually unsuccessful. Some cultural groups place great emphasis on food, developing habits of overeating at an early age. In fact, in some societies obesity is associated with success and even health. Education of individuals, families, and all ethnic groups in society is important to achieve proper understanding of fantastic health benefits obtained in weight reduction, also enabling the provision of emotional support during the transition.

The dietary treatment of obesity constitutes our mainstay for successful therapy. It is crucial to maintain good nutritional balance with any diet chosen, especially limiting the calories sufficiently to lose weight. **Crash diets** should be discouraged, as a weight loss of 2-3 pounds weekly is quite sufficient for most obese patients to regain their healthful profile without looking like a "dried prune." I always emphasize the use of *natural* foods, such as fresh fruits, whole grain cereals, and vegetables. Modest limitations of salt intake helps prevent fluid retention. Avoid as much as possible all rich foods, such as gravies, sauces, salad dressings, and desserts containing much sugar. Be sure to reduce fried foods, as fat contains 9 calories per gram compared with 4 cal./gm. for most carbohydrates and proteins.

For individuals finding it difficult to maintain a low calorie diet continuously, a **fast** one day a week using limited amounts of clear liquids is encouraging. Some find it more satisfactory to restrict their food intake to **two meals a day**, usually with a hearty breakfast and lunch and little or no supper. I teach my patients that being hungry one-third of the time is better than being hungry all of the time. Thus, these people can accept a two-meal-a-day plan and profit thereby. It is not necessary, however, in most sensible reducing diets to be hungry in a physiologic sense at all. The use of natural foods in abundance will satisfy the appetite, particularly if a few olives or nuts are included for "**satiety value**." Snacking should be eliminated. Some commonly used snacks may require a great amount of exercise to burn up the calories taken in this way.

Exercise has also been endorsed as a method to increase caloric loss. Although the stimulus to the circulation, as well as the balancing effect on the emotions are profound, a very minimal caloric effect is obtained with exercise, compared to the reduction in food intake. The *metabolic rate*, however, increases with exercise, sometimes lasting for hours. Obese subjects are prone to more sedentary patterns of behavior and often walk and work more slowly than their leaner counterparts. Motivational factors, goals, and an overall emphasis on physical fitness is important to achieve the very real benefits that exercise can make toward a weight reduction regimen.

The use of appetite suppressants, amphetamines, hormones from the thyroid gland and diuretics, are mentioned only to discourage their use. Their indulgence always upsets the balance of body chemistry and places a false emphasis upon "miracle drugs" rather than **diet** in treating the obese. More radical surgical procedures include the **jejuno-ileal bypass** (creating an unnatural shunt between two parts of the small intestines) and **gastric stapling** (where the stomach size is drastically reduced with a row of staples). Such measures should not even be considered unless a grave medical emergency exists. In such cases there are usually safer approaches, such as fasting or dental wiring. All of these do not reach the underlying cause, namely dietary reeducation, emotional stabilization, and the promotion of overall physical fitness that are so essential to long-term success in weight control.

This more rational handling of obesity can be a challenging and rewarding discipline to both patients and health counselors. A person's victory over appetite often proves the key to unlock many dimensions of fulfillment in emotional, as well as spiritual lines.

MALNUTRITION

Although overnutrition so characteristic of obesity could be considered a type of **malnutrition**, such diagnosis is usually reserved for the deficiency syndromes. In all parts of the world various deficiencies of vitamins, minerals, protein, or calories can be seen. Deficiencies are naturally more prevalent in countries where food supply is limited and poverty abounds. Careful analysis of food intake and any form of intemperance—such as manifested in alcohol consumption, bizarre food practices, food faddism, or the abuse of drugs—are productive to evaluate these conditions. Repeated closely spaced pregnancies and psychological disturbances manifested by a change in food intake should be assessed. Chronic infection, anorexia, or diarrhea likewise may profoundly affect the nutrient balance.

Measurement of **height** and **weight** should never be omitted. These are the most commonly used measurements of growth in children and adolescents. Other body measurements include **skin fold thickness**, head circumference, and biochemical tests measuring blood levels of various nutrients, such as proteins, vitamins and minerals. At times, therapeutic trials of replacement nutrients play a role in the diagnosis of deficiencies. In general, however, nutrient stores must be depleted *before* low blood levels of any nutrients are found. Changes in the body chemistry and functional neurologic defects occur late in the course of a deficiency. Take a careful history for invaluable help in the initial phase of treatment. Then combine this with a high index of suspicion for various nutrient-related disorders.

In spite of modern technology and transportation, there are still large areas in our world where **famine** is epidemic. In fact, the risk of mass starvation in many countries is all too real, and often associated with other diseases. Body changes during the starvation reflect physiologic attempts to adapt to undernutrition. Fat stores are utilized *first* in order to spare structural protein. Thus, body fat diminishes more rapidly than does muscle. Extensive losses occur later in other organs, especially the liver and intestines. Fortunately, the central nervous system and circulation maintain themselves, whatever the cost to less essential parts of the organism.

The person during **starvation** also conserves calories by reducing his output of energy. Voluntary physical activity decreases, as does the metabolic rate. A semi-starved patient complains of feeling tired, irritable, and depressed. He may also show lack of ambition, and narrowing of interests, then develops muscle soreness and cramps. The hair begins to fall out, and cuts and wounds heal slowly. Cold temperatures are poorly tolerated. Ultimately, the individual looks haggard, pale, and emaciated. At times swelling (*edema*), particularly of the eyelids and cheeks appear, masking the degree of weight loss. The pulse weakens and the eyes become dull, looking like unglazed porcelain. Without relief and too often alone, the hapless victim of starvation then dies on the street of some large city.

The **rehabilitation diet** for patients recovering from starvation must begin with *small* quantities of the simplest food, taken at frequent intervals. A natural diet is preferable to the use of "predigested" end products. Vitamin and protein supplementation are ordinarily unnecessary. General dietary allowances should be approximately 100% of those recommended on the basis of the patient's "desirable" weight. Recovery from starvation, however, advances at a very slow pace. Weakness, fatigability and muscle aches, as well as depression, may persist for weeks to months. Recovery of strength and working capacity is slow. Eventually, recovery is sure, and a life has been saved.

Protein Calorie Malnutrition is another type of disorder seen in early childhood. One such syndrome, called *kwashiorkor*, appears most commonly between the ages of one and three years. This tragic disorder occurs frequently in Africa in children displaced from their mother's breast by subsequent pregnancies. Conditioning factors, such as diarrhea, parasites, and skin rash may be seen. Edema is the principal sign. It is associated with low serum proteins. The child's face may appear round and moon-like. The hair changes with lightening of color, straightening of curly hair, and stripes of lightened color that attest to oscillating levels of good and poor nutrition in the past.

The other major type of malnutrition is called *nutritional marasmus*. This compares with severe semistarvation in adults. It most commonly affects infants during the first year of life. The most conspicuous features in marasmus are wasting of muscle and fat, with growth retardation. Affected infants appear prematurely old, and often suffer from vitamin deficiency. Both types of malnutrition respond to a careful feeding regimen of simple foods, given first at frequent intervals, containing both adequate protein and calories.

VITAMIN DEFICIENCIES

Although definite diseases can be associated with the excess intake of certain vitamins, these are seldom seen on a large scale. Much more common are the deficiencies described below.

Pellagra is a disease caused by the deficiency of *niacin*, one of the B vitamins. The name is derived from the rough skin characteristically seen crusting around the hands and neck. Painful burning of the mouth, shaking of the body, and less commonly, mental disturbances can result. Pellagra was common in the United States in the early 1900's. A healthful diet was discovered to be curative. One of the essential amino acids, *tryptophan*, is converted into *nicotinic acid*, a counterpart of niacin. Deficiency of other nutrients sometimes complicates the disease. Individuals subsisting on a diet primarily of corn are predisposed to pellagra, since corn protein is low in tryptophan and most of the milling removes the vitamin.

Classically pellagra is characterized by the "three D's" — *diarrhea, dermatitis,* and *dementia.* Certain earlier symptoms may develop, however, including loss of appetite, indigestion, weakness, burning in the mouth, and insomnia. Pellagra most commonly appears in the spring or early summer, when the dietary deficiencies of winter combines with renewed exposure to the sun seems to precipitate the outbreak. The skin problems begin to look much like a sunburn. Burning may be intense. Sun-exposed areas, such as the neck, arms, and hands are affected most commonly. Later the skin becomes brownish in color, then rough and scaly. Soreness of the mouth is typical, with inflammation of the tongue. Diarrhea may or may not be present. Mental disturbances usually begin with episodes of nervousness and tremor. Later there occurs confusion, depression, or even delirium.

Early replacement of the B-complex vitamin with high doses of niacinamide is recommended. This related substance does not cause unpleasant vascular flushing like nicotinic acid does. Most people can take them orally. As symptoms subside, all vitamins should all be obtained from a well-balanced, varied diet of natural foods.

Thiamine Deficiency, called *Beriberi*, has been known to western medical science since the seventeenth century. Recognized first in the Orient, beriberi has been associated with a deficiency of *thiamine*. It commonly appears when the diet exclusively consists polished rice. Cases are occasionally encountered in the United States, particularly in infants and in alcoholics.

Three main types of this disease are identified. A chronic form called **"dry beriberi"** causes tenderness in the calf muscles and weakness in the legs.

The acute form, "**wet beriberi**", is characterized by cardiovascular changes, with edema, congestion of the lungs, and heart failure. In alcoholics, the brain damage may be irreversible. Beriberi in infants continues to be a health problem in the Far East, where a child may lose his voice, develop heart failure, or gastrointestinal changes with vomiting and constipation. Adequate nutrition for the breast-feeding mother is particularly important for its prevention.

The therapeutic response to thiamine in infants and adults with beriberi involving the heart is dramatic. A rapid transition, however, should be made from vitamin supplementation to a diet containing adequate wheat germ, rice polishings, or whole grain cereals. This disease is entirely preventable, and reflects one of many conditions following the wake of the industrial revolution.

Riboflavin deficiency is still common in many developing countries. In the Unites States there appears to be a correlation between low income and riboflavin intake. Milk and certain vegetables are good sources of riboflavin, However, when the milk is exposed to direct sunlight a considerable amount of this vitamin is destroyed. Riboflavin is reduced when the food is treated with alkali, such as we find in certain preservatives and the use of soda. Lack of riboflavin usually results in sores, developing at the corners of the mouth, inflammation of the tongue, and sore throat. Late findings affect the nerves, as well as the blood, with the development of anemia. Replacement of the vitamin rapidly reduces these changes.

Vitamin B$_6$ deficiency is seen occasionally in individuals who eat very few plant foods. Seizures occur in babies fed formulas deficient in B$_6$. This has especially been a problem when a relatively high kidney excretion develops during pregnancy, while a mother was given high dose supplements. A number of drugs interfere with vitamin B$_6$ utilization, such as isoniazid, used in the treatment of tuberculosis. Eating a natural varied diet, it is not difficult to get plenty of *pyridoxine*. It is the vegetable source of vitamin B$_6$.

Scurvy is another vitamin deficiency with world wide prevalence as well as a colorful history. This condition is caused by a deficiency of *ascorbic acid*, also called *vitamin C*. It was a common cause of mortality in sailors during the fifteenth and sixteenth centuries. James Lind, a British naval surgeon, developed a simple cure in 1747 by giving the sailors two oranges and one lemon every day. Their swollen gums, weakness, and bleeding tendencies responded dramatically, giving rise to the nickname, "Limeys." In more recent times scurvy appears more commonly in alcoholics, food faddists, and the impoverished elderly living on a grossly unbalanced diet.

The principal manifestations of scurvy are hemorrhages in the skin, swollen and bleeding gums, aching muscles, fatigue, and emotional changes. These symptoms appear after two months of depletion. Appearing occasionally in children, scurvy produces tenderness and swelling in the legs. Extreme pain may be present. Finally, after the teeth erupt, swollen gums and bleeding develops. Skeletal changes show signs of growth retardation. In some cases of a vitamin-D deficiency syndrome, rickets, may co-exist.

A carefully taken feeding history is helpful for the diagnosis of *infantile scurvy*. After 46 months of age any infant fed solely with the bottle, using only boiled cows milk or a milk substitute, may develop this disease. Fresh orange juice or another dietary source of vitamin C is rapidly curative. Extremely high supplements of ascorbic acid are seldom necessary. They may produce an abnormal dependency, based on the development of increased excretion originating in the kidneys to compensate for this superabundance. Large doses of vitamin C can also inactivate vitamin B_{12}. That, at times, unfavorably affects reproduction.

Vitamin A is primarily manufactured by the conversion of dietary *beta-carotene* into the active form, *retinol*. One of the first symptoms of vitamin A deficiency is inability to see in reduced light (night blindness). A later change in the eye is the presence of dryness, *xerophthalmia*. The conjunctiva becomes opaque, the secretion of tears decreases, then a sticky secretion appears over the cornea, called the *Bitot spot*. This mark has the appearance of a flake of meringue. Further destruction of the cornea may occur, leading eventually to blindness.

In treating the acute disease, a supplement of vitamin A is recommended. The prevention of deficiency using a balanced diet containing green and yellow vegetables, fresh fruit, and vitamin supplemented milk is entirely adequate. Green and yellow foods such as carrots, cantaloupe, squash, and dark green leafy vegetables are considered excellent sources for this vitamin.

A high intake of carotene appears in adults using carrot juice or a similar food concentrate excessively. **Carotenemia** may color the skin, but should not be confused with jaundice. It is considered harmless and will subside when the carotene intake is reduced. **Hypervitaminosis A**, on the other hand, can produce an acute toxicity. In infants, it presents as drowsiness, vomiting, and other signs of increased intracranial pressure. Adults commonly develop a headache within hours after any injection of a toxic dose. Blurred vision, nausea, vomiting, or drowsiness may also develop. The skin peels and hair loss occurs. With chronic ingestion of high doses, liver changes resembling cirrhosis are seen. Psychiatric side effects manifest themselves, but prognosis is good when vitamin A ingestion ceases.

Vitamin E is the common name of a group of related fat soluble vitamin, called *tocopherols*. They vary in their potency, with the alpha form being thought most active. A number of animals develop a Vitamin E deficiency syndrome, with deterioration in the muscle fibers, impaired reproduction, or anemia. Clinically, these insufficiencies are rare in adults. When the diet contains enough polyunsaturated fatty acids, plenty of dietary vitamin E is usually available. Unfortunately, optimistic expectations of many researchers have been disappointed in spite of the literature proclaiming the miracle-working powers of this vitamin. We do not know for certain whether vitamin E supplementation can favorably affect physical endurance, cardiac status, sexual potency, or longevity in individuals with normal blood levels of Vitamin E (*tocopherols*).

A number of vitamins affect the production of blood or its proper coagulation. **Vitamin K** is present in most edible vegetables, particularly the green leafy ones. A similar vitamin is also produced by intestinal bacteria. The gradual accumulation of vitamin K levels in a newborn baby explains easily why ancient recommendation for an *eight-day* circumcision was made to the Jews. Hemorrhagic disease of the newborn as well as in adults is prevented by proper blood levels of this vitamin.

Vitamin B_{12}, folic acid, and iron are also closely related to blood production and have been discussed in Chapter 4, dealing with the circulatory system.

TRACE MINERALS

Many **trace minerals** are known to be essential to physiologic processes. It is not known in all cases that supplementation of these can cure specific diseases, but a few of the common sources are listed below. **Zinc** is widely distributed in foods, particularly breads, cereals, lentils, beans, and rice. This nutrient is essential to growth, as well as in repair and healing processes. **Copper** is abundant in raisins, whole grain cereals, dried legumes, and nuts. It also plays a role in blood production, tissue metabolism, bone development, and nerve function.

Cobalt is a component of vitamin B_{12} and comes from a variety of sources. Called *hydroxycobalamin*, vitamin B_{12} is a vital ingredient in blood cell formation as well as healthy nerve function. Deficiency of B_{12} produces the disorder **pernicious anemia**. Vitamin B_{12} is found in many animal products, such as milk, eggs, and cheese. It is absorbed in the small intestine (*ileum*), and requires a protein *intrinsic factor* for complete absorption. Intrinsic factor is found in the stomach. It is often deficient in people who have chronic gastritis or those who have had the major part of the stomach removed by surgery. Total vegetarians should be sure that their diet includes some vitamin B_{12}. Many breakfast cereals, soy milks, and meat substitutes are fortified with B_{12}. It is available in tablet form. One microgram is sufficient for daily protection.

On the other hand, many vegans have gone for years without evidence of vitamin B_{12} deficiency. There is a urine test that can determine any presence of B_{12} deficiency. It is called *urinary homocysteine* and *methylmalonic acid*. Both of these substances are metabolites of vitamin B_{12}. Together with serum B_{12} measurements, these analyses are effective in screening vegetarians for any trace of B_{12} deficiency before problems appear.

The anemia of vitamin B_{12} deficiency is *macrocytic*, meaning that the red blood cells are unusually large. More serious are the nerve and spinal cord disorders that develop. Neurologic signs include loss of position and vibration sensation, combined with sensations of numbness and tingling. Later, serious impairment of gait and bladder (*sphincter*) control are seen. Some of these symptoms may persist long after vitamin B_{12} is again replenished. Moreover, this neurologic damage may occur before any evidence of anemia, making diagnosis very difficult in early stages. Prevention is the watchword for vitamin B_{12} disorders.

Selenium, like vitamin E, protects against cellular damage and lowers the risk of cancer. Cereal grains are good sources of this mineral also. **Manganese** and **magnesium** affect a host of enzyme systems. They likewise come from whole grain cereals, as well as many vegetables. **Nickel, silicon, fluorine**, and many other minerals are also important to the body. Whole grain cereals are a major source of **Chromium**. It is also found in Brewer's yeast. This mineral helps to improve glucose tolerance and is an important preventive against the development of diabetes.

OTHER HORMONAL DISORDERS

Finally, we turn to the common endocrine glands that occasionally produce a disease. Many people are concerned about the function of the **thyroid** gland. This endocrine organ, located at the base of the neck just below the "Adam's apple" (*larynx*) is an important regulator of the metabolism of the body. Its overactivity results in characteristic symptoms, such as a rapid pulse, bulging of the eyes, nervousness, tremor, and diarrhea. Tumors of the thyroid gland, as well as the overproduction of the brain hormone stimulating the gland to produce excessive amounts of thyroid hormone may cause these problems. Blood tests are available to determine the level of *thyroxine*, the major hormone, as well as others circulating in the system.

Although stress may be a precipitating factor in the development of **hyperthyroidism**, a failure to respond to the recommended change in lifestyle with increased rest and physical exercise, should lead a person to seek medical counsel, as surgery is occasionally indicated.

Many more people are concerned about *underactivity* of the thyroid gland. This is often blamed for obesity but in reality is seldom the cause. A tendency to fluid retention, sluggishness, drying of the skin, constipation, and fluid retention should lead one to seek the appropriate blood tests and accurate diagnosis. The typical patient with advanced **hypothyroidism**, called *myxedema*, becomes very complacent, with subdued emotional responses and dull mental processes. This so-called "bovine placidity" is much less distressing to its possessor than to the patient's associates.

Neurologic syndromes are occasionally mimicked by hypothyroidism. They normally clear rapidly with replacement therapy. Many different forms of thyroid medications are available, but should not be used unless a definite deficiency is diagnosed. In such case full hormone replacement becomes necessary, usually for life.

The **adrenal** glands are organs of great benefit, often blamed for minor symptoms. It is my belief that although the adrenal glands may play a role in **hypoglycemia**, this syndrome should not be confused with adrenal exhaustion. **Addison's disease** is the medical term for lack of the production of *cortisol* and other steroid hormones. In this case, weight loss, weakness, low blood pressure, and a disturbance in salt balance occurs. Replacement therapy is necessary to avoid life-threatening complications, and with the appropriate hormone, metabolic balance may be achieved and normal life expectancy realized.

Symptoms of excessive cortisol, called **Cushing's Syndrome**, are sometimes seen either from excessive intake of a related drug or from tumor overproduction of the body's own hormone by an adrenal cortical tumor. In this case, the face becomes moon shaped and a "buffalo hump" appears over the shoulders. Blood pressure may be elevated and a diabetic glucose tolerance appear. Eventually the bones become demineralized and may develop spontaneous fractures. Hypertension usually appears, as well as an increased tendency to ulcer formation. For these reasons, the disease should be recognized as early as possible and confirmed with appropriate blood tests. Treatment should be directed toward the cause.

It is well accepted that prolonged stress can cause gradual weakening in these endocrine organs. Exposure to prolonged noise, lack of sleep, excessive worry, dietary indiscretion as well as many emotional factors may precipitate either depletion or excessive production of many endocrine hormones. Numerous cardiac symptoms, menstrual disorders, blood pressure changes, as well as general symptoms of exhaustion, fatigue, and depression stem from hormonal interaction combined with the body's response to prolonged stress. Simple lifestyle measures may be curative, but therapy must be prolonged. Often changes in the entire lifestyle are required in order to effect a cure.

Nevertheless, I believe that the hormonal-biochemical interaction related to nutrition and the endocrine system constitutes one of the most challenging frontiers for investigation. Understanding it may impart to sufferers a long and useful life with ultimately the reestablishment of perfect health.

Data Used to Calculate the Composition of Vegetables		
	CARBOHYDRATE CONTENT	WEIGHTINGS
FOOD	(Starch and Sugar) gm./100gm.	(Based on usual rate of consumption)
Beets	8.0	3
Carrots	7.5	4
Onions	7.2	1
Peas, green	9.0	4
Pumpkin	5.1	--
Rutabaga	6.7	½
Squash, winter	4.9	2
Turnip	4.6	1
Weighted average	7.0	

DIABETIC DIET EXCHANGE LISTS

FOODS THAT NEED NOT BE MEASURED

(Insignificant carbohydrate or calories)

Cranberries (unsweetened)
Clear broth
Lemon
Gelatin (unsweetened)
Pickle, dill
Seasonings:
Chopped parsley, mint, garlic, onion, celery salt.

LIST 1. MILK EXCHANGES

One exchange of milk contains 8 gm. of protein, 10 gm. of fat, 12 gm. of carbohydrate, and 170 calories.

This list shows the different types of milk to use for one exchange:

Type of Milk	Amount to use
Soy milk	1 c.
Whole milk	
(homogenized)	1 c.
Skim milk	1 c.
Evaporated milk	½ c.
Powdered skim milk	¼ c.
(nonfat dried milk)	
Buttermilk	
(made from skim milk)	1 c.

One type of milk may be used instead of another. For example, one half cup of evaporated milk in place of 1 cup of whole milk. Soy or rice milks are much preferred to reduce disease risks from dairy animals.

Skim milk and buttermilk have the same food values as whole milk, except that they contain less fat. Two fat exchanges are added when 1 cup of skim milk or buttermilk made from skim milk is used in place of whole milk, calculated in a diet pattern.

LIST 2. VEGETABLE EXCHANGES: GROUP A

Group A contains little protein, carbohydrate, or calories. *One cup at a time may be used without counting it.*

Asparagus
*Broccoli
Brussels sprouts
Cabbage
*Escarole
Eggplant
*Beet greens
*Chard
*Collards
*Dandelion greens
*Kale
*Mustard
*Spinach
*Turnip greens
Cauliflower
Celery
*Chicory
Cucumbers
Lettuce
Mushrooms
Okra
Radishes
Sauerkraut
String beans
Summer squash
*Tomatoes
*Water cress
  * *These vegetables contain a lot of vitamin A.*

LIST 2. VEGETABLE EXCHANGES: GROUP B

Each exchange contains 2 gm. of protein, 0.7 gm. of carbohydrate, and 35 calories. *One half cup of vegetable equals 1 exchange:*

131

Beets
*Carrots
Onions
Green peas
*Pumpkin
Rutabagas
*Winter squash
Turnip

> *These vegetables contain a lot of vitamin A.*

LIST 3. FRUIT EXCHANGES

One exchange of fruit contains 10 gm. of carbohydrate and 40 calories. *This list shows the different amounts of fruits to use for one fruit exchange:*

Fruit	Amount to use
Apple (2" diam.)	1 small
Apple sauce	½ c.
Apricots, fresh	2 medium
Apricots, dried	4 halves
Banana	½ small
Blackberries	1 c.
Raspberries	1 c.
*Strawberries	1 c.
Blueberries	2/3 c.
*Cantaloupe (6" diam.)	¼
Cherries	10 large
Dates	2
Figs, fresh	2 large
Figs, dried	1 small
*Grapefruit	½ small
*Grapefruit juice	½ c.
Grapes	12
Grape juice	¼ c.
Honeydew melon	1/8 medium
Mango	½ small
*Orange	1 small
*Orange juice	½ c.
Papaya	1/3 medium
Peach	1 medium
Pear	1 small
Pineapple	½ c.
Pineapple juice	1/3 c.
Plums	2 medium
Prunes, dried	2 medium
Raisins	2 Tbsp.

*Tangerine	1 large
Watermelon	1 c.

These fruits are rich sources of vitamin C.

LIST 4. BREAD EXCHANGES

Bread	1 slice
Biscuit, roll (2" diam.)	1
Muffin (2" diam.)	1
Corn bread (1½" cube)	1
Cereals, cooked	½ c.
Dry, flake, and puff types	¾ c.
Rice, grits, cooked	½ c.
Spaghetti, noodles, cooked	½ c.
Macaroni, etc., cooked	½ c.
Crackers, graham (2½" sq.)	2
Saltines (2" sq.)	5
Round, thin (1½")	6
Flour	2½ Tbsp.
Vegetables:	
Beans, peas (dried, cooked)	½ c.
(Lima, navy, split peas, cowpeas, etc.)	
Baked beans, no pork	¼ c.
Corn	1/3 c.
Popcorn	1 c.
Parsnips	2/3 c.
Potatoes, white	1 small
Potatoes, white, mashed	½ c.
Potatoes, sweet, or Yams	¼ c.

LIST 5. FAT EXCHANGES

Margarine	1 tsp.
Avocado (4" diam.)	1/8
Soy mayonnaise	1 tsp.
Oil	1 tsp.
Nuts	6 small
Olives	5 small
Peanut butter	1 Tbsp.

CHAPTER NINE

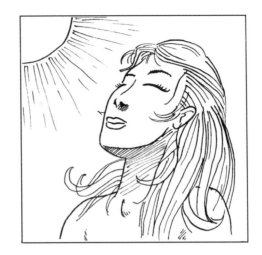

THE

SKIN

AND ITS

DISEASES

The **skin** is the body's largest and most obvious organ. It is a tough yet flexible protective enclosure. Altogether, your skin is the heaviest organ in the body, and also has the largest surface area, over 3,000 square inches. In some places your skin is paper thin, while the soles of the feet and other calloused areas are more durable. Consider the incredible number of structures fitted into an area no bigger than your fingernail: several dozen sweat glands, hundreds of nerve endings, many yards of tiny blood vessels, numerous oil glands, hairs, and literally thousands of cells. In fact, one-third of all blood circulating through the body goes to the skin. This is why it becomes such a valuable organ to help control your circulation. Moreover, your skin is easily influenced by temperature, both heat and cold. This property is used effectively by the hydrotherapist.

Your skin is subject to many diseases. Most anciently feared was leprosy, where the skin appeared as white anesthetic patches. Although leprosy still exists in some areas of the world, many more common afflictions appear today, some resembling the boils of the patriarch Job and causing equal distress. Numerous common diseases will be discussed below, with appropriate treatments that can be rendered in one's home.

First, however, some general principles of the care of the skin are in order. Millions of pores, acting like tiny mouths, cover the visible protective surface. These sweat glands exude a tiny amount of perspiration having cooling properties, as well as eliminative functions. Regular bathing helps to keep the pores clean, but after a hot bath your pores need to be "closed" by finishing with a cool spray or a cold mitten friction. This helps to prevent your catching a cold.

Our garments should be frequently cleansed, particularly underclothes, so that the impurities from the pores are not reabsorbed after the waste matter is thrown off. Regular exercise helps induce the blood to the skin's surface, not only relieving the internal organs, but giving a healthful glow to the skin and distributing the blood more equally to the extremities.

Several nutrients are important in maintaining the health and integrity of the skin. Vitamin A guards against dry skin and helps to prevent blemishes. Vitamin C in the right amounts protects the small capillaries, preventing bruises. The B complex vitamins are very important in the prevention of eczema, and protein helps to form connective and elastic tissue retarding the aging process and wrinkling.

COMMON SKIN INFECTIONS

Many microorganisms normally reside on the skin. The bacterial flora function beneficially by inhibiting the growth of many strains of pathogenic bacteria. Infections develop when the normal surface of the skin is broken by injury or when some disease disrupts the protective "acid mantle" that, in health, protects the skin from colonization by infective germs. These organisms fall into the usual spectrum of infectious agents discussed in Chapter Three.

Impetigo

Impetigo is a common infection of the skin caused by the bacterial germs *Streptococci* (Group A beta hemolytic) and *Staphylococci* (coagulase positive). These organisms are introduced into the skin after disruption of the normal barrier, such as following insect bites or trauma. If there is itching, the subsequent scratching allows the organisms to embed themselves into areas of normal skin and form pustules. This infection becomes contagious and is usually disseminated by direct physical contact. General symptoms, such as fever and swollen glands, are uncommon. The pustules, resembling **acne**, usually have surrounding areas of redness and crust formation, may multiply and spread.

Most commonly involved are the exposed parts, your extremities and face. Cultures are helpful in determining the exact organisms involved. Prompt treatment with hot moist compresses, disinfectant soaps and meticulous cleansing of the surrounding skin can bring rapid resolution of all but the most stubborn skin infection. Your hands should be washed frequently and finger nails kept clean. Conscientious avoidance of scratching or rubbing the offending lesions is important to prevent the lesions spreading to other areas.

The diet that encourages resistance of infection is simple, with fruits, fresh vegetables, and whole grains predominating. Strictly avoid sugar and greasy foods.

Several types of complications can be seen, usually classified as a type of *pyoderma*. *Folliculitis* occurs when the bacteria invade tissues surrounding the hairs. This is more common in the armpits and bearded area. *Cellulitis* develops from the dispersion of the infection along deeper planes of skin. *Lymphangitis*, often confused with blood poisoning, presents itself as a streak of redness, indicating the advancement of infection along the lymphatic channels. Each of these problems responds well to alternating hot and cold compresses, or hot and cold contrast baths described in Chapter 17 on hydrotherapy. Use them in combination with strict antisepsis of the skin.

Boils

Any collection of pus in a localized are is usually of bacterial origin. Small pustules, especially those occurring the beard area, are called *furuncles*. A yellow discharge (*exudate*) will usually drain spontaneously when the lesions open, while pain and pressure are immediately reduced. Occasionally, mild fever and lethargy may occur, but signs of a severe infection are usually absent.

The mature lesion, brought to a head by repeated applications of hot compresses is ready for incision and drainage. After careful cleansing with alcohol or other antiseptic, a sterile needle or sharp blade can be used to open the top of the lesion and allow the pus to drain. The application of a charcoal poultice will also aid in its resolution. Lesions in the central portion of the face are more dangerous, because of the veins that drain in toward the cavernous sinus of the brain. These should be evaluated by a physician.

A second class of localized abscess is the *carbuncle*. These are usually deeper and more painful. Conditions which predispose to developing these infections are high fat diets increasing oil production of the skin, occlusive dressings and cosmetics that block the drainage of oil and sweat glands. Unusual friction rubs or excessive exposure to oil may also be harmful. Reduced resistance to infection transpire in the malnourished, alcoholics, diabetics, newborns, and those with blood diseases. Inasmuch as these germs are contagious in character, hand washing, antiseptic skin cleaning, and other hygienic measure are mandatory.

Erysipelas

This distinctive type of **cellulitis** involving the skin and subcutaneous tissue is caused by the *beta-hemolytic streptococcus*. Beginning as a reddened, irregular, swollen plaque, the lesions spread to reach a maximum size of 15 cm. in diameter. Usually the sores are solitary with a preference for the face, scalp, extremities, or genitalia. Fever, headache, and lethargy are common, with a general physical appearance of toxicity.

Enzymes released by the offending bacteria produce marked swelling of the skin with inflammation. It is occasionally difficult to distinguish between **erysipelas** and severe cellulitis. The former condition, however, develops into "blood poisoning," with bacteria traveling to create abscesses elsewhere in the body. They may even infect the inner lining or valves of the heart. Rest with elevation of an infected extremity are beneficial. Cool, wet dressings or alternating hot and cold compresses are crucial, while in advanced cases specific antibacterial therapy is recommended.

Scarlet Fever

Scarlet fever results from the production of a toxin by the *beta-hemolytic streptococcus*. The rash involves the mouth and throat, and the skin over the body. Usually the patient manifests sore throat, headache, loss of appetite, and fever for two to five days before the skin rash appears. The latter begins as a patch on the posterior neck, chest, or axillae. It then extends to involve the abdomen, extremities, and face with a pin point type of redness. The involved skin feels and looks like sandpaper, and the rash blanches with pressure. Pallor is present around the eyes and on the end of the nose. The tongue is often coated white with the edges appearing red, as a strawberry. Peeling skin over the hands and feet frequently evolves.

Untreated, the condition may last from four to six weeks. Severe complications, such as mastoiditis, sinusitis, arthritis, and even carditis may occur. Specific antistreptococcal therapy is usually indicated in the prevention of these complications. General hydrotherapy treatments and a spare diet during the acute phase are valuable to hasten rapid convalescence.

Acne Vulgaris

A very distressing condition that occurs primarily among adolescents is **acne vulgaris**. Although the exact *cause* of this troubling affliction is not completely known, acne is definitely associated with hormone changes. These include those that cause sexual maturation and growth during the teenage years. Skin variations take several possible courses. Frequently, around the face, neck, and back ones hair follicles will become plugged with a waxy secretion that appears as the typical **blackhead** (*comedone*). These plugs can be removed with a "comedone extractor." The device can be purchased at any pharmacy. Using this instrument is much preferable to pinching the pimple. Traumatizing the skin can spread infection.

Obstruction to drainage of this material can develop a bacterial infection, producing the typical **whitehead** or pustule. These may be large and extensive. In more serious forms, called **cystic acne**, infection may produce permanent scarring. A high fat diet, rich in fried or greasy foods, or meat and cheese, frequently changes the oil secretions on the skin and thus aggravates this tendency. Average teenage diets are often low in natural seed oils, nuts, fruits, and grains. This further enhances the development of acne. Poor diets may perpetuate it for several years.

Combined with high–fat dietary patterns is the increasing use of fashionable cosmetics. Most of them block the pores and prevent the skin from breathing. There are dozens of skin remedies available in pharmacies today. However, I find the following remedial agencies important, both in prevention and treatment of acne.

The skin must be cleansed once or twice daily with an antiseptic soap. This reduces the germ count and prevents the bacterial colonization in deeper pores that may be plugged. **Blackheads** and other lesions should *never* be squeezed or picked at, particularly with dirty hands or fingernails. **Whiteheads** can be treated, as mentioned above for furuncles, with incision and drainage after appropriate antiseptic preparation. Sunlight exposure is important, not only to curtail bacterial colonization, but for general toning of the skin to resist disease.

Teenager's diets should be simple but varied, with adequate vitamin and mineral composition, and a strong emphasis on fruits, whole grains, nuts, and vegetables. Butter fats, cocoa, coconut, meat, and fried greasy foods should be strictly avoided. Most saturated fats tend to clog the pores. Soy milk is valuable to further reduce any dietary source of cholesterol or saturated fat. Sugar intake should be restricted to aid general resistance to infection. Habits of adequate rest, daily exercise, and frequent bathing are most advantageous.

Cold Sores

Painful ulcerating lesions around the mouth, on the face, and in the genital region are usually caused by a virus, called *Herpes simplex*. These lesions, frequently called **cold sores** or **fever blisters**, may follow an infection. Respiratory illness, influenza, or serious bacterial diseases are some of the common triggers. Nearly everyone is exposed to the *Herpes simplex* virus during childhood or young adult life. In most individuals a gradual immunity develops. In the unfortunate others, the Herpes virus invades a regional nerve. From this protected position it periodically spawns the skin reaction. A second type of *Herpes simplex* virus involves the genital organs. Transmitted usually by sexual relations, Herpes ulcers may become extremely painful. If present during late pregnancy, Herpes can provoke a serious, occasionally fatal, viral infection of the newborn.

Herpes simplex is frequently triggered by prolonged exposure to sunlight. Fever, trauma, menstruation, and cold exposure, as well as anxiety may be contributory causes. Because a sensory nerve is irritated, numbness or tingling may be present, associated with the skin lesions. Involvement of the brain (*meninges*), the cornea, or *Herpes* infection superimposed on eczema are more serious diseases. They should be evaluated by a skilled physician. Specific antiviral agents are somewhat experimental, all with potential side effects. The treatment of **keratitis** (infection of the cornea) is urgent, to prevent ulceration and blindness.

Several simple treatments are most helpful for cold sores about the mouth or other skin locations. They act as drying agents to the skin, including *camphor*, alcohol, and similar proprietary medications. Topical hydrocortisone containing creams *(corticosteroids)* can be applied for temporary symptomatic relief.

Varicella

Chicken pox or *varicella* is caused by a virus in the same family as *Herpes simplex*. The virus produces in adults a disease called *Herpes zoster* or **shingles**. The childhood variety is quite typical with a reddened rash, becoming raised and developing small blisters. These evolve in various stages and eventually form crusts. This disease is contagious and is probably transmitted from one person to another through the skin or respiratory tract. Severe itching, however, can lead to secondary bacterial infection. Sometimes deep scabs produce permanent scarring. Topical drying lotions can give relief of itching, while specific treatment of secondary bacterial infections is essential.

Zoster or *shingles* is a second disease caused by the same Herpes virus. The first manifestation of this condition is usually severe pain, localized to one side and following a nerve distribution in the face, neck, or trunk. At this early stage of the disease the condition may be misdiagnosed as a heart attack, hiatus hernia, migraine, or other pain syndrome. Several days later, however, the eruption appears as grouped reddened papules that rapidly evolve into tiny blisters distributed on the skin over the nerve (called the *dermatome*). Diagnosis is usually simple at this stage, while therapy is more difficult.

Although complications are rare and contagion is uncommon, in elderly people severe pain may persist. This is called "postherpetic neuralgia." It is rare in patients younger than 50 years, but may be quite disabling to the elderly. The shingles infection itself is self-limited. Topical drying lotions are helpful. A relatively new cream is now available for pain control. Called *Zostrix*, it is actually based on cayenne pepper, containing the ingredient capsicum.

In our institution I have seen relief from a series of steam baths, producing a mild fever. Just as the fever helps fight the childhood viral disease, I find fever effective in reducing the sequelae of this disease and hastening the clearing of the rash. Moist compresses, such as the use of a charcoal poultice, can also reduce the pain and local inflammation over the involved nerve. Sprays, such as Dermaplast, may produce temporary relief for the pain and irritation. Experimental treatment using the smallpox vaccine for shingles patients was studied and found ineffective.

Molluscum Contagiosum

This viral disease affects the mucous membranes as well as the skin. It produces multiple raised reddened lesions, each having a small central crater. The size is less than ¼ inch (2 to 4 mm). Clusters of lesions tend to erupt in groups or lines. These papules emit a thick white material with pressure. They spread by contact. In order to remove them, a method must be chosen that minimizes scar formation and pain. Freezing with liquid nitrogen, the use of a comedone extractor (see page 136), or disruption of the central core with a scalpel or sterilized needle can produce rapid relief with insignificant scarring.

Warts

The **common wart** is caused by a virus which invades the skin, producing the characteristic elevation of the skin or mucous membrane. Several forms occur. The common rough thickened plaques (*verruca vulgaris*) occur frequently in childhood. They are most familiar on the hands, fingers, and around the nails. Satellite lesions may occur, or they may appear in areas of trauma. Small capillaries, when thrombosed, may exhibit black dots, resembling seeds.

Flat warts are multiple skin-colored papules on the face, neck, or the back of the hand. Around the eye or mouth small pointed (*filiform*) warts may appear like soft pliable tags. A most difficult wart to eradicate is the one found on the sole or **plantar wart,** occurring in the thick calloused skin of the feet. It is important to differentiate these from corns or calluses. A final type of wart is seen in the genital area, called **condyloma accuminata**. These cauliflower–shaped, warty clusters may extend into the vaginal or rectal mucosa. Usually related to sexual contact, they may become quite painful.

There are several acceptable methods of treating warts. Electric needles can be used to dry up the warts, but this usually requires local anesthesia. Chemicals such as *bichloracetic acid* can destroy the wart tissue and, when carefully controlled to depth of penetration, it is usually successful. More recently *cryosurgery* is used, freezing the lesion with liquid nitrogen or with a special instrument utilizing carbon dioxide as the cooling agent. Most treatments of warts work by liberating the virus into the circulation, thus exposing it to antibodies. The usual type of warts on the hands should be frozen with liquid nitrogen or treated with chemicals, such as salicylic acid and lactic acid (*duofilm*), trichloracetic acid, ammoniated mercury ointment, or *cantharidine* (Cantharone). These treatments will not usually leave a scar.

Electrosurgery is also effective, and for most lesions the remaining scar will not be too visible. Approximately 20% of the warts resolve spontaneously within one year. Plantar warts should be treated carefully with a nonscarring procedure. Permanent scars may be painful. Gentle excavation of the wart with a scraping instrument (*curette*). Also, the use of chemical irritants or freezing measures are usually quite effective. The **venereal wart** (*condyloma accuminata*) can be a real therapeutic challenge. One treatment involves an application of a special solution, 25% podophyllin in tincture of benzoin. Caution is required, because of skin irritation risk. This treatment should NEVER be used during pregnancy!

The study of warts can be challenging, because of the antigen-antibody relationships of this ubiquitous virus. It has provided a model for understanding the production of tumors. This some day may help us develop safer and more physiologic ways of fighting other viruses, such as those which cause various types of cancer.

Yeast Infections

A number of distinct species of yeasts or fungi can infect the skin and its appendages. Although some are always disease producing (called *pathogenic*), many are *opportunists* and live normally on the skin, causing infection and symptoms only when conditions prevail that allow excessive growth or an imbalance in normal body flora.

Ringworm is a common and very distressing fungal infection. It is classified sometimes by location and also biologically to describe different organisms which can be cultured. Small red, itching, scaling spots develop on the skin surface, then grow outward. The margin gradually increases in size, while the central portion of the eruption begins to heal spontaneously. Occasionally, after shaving their legs, women can develop deeper fungus infection of the hair follicles, characterized by redness, itching, and granuloma formation.

Another location for infection with the ringworm (*Tinea*) organism is the nails. Called **onychomycosis**, this infection usually involves single nails, more commonly on the toes. As fungal organisms grow in the nail plate, the nail becomes opaque, brittle, cracked, and partially separated from its bed. Occasionally an associated fungus infection occurs in the surrounding skin.

The third type of ringworm, *Tinea cruris*, occurs in the groin. This may itch and exude some fluid. It slowly spreads until treatment is instituted. The hands, feet, and scalp can also be involved with the *Tinea* family of organisms. Formerly occurring as an epidemic in children, *Tinea capitis* is now less common. These round or oval, sharply defined lesions cause breaking of the hair, patchy baldness, and occasionally drain a pus-like material. A special fluorescent (Wood's) light may illuminate the lesions, producing a bright yellowish-green fluorescence.

The most superficial infection, *Tinea versicolor*, occurs in hot humid climates. Slight scaling patches usually involve the trunk, neck, and upper arms. Gentle scraping may make the scaling more evident. Confirmation of the diagnosis in these fungus infections involves scraping the scaling lesions into a glass slide. After applying a 10% solution of potassium hydroxide and heating the slide gently, the characteristic fungus organism can be seen under the microscope. They usually appear, like most yeasts and fungi, as branching strands, called *hyphae*.

Treatment of superficial fungus infections is quite effective, using a number of common antifungal preparations. The application of sulfur ointment, painting with tincture of iodine, or half strength of Whitfield's ointment is usually helpful. Topical salicylic acid, or the use of newer creams, such as *Tinactin* can prove beneficial. Most are over–the–counter items available at any pharmacy. Toe nail involvement is often resistant to therapy. It may require the surgical removal of the nail, or periodic trimming and tolerance of a slow, ever present infection.

Many yeast-type organisms can infect the skin. The most common infection, however, is produced by the yeast *Candida albicans*. Formerly called *monilia*, this infection still is described occasionally as **Moniliasis**. When seen in the mouth, the disease is called **thrush**. Cottage cheese-like growths are seen along the surface of the cheeks, in the tonsillar area, and coating the tongue surface. Frequent in infancy, this lesion responds well to specific antifungal therapies, such as *nystatin*, or the painting with Gentian violet.

Vaginal involvement with yeast is also a common occurrence. Often producing inflammation, pain, or a cheesy discharge these **vaginitis** infections are easily treated, but seldom completely eradicated. Aggravating factors include the use of hormone agents, birth control pills, and elevated blood sugar, as in uncontrolled diabetes. It is a troublesome affliction of pregnancy, also seen commonly in times of stress, and immune deficiencies. Common hygienic measures, such as the use of cotton undergarments, frequent bathing, and the avoidance of panty hose can allow necessary aeration, to reduce the moist and warm environment that favors growth of Monilia. **Douching** with one table-spoon of white vinegar in a quart of warm water or the topical application of specific yeast inhibitors may give rapid relief of symptoms and reduce the risk of recurrence.

A third type of yeast infection is seen in babies, occurring again in the moist diaper area. Appearing as pinpoint red papules, then coalescing to a red **diaper rash**, the yeast grows and spreads. Plastic "disposable" diapers contribute to this predicament. Careful drying, cleansing, and the topical use of mild ointments, such as *A & D ointment, Desitin*, or a powdered corn starch can allow improvement of most cases. Ultraviolet light from the sun is helpful, not only in drying involved skin, but killing the offending organism.

ECZEMA

The terms **dermatitis** and **eczema** are used for a variety of inflammatory changes involving the skin. These can be produced by a variety of irritants, allergens, and other factors. Characteristically, the skin changes consist of reddening, swelling, moist "weeping," and mild to severe itching. Later stages exhibit scaling with crust formation and eventual scarring. Several types are described below.

Contact Dermatitis

Skin changes in this category of inflammation start in areas of contact with the irritating or allergy-producing agent. The reaction is usually localized, and limited to the area of exposure. There are two main types. **Primary** or **toxic dermatitis** may occur in any individual without prior exposure. The **allergic** type occurs only in *sensitized* individuals. Some of these will be considered in the next chapter.

Substances which contact the skin and produce this rash are found in clothing, soaps or detergents, cosmetics, industrial chemicals, or the outdoor environment. An example of the latter is the distressing rash produced by *poison ivy, poison oak*, and *poison sumac*. The causative agent is a plant resin, called *urushiol*. Certain exotic hardwoods resins, and the sap from the mango tree can produce a similar rash. *Formalin* and certain flame retardant chemicals may be impregnated in garments and cause the same rash described above.

Occupational dermatitis may be due to cement (*chromics*) in bricklayers, to wheat in bakers, to adhesive tape, anesthetics, sunscreen lotion, and many other substances. Most important, first eliminate the offender as soon as it can be identified. Then apply soothing lotions to relieve the itching and prevent further spread. Needless to say, it is imperative to avoid scratching these lesions or otherwise irritating them during the healing phase.

Seborrheic Dermatitis

Areas of the body richly supplied with sebaceous glands may develop this skin condition. Scaly, somewhat greasy material is produced, which can vary from the **dandruff** of scalp involvement to the **cradle cap** seen on babies. Redness around the face is common, with specific involvement of the eyebrows, scalp, and other areas rich in oil glands. Dietary changes to reduce the fat intake in conjunction with adequate sun exposure, frequent shampooing, reduction of stress factors, and improvement of skin hygiene are all important in relieving these conditions.

Atopic Dermatitis

Called at times **infantile eczema**, this condition typically begins early in life. Usually there is a strong family history of various allergic conditions.

Dryness, cracking, and scaling produces the characteristic lichen-like (*lichenification*) appearance that is the hallmark of atopic eczema. The disease reaches its maximum severity during the second and third decades of life, then gradually subsides. Each episode starts with violent attacks of itching, probably related to excessive dryness of the skin. These attacks frequently occur at night, and provoke furious scratching, which often leads to infection.

Treatment is difficult in this chronic condition. It is important to avoid measures which produce excessive drying of the skin, such as harsh soaps, frequent washing, or scratching involved lesions. Special nondrying soaps, such as *Neutrogena*, or *Cetaphil lotion* can be soothing. Reduction of all known stress factors, careful examination of the diet, and general habits of temperance are important to control this troublesome condition. The itching can often be relieved temporarily with the use of a moist oatmeal paste applied to the skin. *Aveeno* baths are also beneficial in this regard. The challenge of eczema is well worth further study for physicians or families interested in granting relief for these highly visible problems.

Psoriasis

Psoriasis is a common, chronic, and recurrent disease of the skin. It affects people of both sexes and is most frequently seen from youth to middle-age. Typical lesions appear commonly on the elbows and knees, as well as the scalp and the lower part of the back. These patches may be thick and tough. In early stages they are red with a dry, silvery scale. Coin-shaped lesions are common. Scrapings of the scales resemble scrapings of a candle. In acute stages of psoriasis the characteristic lesions may develop in areas irritated by scratching or from contact with other nonspecific irritants. The nails may be involved and are usually pitted.

Occasionally, *psoriatic arthritis* is seen in conjunction with this rash. Tension and stress in the home, tobacco usage, and a diet high in fat, greasy foods, and particularly meat will aggravate the condition. Sedentary indoor workers may carry these lesions for years. Sunlight, especially the natural ultraviolet rays, has been very helpful in treating psoriasis. Most lesions gradually clear where exposed to the sun. Even severe scalp involvement may respond if the hair is cut short.

Although steroids, such as Cortisone, are often used in treatment of psoriasis, the side effects are such that I advise real caution. A mixture of lanolin, zinc oxide paste, and *Burroughs' solution* (see Appendix) helps soothe the irritated, inflamed areas. Toxic mineral elements, such as mercury and arsenic, or the use of coal tar are all quite irritating and should usually be avoided. With a combination of hygienic remedies, careful diet, and a liberal use of sunlight, this difficult condition can be improved and in many cases arrested.

THE AGING SKIN

Characteristic skin changes occur as a person grows older. In most individuals there is a loss of subcutaneous elastic tissue and wrinkles appear. Sometimes these are distressing, and many plastic surgery operations have been devised to lift the face, correct baggy eyelids, or otherwise make a person look younger. More important are the changes that can lead to disease. Chronic exposure to wind and sun with other forms of irritation to the skin may produce dry, scaling plaques, particularly on the face or exposed areas. A premalignant skin irritation known as **senile keratosis** may occur under these circumstances. The lesion should be removed or otherwise treated to prevent skin cancer.

Common raised pigmented waxy looking plaques occur in aging skin, both on the face, extremities, and trunk. These **seborrheic keratoses** are completely benign and are normally quite superficial. Freezing with liquid nitrogen, electrodesication (cautery), scraping, or curetting of the lesions may remove them completely and allow for the return of normal skin in that area. Thinning of the hair and eyebrows are also common in the aging process. Individuals should anticipate the waning of youth with an acceptance of certain changes and the cultivation of a disposition that will produce "happy wrinkles" and an adjustment to the golden years that preserves maximal health and interests in life.

The low fat vegetarian diet greatly improves circulation. Its influence on the skin is beneficial as well. Many are promoting the use of **Vitamin E** to retard aging. While this oil is helpful in certain topical applications, wholesale supplementation is seldom necessary, In preference, I recommend the use of nuts, whole grains, fruits, and vegetables as the diet best calculated to promote longevity and insure good health of the skin. Cleansing baths, exercise, and regular changing of clothing are just as helpful to the senior citizen, as they are important for the baby.

ITCHING SKIN

Although the symptom of **itching** (*pruritis*) has been discussed in connection with some of the above disorders, this symptom warrants separate discussion, because it is so common and there are many approaches to therapy. Most normal people have some irritated places that they scratch every day. Often the sensation is so mild that it is barely noticed. There is no harm in an occasional scratching, but constant itching is different. It is typically a distress signal indicating specific trouble.

With about 20 square feet of skin covering our bodies, there are literally millions of nerve receptors. Many of these can convey the sensation of itching, at times becoming so sensitive as to be almost beyond control. Allergies may produce itching and are described in Chapter Ten. Insect bites, pinworms, nettles, plant juices, chemicals, metals and many body secretions can produce similar distress. Excessive sweating, as well as unusual dryness, can provoke itching. In the winter season, many people suffer from **dry skin**. Often this is made worse by bathing, especially with soap or worse yet, the bubble bath, a detergent bath water that removes most natural body oils. Mild soaps such as Dial, Aveeno, Neutrogena, and AlphaKeri are good for sensitive skin. Occasionally, the *habit* of scratching can develop. When present, this should be overcome. Nervous tension often aggravates itching, as does anxiety.

Relief can usually come by breaking the "itch-scratch cycle," and simply **refusing** to scratch. If this is impossible, careful trimming and filing of the nails, or the wearing of soft gloves at night may be necessary. Starch baths are useful using either corn starch or powdered oatmeal. It is important to avoid soap, except in cleansing the groin, armpits, or feet. Avoid all excessive washing. Hydrotherapy employing moist, hot packs or the contrast shower acts as a *counter irritant* and relieves the itching. Further examination, laboratory tests, and hormone analyses can become worthwhile in difficult cases. In all these conditions the **cause** should be ascertained. Then nature can be assisted in restoring health again.

HAIR LOSS

Hair is present over most areas of the body. Our *follicles* are the source of these hairs. Although most of them are very fine, the top of the head, the eyebrows, the eyelashes, and the groin are sources of coarser pigmented hair. A tiny muscle is attached to each hair follicle, and can literally make the hair stand on end! *Goose flesh* is an example of this, when the muscle contracts in an attempt to reduce heat loss and generate body heat. This same muscle (the *arrector pili*) helps to compress the oil glands, lubricating not only the hair but the surrounding skin. Specialized hairs, such as eyebrows and eyelashes, prevent dust from irritating the eyes and give symmetry and shade.

When hair loss occurs over the scalp, varying degrees of baldness may develop. Some types are hereditary, others are related to hormonal changes, aging, or the presence of disease. It is important to exclude fungus infections and carefully examine the hair shaft and follicles for signs of disease. Meticulous evaluation of the diet, together with hygienic care of the scalp and the use of appropriate bathing aids can reduce the amount of hair loss and its associated distress. When unusual necessity requires, transplants are even available to restore hair to bald areas. Because of significantly increased heat generated over the scalp, the employment of wigs and hair pieces is best avoided. Contentment with our appearance is a great gift. When all natural health measures are being encouraged, we can certainly be at peace and trust our countenance to the Creator.

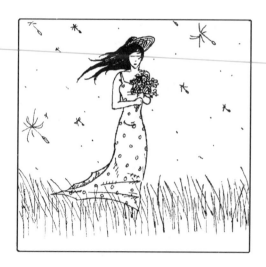

CHAPTER TEN

ALLERGIES

The number of people suffering from various types of allergies is tremendous. These disorders range from the sniffles during certain pollen seasons to a danger of sudden death from shock after one bee sting. A number of body organs are affected by allergies, including the gastrointestinal tract, the lungs, the nose and sinuses, the eyes, the skin, and even the bladder. In fact, almost all membranes and mucous linings of the body can be target organs for allergic manifestations.

Literally hundreds of different remedies are sold across the counter and by prescription in neighborhood pharmacies. Similarly, hundreds of skin tests are performed to try and determine the exact cause. Specialists devote their lives in an attempt to understand the nature of allergies. Yet with all of this light and scientific research focused on the problem, a *cure* has not yet been found. We will consider some of the more common types of allergy and a few simple treatments that anyone can do in his or her home to either avoid the cause or provide relief.

Asthma

This allergic disease of the respiratory system primarily affects the lungs. At the end of each tiny air tube that reaches the lung is the alveolus, where gas exchange occurs. Here oxygen enters the red blood cells to be exchanged for carbon dioxide, which is then exhaled. The bronchial tubes that form the large and small air passages have specialized smooth muscle in them that constricts under certain conditions. In contrast, with the smooth muscle of the artery walls, these bronchial muscles dilate in response to adrenalin and constrict in the presence of histamine as well as other chemical mediators of allergies. A

146

condition described as bronchial asthma occurs when there is spasm of the bronchial tubes, leading to obstruction in the airway. Usually there is also excess mucus accumulation and thickening of the mucus, making it more tenacious and difficult to clear.

The asthmatic patient, then, primarily has an air hunger, with musical wheezes in the lung. These can be heard easily with a stethoscope over the chest and in more severe asthmatic crises becomes audible to the unaided ear.

A number of conditions can produce these symptoms. There are certain drugs which can create an allergic reaction, as well as many industrial inhalants that irritate the lungs. A few people react to food allergies with the production of asthma, though this is less common. Most frequently, the asthmatic sufferer reacts to inhaled particles in the air, called *allergens*, which may be of a biologic nature or inanimate particles. House dust is an example of the latter. Danders from cats, dogs, horses, feathers, or down also can produce wheezing.

Commonly seen in the spring, summer, and fall are allergies to various inhaled pollens. Although some people primarily suffer from hay fever (discussed below), others are affected in their lungs. The inhalation of pollens, such as those from pine trees in the spring, wildflowers in the summertime, ragweed or goldenrod in the fall, may produce characteristic responses. These are related to the number of particles inhaled and the efficiency of the nasal filtering mechanism.

Emotions can also trigger allergies. I remember vividly the experience of a teenage girl who suffered a violent asthma attack in a hospital when she remembered with nostalgia her dear pet cat at home alone! Moreover, numerous infections in the lung are seen in conjunction with asthma. These are usually termed **asthmatic bronchitis**. Frequently seen in childhood, they are often associated with an upper respiratory infection.

A physiologic approach to asthma then involves several factors. The secretions should be thinned with a copious fluid intake, preferably by the oral route. Inhalations of cool moist air can often help in the clearing of secretions and the thinning of this very sticky mucous material. Gentle coughing assists in expelling of the mucous plugs, but this should be done in combination with the inhalation of humidified cool air. The use of a stem vaporizer is to be discouraged, as this often adds to the swelling and edema formation in the bronchial tubes.

Hydrotherapy is important in the treatment of asthma. Often the adrenal glands can be stimulated early in the disease by a quick ice rub to the spine in the upper back, associated with brisk tapping (*percussion*) over the adrenal area (see Chapter 17). This stimulation of the sympathetic nervous system results in the discharge of enough adrenalin to counteract the acute effects in beginning stages, as well as induce dilation of the bronchial tubes.

Prolonged hot packs to the chest can sometimes be effective in relaxing both the respiratory muscles and the patient's nerves. This must be repeated several times, and will often abort the acute asthmatic attack and eliminate the need for medication. Inhalation therapy with the use of bronchial dilators and theophylline derivatives are often used in a hospital setting. Sometimes *mullein tea* (Chapter 18) or other teas containing theophylline can be used with some effectiveness to further aid in combating the bronchial spasm. As in any disease, a thorough attempt to discover the cause, then as far as possible eliminate it, will reward the asthmatic sufferer with an increase of comfort and removal of those conditions that progresses in the advanced case too often leading to emphysema.

Hay Fever

Hay fever or *allergic rhinitis* is a hypersensitivity disease involving the nose and sinuses. The mucous membrane becomes inflamed in response to an allergic substance and produces a watery, profuse discharge associated with increased tearing, itching of the eyes, and sneezing. This condition is usually seasonal, with the peak incidence corresponding to the presence of the offending allergenic inhalants. Pollens of trees, grasses, wildflowers, and other weeds are the most common culprits in producing this allergy. Some people are affected by danders, the particles produced from the skin of animals or hair from cats, dogs, horses, etc. House dust, molds, feathers, and even certain foods can produce hay fever. The appearance of the inner mucous lining of the nose is usually pale and thin, as opposed to upper respiratory infections where the mucus becomes thick, and the mucous membrane reddened and swollen.

Usually it is quite helpful for the allergy sufferer to know and identify the offenders. Scratch tests are usually helpful in evaluating the type of sensitivity. Intradermal injections are more commonly done by ear, nose, and throat specialists or allergists. However, the simpler and less expensive scratch tests are usually sufficient to establish the cause and initiate desensitization therapy. Recent advances in the use of allergy shots have allowed a more rapid desensitization procedure that is replacing the traditional year-round technique. The hay fever sufferer will find relief from the plentiful use of tissues, by placing cool compresses over the nose and sinus areas. Frequent nasal irrigation with cool saline (sniffing or spraying the salty solution) will help remove entrapped pollens and other particles, and clear the nasal passages of the allergy–producing substances.

When the allergy is due to *Bermuda grass* or *ragweed*, activities outdoors such as yard work and lawn mowing may require the use of a mask. An appropriate respiratory filter can trap these pollens and minimize the symptoms, while still allowing work outside. Botanical identification of certain plants, such as ragweed, goldenrod, and various trees, grasses, and wildflowers will interest the pursuit of further nature study, while cautiously avoiding fields and forests where the prime offenders abound.

The chronic use of antihistamines and nasal sprays is to be discouraged, as side effects are frequent and troublesome. Excessive drowsiness, disturbance of digestive secretions, and the "rebound phenomenon" associated with nasal reaction to decongestants are all avoidable with this emphasis on natural remedies. Further attention to the diet, or in unusual cases, the relocation to a different climate may be necessary to bring hay fever and its troublesome symptoms under control.

Hives

A number of allergic conditions affect the skin. Some of these, such as *eczema* are mentioned in the previous chapter. **Hives**, or *urticaria*, is a very common manifestation of hypersensitivity. Many causes for this exist.

The disease itself is manifested by the sudden appearance of reddened areas, which rapidly become welts, being distributed generally over the body or localized to the face, neck, or extremities. Intense itching is usually present. The lesions often migrate and change their appearance rapidly. The rash, however, usually does not blister or weep unless scratching has abraded the skin and allowed the entrance of germs.

Food allergies can sometimes cause hives. Very frequently an allergy to strawberries, shellfish, or some less common food can trigger a sudden onset of this rash. Reaction to substances such as wheat, milk, or eggs is more rare. It is necessary to avoid the food if one wishes to eliminate the symptom.

Several drugs can also cause hives. This condition is usually termed a **drug allergy**. The most common producers of this drug reaction are Penicillin and related antibiotics. Sulfa drugs and pharmaceuticals from nearly every major class of medicinal agent can produce an urticarial reaction in the sensitized individual.

Babies seldom get hives unless a drug has been present in the milk or they have had previous exposure. But it is frequently seen in children and adults with no particular preference as to age, sex, or race. The result of stress at both conscious and subconscious levels may trigger a sudden onset of urticaria. However, in up to 50% of the cases the exact source cannot be detected with certainty. It is very worthwhile to **look** for the cause, however, and consider any substance that is inhaled, ingested, or contacted by the skin as a possible factor to exclude.

Treatment of hives should first begin with reassurance. This condition is self-limited and is usually neither life threatening nor contagious. The intense itching can be relieved considerably by cool baths with the addition of one cup starch or oatmeal powder (*Aveeno*), or alternately using ½ cup baking soda. Lotions may be helpful to reduce the symptoms. Try ice packs for local lesions. Antihistamines seem to counteract the reaction, but usually are not necessary as the condition commonly disappears within hours.

An exception to this may occur with bee sting allergy. If an individual is highly allergic to the sting of a honey bee, wasp, hornet, or yellow jacket, the reaction with hives will be immediate and generalized. Not only should ice and/ or moistened charcoal be applied to the site of the sting, but in emergencies the administration of adrenalin or a similar substance is necessary to prevent rapid progression into the swelling of the respiratory passages or the sudden development of shock. Since bee sting hypersensitivity can be lethal, careful diagnosis and prompt treatment is essential. Moreover, in such cases, desensitization injections can permit greater freedom in outdoor life and remove the fear that often grips parents as well as children who live with this threat of danger.

Food Allergies

There is probably no area more controversial and perplexing as suspected allergies connected with food. These range from sensitivity to food additives, such as coloring, preservatives, and other foreign chemicals, to plant sources, to actual hypersensitivity to protein and other constituents of fruits, grains, nuts, vegetables, or animal foods. Careful detective work and long-term adherence to dietary regimens are frequently necessary to first diagnose and then live with food allergies.

It is my belief that the stage is set for many food allergies by feeding patterns in infancy, such as the early introduction of solid foods, the widespread use of cow's milk in prepared formulas, and the relative lack of mother interest in prolonged breast feeding. Maternal use of drugs which sensitize the babies *in utero* or during the breast-feeding period can also prepare the way for allergic responses to develop.

The most common allergy that occurs in infancy is a sensitivity to cow's milk. This is often manifested in diarrhea, unusual regurgitation, excessive gas or colic, or a "failure to thrive." Usually a change to soy milk formula if breast feeding is not available will stabilize the situation, although rarely more restricted and specific formulas have to be devised.

A majority of the black and oriental races and lesser percentages of Caucasians are sensitive to cow's milk even in adult life. This, however, is due to the deficiency of **lactase**, an enzyme which helps to split milk sugar (lactose) and render it available for absorption. Diarrhea, excessive gas, and an acid stool are produced. Simply abstaining from milk is curative. You must always suspect the diagnosis in order to apply the proper remedy at once, thus removing the cause.

Other people are truly allergic to the proteins of cow's milk and find unpleasant symptoms, such as frequent sinus or nasal congestion, related to the intake of milk. Please note, however, that skin scratch tests for food allergies are notoriously unreliable as indicators of an individual's sensitivity to the **eating** of these foods. It appears that the skin is just not a parallel indicator with the gastrointestinal tract. The only way to be certain in diagnosing food allergies is through trying an elimination diet.

Next to milk as a cause of allergy, chocolate and wheat lead the list. Usually the grains are less common allergens, but berries (such as strawberries), nuts, shellfish, eggs, and many other foods can produce similar symptoms. It is believed by some that symptoms resembling hypoglycemia, such as episodic weakness and certain mental aberrations (anxiety, panic attacks, depression, etc.) may be related to food allergies. It must be acknowledged, though, full proof is lacking to completely confirm this theory as yet. Nevertheless, eliminating the offending food, then gradually progressing from a limited diet to a more liberal intake of varied foods **will** help bring a return of health and strength, with fewer physical symptoms and more emotional stability.

Sulfites are added to foods to serve a variety of purposes. They preserve food by killing bacteria and yeasts. They retain color and apparent freshness by acting as antioxidant. They may also be used to sterilize containers and arrest fermentation in alcoholic drinks. The label may contain any of the following listings, all various types of sulfites: *sulfur dioxide, sodium sulfite, sodium bisulfite, potassium bisulfite, sodium metabisulfite* and *potassium metabisulfite*. Many people are allergic to sulfites, reacting with skin rash or asthmatic wheezing.

Carefully test for allergies with a medically approved method. **RAST** (Radio Allergo Sorbent Test) testing offers an easy way to evaluate the blood for immediate immune reactive (IgE) factors. The more definitive, though expensive, **ELISA/ACT**™ (Enzyme Linked Immune Sorbent Assay / Advanced Cell Test) measures both immediate and delayed responsiveness to over 300 foods and environmental chemicals. Additional detailed evaluations, however, may require a period of observation and careful dietary therapy in a sanitarium or preventive lifestyle institution to isolate specific factors or undertake dietary trials.

Anaphylactic Shock

Anaphylactic shock is a highly dangerous allergic manifestation that occurs when an individual has an immediate life-threatening reaction to contact, ingestion, or injection of an allergen. This rarely occurs with food allergy, but is most commonly associated with drugs. Penicillin injections have periodically produced this severe type of anaphylactic shock.

Stings from hornets, honey bees, bumble bees, and yellow jackets in sensitized individuals can provoke anaphylactic reactions. Even inhalation of allergens, such as antibiotic powder, or caster bean flour, may cause anaphylaxis. Symptoms occur within seconds to minutes after the substance enters into the body, when precipitous drop in blood pressure occurs. Frequently there is difficulty breathing, profuse sweating, and sudden generalized vascular relaxation that causes faintness. In fatal cases stoppage of the heart or respiration follows.

151

Prompt emergency resuscitative measures are necessary to save the life of a victim in anaphylactic shock. Subcutaneous injection of adrenalin in the appropriate dosage (based on body size) is life saving in such a situation, while general first aid measures involving adequate **airway**, artificial **respiration**, and closed chest **cardiac massage** are instituted. Increasing anaphylactic cases of this nature has brought physicians to adopt a more conservative attitude in the administration of antibiotics by injection. **Bee sting allergy kits** are available for those sensitized individuals who live with this ever present threat of danger.

Specific Hypersensitivity

Several other types of allergies manifest themselves in inflammatory states of various body organs. Allergies have been implicated as the cause of **cystitis** or inflammation of the bladder, and this typically resembles a urinary tract infection. The joints can be affected by allergies, with ensuing pain, swelling, and disability. Allergies in the bronchial tree, the sinuses, and the upper respiratory tract are likewise common.

Most commonly seen is hypersensitivity to substances contacting the **skin**. Nickel, as in watch bands, elastic in undergarments, various cosmetics, dyes, creams, lotions, medications, and plant substances all can produce the skin rash of allergic dermatitis or aggravate an existing **eczema**. All known offenders must be avoided to regain health. Allergy as a medical specialty is growing, with the increasing number of chemical, biological, and food sensitivities that send more people for testing and treatment each year. While cures are illusive, control is frequently possible, offering considerable hope, especially good news to allergy sufferers.

CHAPTER ELEVEN

HEALTHY

BREATHING

AND

RESPIRATORY

DISEASE

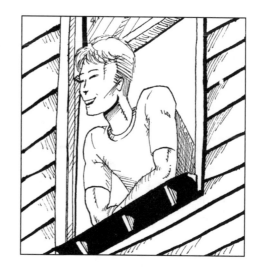

When it comes to the lungs, everyone needs a healthy pair, for without air no one can live more than a few minutes. Of all the elements in nature, **oxygen** has to be most constantly supplied to the human system. With rare exceptions, more than 4-5 minutes without oxygen will result in irreversible damage to the brain and other vital organs. For this reason, our bodies have been designed with a mechanism for constant exchange of air. Furthermore, the respiratory tract has been provided with marvelous safeguards to cleanse the membranes and prevent any entrance of infectious agents.

The rapid growth of urban populations, as well as the use of tobacco, has produced a large number of respiratory diseases. Still, most of the diseases of the respiratory system are of an infectious nature. In studies of mortality, the deaths due to pneumonia and tuberculosis have been replaced by an increasing number from lung cancer and emphysema. A few of the more common conditions will be dealt with below.

First, it is helpful to include a brief description of the proper mechanics of breathing. Correct **posture** is invaluable in allowing complete expansion of the lungs. It is proper to avoid tight-fitting garments, such as elastic bands about the chest and waist, all habitual stooping or a slumped sitting posture, all of which can prevent complete chest expansion. The most efficient respiration utilizes the diaphragm. This is a large flat muscle that separates the chest from the abdominal cavity. Contraction of the diaphragm creates a vacuum within the chest, allowing entrance of air concurrent with the moderate protrusion of the abdomen. Sitting erect and standing with the shoulders back and the head up, together with a straightened position of the spine are all essential to deep, full diaphragmatic breathing.

The **vital capacity** is a measure of the greatest volume of air one can take into the lungs in a deep breath. Pulmonary function tests can also measure the **timed vital capacity**, which shows the degree of elasticity of the lungs, which is impaired early in the development of emphysema. Other breathing capacity measurements can be made and serve as predictors of the development of diseases such as asthma, emphysema, or other chronic conditions. The examination of the chest and lungs, as well as brief comments on diagnostic x-rays are described in chapter one.

Lung development just before birth coincides with the production of a detergent-like substance called *surfactant*. This is deficient in a premature baby and is one of the reasons why *hyaline membrane disease* may develop. Another enzyme which is usually present in the bronchial tubes is called *alpha-1-antitrypsin*. Congenitally deficient in some people, this can lead to the development of early emphysema, particularly in smokers or people exposed occupationally to inhaled particles, such as asbestos or coal dust. A simply performed blood test can determine the existence of this hereditary enzyme deficiency. We turn now to consider some of the common diseases of the respiratory tract.

Emphysema

Pulmonary emphysema takes the lives of increasing numbers of people each year. Called *chronic obstructive pulmonary disease*, this condition develops insidiously in people exposed to heavy pollution of the airways. The commonest cause of emphysema today is tobacco smoking. Unfortunately, most individuals do not know that their disease has developed until it is too late to cure the condition. The basic process involved in the development of emphysema first involves the destruction of elastic tissue in the bronchial tubes. Respiration becomes increasingly difficult. Then in later stages many tiny air sacs, called alveoli, lose their walls and coalesce, forming large air sacs or *emphysematous blebs*.

The earliest symptom in developing emphysema is shortness of breath. This is commonly associated with exertion. This exhibits disease risk with decreased ability to carry packages, climb stairs, walk rapidly, or engage in the usual sports. Advanced sufferers of emphysema may develop *cyanosis*, a bluish tinge around the mouth with a dusky appearance of the nail beds. This sign indicates advanced impairment of oxygen intake with a chronic deficiency in the blood. There is abnormal shunting of blood across the lungs, with resultant deficient oxygenation.

When chronic bronchitis or pneumonia are superimposed on the underlying condition, **respiratory failure** can develop. Heroic efforts are being made today in intensive care units to salvage individuals who would otherwise die in such a respiratory crisis. Unfortunately, some hapless victims continue smoking after surviving an acute crisis. I have seen individuals who unfortunately were completely resistant to heroic educational efforts for improving their lifestyle and thus failed to avoid additional relapses.

There is good news, however, for many people with mild to moderate emphysema. Not all need to progress to the end stage, sitting beside an oxygen tank just to support life. Proper diaphragmatic breathing with learning to exhale forcefully through pursed lips constitutes a valuable way of retraining the respiratory muscles and improving the oxygen delivery to the blood and distant tissues. Exercise programs with gradually increasing walking distance has, in my experience, enabled many patients again to return home, climbing stairs, mowing the lawn, working in the garden, or engaging in moderately active sports. It is certainly worthwhile to attempt rehabilitation of a patient with emphysema, at any stage. These efforts, in combination with a strict avoidance of tobacco and air pollution, will add quality to the life of many.

Pulmonary Hygiene is also important. The individual with fragile or delicate lungs must avoid contact with people who have colds or other respiratory infections. For those producing large amounts of mucus, postural drainage treatment is a daily necessity. This can be done in the morning, usually after a few minutes of steam inhalation. Bend over or lie with the head down, allowing gravity to help drain mucus from the chest. The side of a bed is a good place to do this drainage procedure. Calculated to drain the affected segments of the lung, these postural maneuvers are very effective. Clapping of the chest, inhalation therapy, and other specialized procedures may be prescribed by a physician to aid in the home care of the emphysema victim.

Pneumonia

Infection of the lungs is usually called **pneumonia** or **pneumonitis**. This results when harmful germs invade the upper respiratory tract and find their way down to the deeper bronchial tubes and alveoli. When the infection reaches the level of these air sacs (alveoli) pneumonia has developed. Sometimes the infection is very mild and may not even appear as a shadow on x-ray. Coughing is the most common symptom. However, usually the individual will have fever and some shortness of breath also. Generalized chills, malaise, and apprehension appear frequently.

Chest pain is of a pleuritic nature, involving the membrane lining of the lung. It is a sharp pain, well localized, and aggravated by breathing, coughing, or moving. Usually pressure against the area, as well as moist heat is extremely useful in relieving the pain of *pleurisy*.

Investigation should begin early to determine the **cause** of the pneumonia. The sputum can be cultured in the laboratory. If germs are present, a gram stain or bacteriologic culture will give the clue as to a cause. Viral pneumonia usually shows a normal blood count with negative cultures, while bacterial pneumonia germs can frequently be cultured from the sputum.

Unfortunately, the expectorating of cough material usually contaminates the culture with normal organisms resident in the mouth. Doctors therefore attempt to aspirate the tracheal secretions, although this invasive procedure is not without hazards. The chest x-ray can be most helpful, as certain bacteria produce characteristic patterns in the lung. Alcoholics commonly develop *pneumococcal* pneumonia, while children are more likely seen with *Hemophilus influenza* or *Staphylococcal* organisms.

Individuals who are routinely taking broad-spectrum antibiotics may develop pneumonia caused by less common organisms such as *Pseudomonas*, *Klebsiella*, and *Candida* species. The latter is a fungus infection that is particularly difficult to treat and is often seen in those whose normal organisms have been artificially suppressed, or whose immune system was compromised by drugs such as Cortisone derivatives. Even worse is the *Pneumocystis carina* pneumonia found in AIDS patients or HIV carriers.

Once the diagnosis is established, specific treatment should be instituted promptly. Cooling measures can be used for high fevers. Pneumonia patients must be adequately hydrated. Usually this can be done by mouth. Water, fruit juices, and diluted soups are most helpful to maintain hydration. These also enable the mucus to be thinned, making expectoration less difficult. Steam inhalation with a moist steam vaporizer is helpful to bring up the secretions. Eucalyptus oil or other inhalant additives can be used to enhance its value.

Hot packs are extremely useful when applied to the chest in a manner similar to the general hydrotherapy approach described in chapter seventeen. These alternating hot and cold treatments may be repeated two to three times daily. In critical cases fomentations may be given more often for brief periods to enhance the circulation and clearing mechanism inherent in the lungs. Postural draining helps to clear secretions.

A spare fruit and juice diet is advantageous in the early stages to enable the body to concentrate on attacking the invading germs and winning the battle for survival. It is important to note that viral pneumonias are entirely unresponsive to antibiotics and most fungal infections respond poorly also.

Because pneumonia is typically contagious, it should be diagnosed whenever possible and isolation measures instituted. Cough into a tissue and dispose of it immediately. That is usually sufficient to trap the expectorated germs and prevent contagion. Adequate sunlight in the sick room helps to kill germs, as well as purify the air. Some fresh air should be circulating in the sick room, even if this means utilizing a little more heat. Cold drafts, however, should be kept away from the sick individual, as a chill may provoke a relapse more serious that the first infection.

Persisting in these measures for many days can cure all but the most stubborn cases of pneumonia. When complications such as advanced asthma, emphysema, or other chronic lung disease are superimposed on the underlying pneumonia, a physician should be consulted to perform the appropriate laboratory tests and supervise the treatment of any serious illnesses.

It is so very rewarding to see these infectious diseases improve with the use of these simple treatments. I have been impressed many times that patients treated naturally develop better resistance and more healthful, long-term consequences in their lungs that comparable cases where antibiotics and other drugs are used prematurely and without adequate consideration of the causes and abnormal physiologic mechanisms involved.

Tuberculosis

At one time a dread killer affecting most (80%) of the population, **tuberculosis** is thankfully less common, at least in the United States. Because of its profound influence on body metabolism, with a general wasting of flesh and muscles in the advanced states, this disease was early called *consumption*. In spite of modern public health control with its improved sanitation, quarantine, x-ray screening, skin testing, and drug therapy, tuberculosis is still a problem in the United States and is a leading cause of death worldwide. Recent reports of resistant strains have caused renewed public health concern, especially in the ghettos and prisons of large cities.

The tuberculin skin test has become a very valuable screening test, demonstrating clear immune response to the tubercle bacillus after contact by a person. This does not imply that the condition is active. Many childhood infections heal with sufficient antibodies produced to prevent reinfection throughout the lifetime.

Circumstances, however, that cause an individual to lose the natural immune resistance may allow a tuberculosis carrier to become reinfected and contagious. Such habits as tobacco smoking and the occupational exposure to coal dust and other industrial pollutants produce a condition of lowered resistance in the lungs that makes active tuberculosis more likely. Crowded living conditions may coexist with an infected carrier in the family. Exposure to contaminated air, as in hospitals, tuberculosis treatment centers, or large clinics in the underdeveloped nations where infected patients are frequently seen, carrys with it a higher risk of contact and exposure.

The symptoms of tuberculosis are multiple. Most infections begin silently with a slight cough or fever, resembling a cold or flu-like illness. The presence of tuberculosis in the lungs, however, nearly always produces a cough. At time the erosion into a blood vessel may produce **hemoptysis**, the coughing of blood-streaked material, or actual pulmonary hemorrhage. Lung abscesses can develop, while the residual germs multiply slowly in these pockets. Mucus is eliminated by coughing, thus cleansing the lungs of germs.

Often the sputum is swallowed. Since tuberculous germs are quite resistant to acid, these may then pass into the intestinal tract and create infection there. Formerly, in the United States a large amount of tuberculosis involved the small intestine, being acquired through the infection of contaminated milk. Modern pasteurization has eliminated most of this risk, but some intestinal tuberculosis is still seen. The organism can also involve the lymphatic organs or the bones. In less common cases nearly every vital organ can be infected. Meningitis, kidney involvement, and draining sinuses from the skin can all be seen in advanced TB.

It is important to recognize this illness as early as possible, since it is contagious. The use of prolonged moist heat over the lungs can aggravate tuberculosis. Cold compresses, on the other hand, can be much more helpful. Strict rest is necessary, while the body heals this invader. No simple measure is more helpful in the treatment of tuberculosis than the liberal presence of sunlight. The tuberculosis germs are killed on contact with the ultraviolet rays. Even in widespread infections involving the bone, exposure to sunlight has been helpful in effecting a cure.

Fresh air, proper diet, and public control measures of quarantine can also aid in the eradication of this difficult germ. Many antituberculosis drugs are being used by health authorities. They certainly arrest the multiplication of germs so that recovery can be made possible. As with all drugs, these too have side effects, many of them serious. So the further exploration of natural approaches will be utilized to the utmost by those maximally interested in promoting comprehensive health.

Bronchitis

Inflammation of the bronchial tubes may be acute or chronic. A sudden onset of cough is frequently due to bronchitis. This is usually of viral or chemical origin. It affects the upper airways from the larynx down to the secondary divisions of the major bronchi. The cough is termed "brassy" and is usually not productive of mucus.

Prolonged coughing can irritate the bronchial tubes enough to cause bleeding. If hemoptysis occurs, further investigations should urgently be performed. With persistence of a bronchial cough, the upper chest may become sore, with pain on inspiration. There is seldom any fever or general symptoms. However, fatigue and sleeplessness may develop if the illness is prolonged. Hot, moist compresses or *diathermy* treatments over the upper chest are helpful. They work best when combined with expectorant cough syrups such as honey–eucalyptus (see Chapter 18) and the use of steam inhalations. The earlier these treatment are started, the less severe the illness will be.

Chronic bronchitis is common in smokers. It results from the accumulation of tar and numerous respiratory irritants over a prolonged period. The typical "smoker's cough" is an example of chronic bronchitis, which is typically productive of mucus. The sputum is usually white or gray, but at times may become infected. Then it would be thick, tenacious, and greenish or yellow in color. As in acute bronchitis, fever is seldom present.

Many people "learn" to live with a cough when they could be healed, and live enjoyably without it. Strictly avoid all tobacco. Then combine deep breathing exercises in combination with other pulmonary hygiene measures. The treatments mentioned under the treatment for pneumonia will bring considerable relief to bronchitis sufferers. The coexistence of emphysema naturally complicates the situation. However, with appropriate steam inhalation, postural drainage, and other hydrotherapeutic measures the bronchitis can usually be cleared without residual damage.

Bronchiectasis

A chronic condition of the lungs resulting from acute infection results in the disease called **bronchiectasis**. This involves the more distant bronchial tubes and consists of a *tubular* or *saccular* dilation of the terminal air channels. The copious production of mucus sputum, often pus-filled, may severely cripple a person's efforts to speak in public, sing, or use the voice as formerly.

The above described pulmonary hygienic measures are helpful in both the control and treatment of this disease. Postural drainage, with manual *clapping* (percussion), are especially valuable. Many of these sufferers develop chronic changes which make long-term treatment mandatory. Lifelong adherence to a nonsmoking pattern, and a rural home location may be necessary.

Lung Cancer

The specific symptoms, signs, and diagnosis of lung cancer are well covered in Chapter 6 and will not be discussed at length here. Remember, however, that **cigarette smoking still constitutes the largest single cause of this disease!** Very little improvement has been seen in survival statistics over the past twenty years. In this largely preventable disease, the "ounce of prevention" is certainly appropriate.

MISCELLANEOUS CONDITIONS
WHICH MIMIC LUNG DISEASE

Several diseases may affect the respiratory tract or cause symptoms in the chest. A **hiatus hernia** may mimic the pain of pleurisy or lead to expectoration of mucus. This occurs when the upper portion of the stomach protrudes into the chest cavity through a dilated portion of the diaphragm. Heavy meals, supine posture, tight garments, and obesity are predisposing factors to the symptoms of a hiatus hernia. Characteristically called "heartburn," these symptoms respond well to careful dietary measures, which will be described in detail elsewhere.

Tracheobronchitis, also called **croup**, may be seen in children. It is often a source of deep concern to their parents. Considerable difficulty in breathing may occur, associated with an uncontrollable cough and the rapid development of fatigue. Usually of viral origin, this croupy cough responds to the use of cold vapor, utilizing a humidifier. Moist steam packs on the chest are also helpful in rapidly restoring health to the irritated respiratory tract.

Upper respiratory infections are frequently precursors to the lung diseases mentioned above and should be promptly treated to avoid complications. Consult frequently the chapters on hydrotherapy and the specific discussion of these infectious diseases. This can aid in the home treatment of these annoying, but usually self-limited conditions. Furthermore, the prompt recognition of pulmonary complications in otherwise mild illnesses can be life saving when rational treatment is instituted in the home. Nature is thereby aided in her valiant efforts to combat disease and restore right conditions in the system.

CHAPTER TWELVE

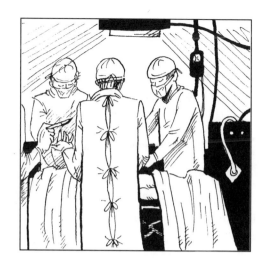

SURGERY

It may seem strange to some readers to include in a book on home treatments this chapter on surgical conditions. Nevertheless, there is a great need in underdeveloped nations for laymen trained in surgical skills. And because of the necessity for a deeper understanding of the indications and basic methods of surgery, I am writing this section. It is also presented with the hope that individuals actually needing a surgical operation may better prepare themselves for it emotionally, as well as physically, and choose wisely their surgeon. You must properly understand the role of various services and know more about proper nutrition, postoperative care, and other factors pertaining to recovery. This can result in considerable savings, not only in the cost of this expensive type of care, but also that which is even more important, the speedy return of health, essential to survival and quality of living.

Antisepsis

One of the outstanding advances that medical science has made in the past hundred years is the establishment of antiseptic principles in the practice of surgery. Milestone discoveries were the germ theory by **Pasteur** and **Koch**, the emphasis on hand washing by **Semmelweis**, and the principles of antisepsis by Lister. To understand the relationship between infective agents and disease has allowed the art and science of surgery to develop many new techniques, as well as life-saving procedures.

Fundamentally, the principles of antisepsis deal not only with the presence or absence of germs, but also with the resistance of the person (host) to their invasion. We have already suggested in Chapter Three concerning infectious diseases that a healthy individual **rarely** gets an infection. The *acid mantle* of the skin and our body's resident normal flora constitute an important barrier to the growth of disease-producing germs. Enzymatic protection by *lysozyme* in the nasal secretions, tears, saliva, and other mucous membranes affords a defense of marvelous significance and complexity.

From simple wound care to most complicated surgery, every individual should know how to avoid contamination by harmful germs. During the 19th century in Austria, Doctor Semmelweis began to encourage hand-washing, requiring this of his residents after each post-mortem examination and before contact with maternity patients. The death rate from infection dropped precipitously. Although this brilliant physician was persecuted by his own profession for these "strange" doctrines, decades later he was acclaimed a medical trail blazer. Without doubt, the washing of hands is as important to safe surgery, as the use of water internally is to fighting fever.

It is especially important to know how to wash the hands and prepare them to handle diseased or injured tissues. Usually before surgery, a soft disinfected bristle brush is used to scrub the hands starting first around each finger, the ends and sides of the fingernails, the palm and backside of the hand, the wrist, and then the forearm. To prepare for a delicate operation, ten minutes of this type of scrubbing is required, typically with an antibacterial soap. Sterile rubber or latex gloves should then be worn. Disinfectants such as organic iodine (*Betadine*), hexachlorophene (*Phisohex*), or other antibacterial soaps are used to prepare the patient's skin for the incision. Where this is not available, soap and water are employed, however the scrubbing must be prolonged. It is well to remember, moreover, that the mere washing of the hands with any substance does not **guarantee** a totally germ-free skin. Sweating is especially common under rubber or latex gloves, with the natural bacteria present in hair follicles and around the nails. Thus the bacterial count is only transiently suppressed, while our real line of defense is our body's resistance. Several routines and techniques of skin preparation will be described in the accompanying table.

In the treatment of skin wounds, copious irrigation with water is essential. With some force, the stream of water is directed at the contaminated areas. The wound is thereby cleansed, allowing germs, foreign debris, and blood clots to be washed away, making the area clean for closure or suturing. Preparation of the skin with appropriate antiseptics is also helpful. Proper nutrition to the injured area includes abundant oxygen and vitamin C to aid wound healing. Elimination of refined sugar assists in fighting infection. These measures, together with the avoidance of tobacco and other harmful substances that impair oxygen supply, will enable healing to occur rapidly.

Wound Care

There are three basic methods by which a wound heals itself. **Primary Intention** is the usual type of healing when an incision or laceration is closed immediately to allow close adherence of the opposing skin edges and subcutaneous layers. This permits healing from side to side with the least amount of scarring and pain. The rate of healing of our skin depends on its blood supply and the presence or absence of pressure, tension, and infection. The facial skin, with its rich blood supply, can heal in 3-5 days, while a thickened area of skin with less nutritive potential, such as the back or feet, may require two weeks or more. If sutures are placed, it is important to know how long healing will require to avoid too early removal and wound separation.

Secondary healing of a wound occurs when the laceration is too large to be closed or is infected and must be left open. A general principle of laceration treatment is this. A wound that has been open more than 8-12 hours is never sutured, since infection may already have developed. In such case, *granulation* occurs with the formation of a specialized tissue across the wound, and later coverage with new skin. Some deformity and scarring usually occurs. Nevertheless, with the exception of very large ulcers, the skin healing is usually complete. Understandably, this takes longer. Proper care of the wound to prevent or treat infection will serve to hasten the healing process.

The **third** method involves the initial formation of granulation tissue, then a secondary closure of the wound with sutures. This accelerates the healing in large open lesions and is usually used when a surgical wound, for some reason, separates and must be closed again. Even more scarring takes place as a rule, but the healing is usually complete.

Some essential factors in wound healing are the presence of adequate protein, vitamins, oxygen, and the prevention of infection. It is generally recognized that the *normal* rate of healing in a perfectly healthy patient is the *optimum* rate that can be obtained. Wounds do not heal as well in anemic patients. With a normal complement of white blood cells the healing of a sterile wound is not impaired. However, when infection is present delayed healing does occur. Swelling (*edema*), whether local or general, appears to interfere with the healing process. Older individuals take longer to heal than the young. Endocrine factors, such as the possible deficiency of thyroid or growth hormone, or adrenal dysfunction, may retard or interfere with the healing process.

Local factors are important. According to Van't Hoff's law, reactions occur more rapidly when the temperature is increased. Conversely, hypothermia will delay wound healing in most areas, although cold is sometimes used for pain control. The areas of the skin which have the best blood supply, such as the face and neck, normally heal the fastest. Fat persons tend to heal more slowly, and their wounds tend to separate more often than in people of normal weight. Skin sutures are usually left in longer. Cleanly incised wounds will heal more rapidly than irregular jagged lacerations. The presence of a blood clot or hematoma may interfere with proper wound healing by preventing close contact of the walls of the wound, and thus there forms a pocket, called "dead space." Infected fluids, pus, and foreign bodies will all retard the healing of these wounds.

It is critical to cleanse the wound of all foreign debris, irrigating it thoroughly before any suturing is attempted. Suture material is also important in the care of wounds. Although stainless steel is the least reactive, it is difficult to handle and remove. The absorption of foreign material, such as gut, silk, cotton, and nylon will occur slowly, in the order that they are here mentioned. Newer sutures of nylon, Dacron, and teflon last longer and cause less reaction, but are not suitable everywhere. A suture use manual may be consulted to aid in selecting appropriate materials. The suture manufacturer's suggestion of needle size, type, and techniques should also be consulted.

Suturing

Considerable practice is required to suture incisions and lacerations quickly and accurately. Yet these skills are not beyond the reach of the average layman gifted with manual dexterity or an interest in mastering the art. If possible, practice your suturing techniques on a piece of sponge rubber, upholstery, or even a pillow. Some surgeons become skilled in knot tying, practicing on door handles or in the automobile while traveling. The accompanying diagrams, located on pages 178 to 189, help demonstrate the principles of the three basic methods of surgical knot tying. The one described as an "instrument tie" utilizes a hemostat or needle holder, while the others require only skillful fingers for proper use. I would suggest that a novice begin with the two-handed tie and instrument tie, adding more complex forms as skill is gained.

Avoid tying the sutures so tightly that insufficient blood flow to the skin edges results. This would cause delayed and incomplete healing of the wound. "Approximate, don't strangulate" is the watch word for closure of lacerations with sutures. As described in the following chapter, there are certain injuries that are never sutured. Human bites, animal bites, and lacerations opened longer than 12 hours, or those grossly contaminated are not sutured, but allowed to granulate and heal by secondary intention.

The placement of sutures and selection of suture material will be described in the following sections, as the various types of lacerations and their special care are considered. In a home-like setting it is possible to make the appropriate needles, like bending a sewing needle, sharpening the point in a chisel fashion to better penetrate the skin. Silk or cotton can be boiled along with the needle, thus sterilizing it for use in suturing. Prepared packages, that come already sterile, are available from suture manufacturing companies and can be obtained in various sizes and needle styles. Remember to consult the suture use manual for aid in selecting the appropriate sutures.

Anesthesia

One of the oldest forms of medical treatment is described in Genesis 2:18 , 21-23, where the **Creator** Himself *"caused a deep sleep"* to come upon Adam while He took out the rib, closed up the incision, and made a "help meet for him." Relief of pain is intimately associated with the rendering of needful medical care. This is one of the physician's cardinal responsibilities. For certain patients, some forms of severe pain may be life threatening. However, in the case of most effective pain relieving medications, addiction can occur, with distortion of mental imagery to the point of serious impairment. Thus, it is wise to look for the simplest methods of relieving pain when attempting to perform surgery.

Probably the oldest form of pain relief is **refrigeration anesthesia**. Extremities can be rendered pain free with ice packs. This is particularly valuable in the case of vascular disease where cardiac and circulatory impairment makes general anesthesia risky. During the World War II, army medics discovered that troops suffering from frostbite might save their limbs if the extremity remained *frozen* until medical care could be secured. This observation influenced all currently accepted first aid for frostbite used in our country.

In order to properly administer refrigeration anesthesia, the extremity needs to be cooled to the point of numbness, while keeping the remainder of the body warm to avoid a general drop in temperature, chilling, or agitation. Ice packs or snow can be used to progressively cool an extremity, either a hand or foot. If the surgery is to be localized to the arm or leg, place the pack just above the site of amputation. This reduces blood loss and allows for a careful, meticulous dissection of the tissue. Broken bones can be set with refrigeration. In the case of a simple fracture of the hand or wrist, immerse the extremity in ice water for one-half hour or more. This will allow manipulation and bone setting to be done quite painlessly.

Refrigeration can also be used topically in the removal of warts, moles, and other skin lesions. Dry ice or liquid nitrogen can be applied with a cotton applicator to freeze a small area and render it numb to pin prick.

A second method of anesthesia is the application of gradual **pressure** on a nerve. The ulnar nerve at the elbow (funny bone) is quite amenable to pressure. Quite often in certain positions a foot or a hand has been known to "go to sleep" due to stretching or pressure on an affected nerve. A knowledge of neuroanatomy can utilize this principle favorably for surgery to an extremity.

Counterirritation can also be applied with electric stimulation near the point of incision. This can utilize DC current, but it is more effective with a pulsed generator, such as rehabilitation centers employ in treatment of chronic pain. **Desensitization** can be obtained with liniments and ointments, mustard packs or plasters. Even animal surgery has been performed using counterirritation, e.g., the "twitch" on the nose of horses.

Finally, it is helpful to understand some of the common injectable anesthetics that are used locally for the relief of pain. These are used both in dental and surgical care. But they have some side effects and potential allergic reactions. Injectable narcotics should *always* be avoided, as they leave behind serious effects on the brain. They are not only difficult to metabolize, but because of their tendency to produce euphoria can become rapidly addicting.

On rare occasions for major procedures, **general anesthesia** may be necessary. The gaseous agent used in these cases should be that which is most rapidly metabolized and least toxic to the system. Nitrous oxide and oxygen are commonly employed together to relieve mild pain. Although *ether* is quite flammable, it still remains the safest form of general anesthesia, due to its rapid clearing from the blood by the way of the lungs and relatively low toxicity to the liver and other organs. Open drop techniques in a well ventilated area can be used, but for safety reasons general anesthesia ideally should be performed in a hospital. Newer anesthetic agents (Halothane, Ethrane, etc.), although more likely to cause toxicity, are less dangerous to the heart and usually nonflammable. Regional blocks, local nerve blocks, and spinal anesthesia have their places in hospital settings but it is beyond the scope of this book to detail their applications.

Biopsies

The removal of a tissue for accurate pathologic diagnosis is called **biopsy**. If the lesion is large and only a small part is to be removed, the surgery is called an *incisional* biopsy. Usually a small portion of normal adjacent skin is excised with the lump under question. When it is possible to completely remove the growth and obtain a margin of normal tissue around it, the procedure is termed an *excisional* biopsy. These are very useful procedures, not only for the diagnosis and treatment of blemishes and abnormal growths of the skin, but also for lumps beneath the skin in accessible organs, such as the breast.

A breast biopsy can often be performed without general anesthesia or hospitalization when the surgical skills are present and the necessity for tissue diagnosis exists. More commonly, skin biopsies are used to determine the presence or absence of cancer and to excise unsightly or irritating growths that have developed in areas amenable to their removal.

On certain parts of the face, such as the alar portion of the nose, the lips, and ears it may be necessary to cover the removed skin with a **graft**. "Split thickness" skin grafts can utilize a very thin membrane of excised skin that matches in color and texture the area requiring the covering. Specialized plastic surgery procedures under local anesthesia can at times be used to enhance the cosmetic results of these operation.

The **technique** of a skin biopsy utilizes an elliptical incision with the ends pointed to permit easier closure. The incision is made perpendicular to the plane of the skin to avoid bevel edges that will increase scarring of produce puckering when the wound is closed. "Undermining" the edges with blunt dissection will enable the skin areas to come together without undue tension and permit suturing with the least likelihood of wound separation. When malignancy is suspected, the margins should be wide enough to prevent possible early penetration of them with abnormal cells, and thus prevent the necessity of a second operation. Appropriate spacing of sutures and their removal in as short a time as wound healing will allow will minimize scarring and improve the cosmetic result of these surgical procedures.

NURSING THE POSTOPERATIVE PATIENT

Because most operations today are performed in hospitals, it is well for family members to know how best to aid the recovery of their convalescing relatives. Undue visiting should be discouraged. The frequent recital of a person's own operation and details of hospitalization can help to depress and confuse the individual recovering from surgery. Visiting just to "chit chat" in the hospital should be kept to a minimum. Well wishers should either send cards or reserve their condolences for later. A devoted family member or trained nurse, however, can be of incalculable value to the convalescing surgical patient.

Immediately after major surgery the incision should be cooled with an ice pack applied over the dressing. This will reduce swelling (edema fluid), lessen the likelihood of bleeding, and modify impressively the pain responses. Avoid excessive movement of the involved area, while maintaining activity in remote portions of the body. And especially encourage deep breathing. This will aid the rapid emergence from anesthesia, while minimizing the sensation of severe pain.

After the initial recovery phase is ended, moist warm compresses can be applied over most incisions, except in areas where the blood supply is compromised or at the distal extremities. In the latter case cold packs may be used. Over the chest and abdomen, however, frequent applications of moist warm packs, such as fomentations or electric heating devices will significantly reduce the pain, while promoting rapid healing of the involved area.

At this stage the healing processes will occur more rapidly in the presence of warmth, since all enzyme reactions as well as the growth of new cells are speeded up by mild heat. Usually the moist hot pack can be applied every three to four hours, enabling the convalescing patient to relax in between, gaining the necessary rest that promotes recovery. From the very first, the incision should be protected from undue moisture and kept clean and dry. Daily changes of the sterile gauze dressing are helpful in allowing air to reach the incision and dry the sutured area.

Adequate fluid intake is important. After abdominal surgery intravenous feedings are often used until the intestinal tone returns. This manifests itself by the passage of gas, and a sensation of hunger. One can hear "bowel sounds" when listening to the abdomen with a stethoscope. At this stage, the patient may be given sips of water or ice chips. If these create no problem, clear liquids such as herb teas, apple juice, vegetable jello, grape juice, and vegetable broth may be added.

After a meal or two in which these clear liquids are well tolerated, the diet can be enriched with the addition of creamed soups, diluted cereals, other fruit juices, milk, or pudding. As rapidly as possible, the diet should be advanced to foods which can be thoroughly masticated, always prepared as attractively as possible. This variety of natural foods can promote tissue healing and emotional satisfaction in the most positive way.

If the patient is in the average community hospital, it is advisable to supplement his diet with some form of whole grain cereal, such as home-made crackers, as well as extra amounts of fresh fruits, dry fruits, or nuts. These should be kept, of course, in plastic containers to avoid attracting roaches, rodents or flies. Nevertheless, the addition of some whole grains and fresh fruit to the average hospital dietary will help provide the extra vitamins and minerals that are essential to a prompt recovery.

Consultation with a dietitian and permission from a physician may be necessary. The natural foods will help to accelerate the healing process and improve the nutritional value of the highly refined "popular" diet usually served in public medical institutions. An individual who requires prolonged feedings with intravenous fluids should ask his physician about the addition of vitamins, as this often neglected measure can be helpful in meeting nutritional needs during a critical illness.

Simple hygienic measures which will aid in convalescence from surgery are adequate water-drinking, exposure to sunlight daily, and availability of fresh air in the sick room. All of these are hard to find in large hospitals. It may demand the selection of a facility for major surgery that recognizes these essentials and provides them.

It is very important to obtain adequate rest at night, and this should be insisted upon. Not uncommonly, hospitals perform at night many routine tasks that do nothing but disturb a patient. An atmosphere of tranquility should be insisted upon. Bedside telephones and the frequent taking of unnecessary vital signs may be intrusions into your peaceful rest that promotes a rapid recovery. It is wise to avoid much television viewing. This distraction puts the mind in "neutral" (or reverse), and stifles creative thought patterns and positive emotions that aid in recovery. Windows with an outdoor view and a stream of fresh air that can enter without hindrance will make convalescence pleasant. Where hospitals do not provide these essentials, early discharge should be advocated, securing the appropriate nursing care in a more home-like setting.

Finally, it must be recognized that exercise is not detrimental to the convalescing surgical patient. Early ambulation will help prevent such complications as pneumonia and clots in the veins. It also aids the general circulation. Activity establishes a feeling of well being that promotes recovery in the most unequivocal way. A short walk within the room, down the corridor, or even, with appropriate clothing, in the out-of-doors, will aid healing for surgical patients in record time. I have seen in my institution patients recovering from surgery of the gallbladder, female organs, or orthopedic procedures taking deep breathing exercises, stretching the limbs, and ambulating considerable distances in the first few days. Complications are almost nonexistent in these patients. Cheerful mental attitudes, good nutrition, and fresh air, combined with physical exercise support a rapid recovery. The gastrointestinal and digestive tone in such cases usually returns earlier, too.

COMMON SURGICAL CONDITIONS

Hernia

There are several types of **hernias**, sometimes called ruptures, that arise from weaknesses in the abdominal wall. These out-pouchings of the abdominal (*peritoneal*) lining occur primarily in the groin, but are also found on the front wall of the abdomen and in the area of the diaphragm. The typical groin hernia occurs from a congenital weakness in the structures comprising the *inguinal ring*. That is the connecting opening between the abdomen and the groin canal. The hernia first presents itself with a bulge in the groin. They frequently occur in infancy or early childhood. Although some hernias may disappear, it is critical to have infant hernias evaluated. Usually they need prompt surgery to avoid complications.

When an intestinal loop enters the hernia sac a bulging occurs, often associated with pain. If it is impossible to replace this protrusion within the abdominal cavity, the bowel is said to be *incarcerated* or trapped. Prolonging this hazard may lead to *strangulation*, in which the blood supply is compromised. Unless prompt surgery is done, rupture or abdominal (*peritoneal*) infection may ensue.

Hernias also occur in association with pregnancy, due to the increased abdominal pressure. Adult men may get hernias when they lift heavy objects, while subjecting the abdominal wall to sudden unusual strain. With continued pressure, the hernia tends to enlarge. Mechanical support for a groin hernia with the **truss** may prevent further enlargement, but usually a surgical repair is indicated. Newer techniques involving one day in the hospital and the use of local anesthesia permit much more rapid convalescence. They are the safer methods of surgery, being especially for the more stoical.

Hernias that occur in previous incisions are called *incisional* or *ventral* hernias. Sometimes these result from infection, complicating previous surgery, where the wound has healed with residual weakness. **Umbilical hernias** are present in the navel. They are frequently seen in newborns. The newborn or young child with an umbilical hernia needs so special care. Applying pressure or taping a quarter over the defect does no good at all. Unless the hernia is extremely large, however, it will gradually close, usually within one to two years. Should it exist beyond the early period of infancy, surgical repair is indicated, primarily to avoid undue awareness to the area when your child enters school.

Diaphragmatic hernias may occur congenitally, but are usually acquired during adult life. The most common is called a *hiatus hernia*. It occurs when excessive food intake, obesity, tight-fitting garments, or undue straining produces a weakness in the diaphragm—the opening where the esophagus leaves the chest to connect with the stomach. Nearly half the cases treated surgically are unsuccessful, so medical therapy is usually advised. This consists of a special diet, taking very little fluid intake with meals, and thoroughly chewing solid food. Lying down, bending over, or stooping after a meal is unwise. Supper should be a light meal, eaten several hours before going to bed. Tight-fitting belts and girdles are avoided. If one experience nighttime heartburn, the head of the bed can be elevated on six inch blocks, allowing gravity to aid in preventing regurgitation of gastric contents during sleep. Persistence of symptoms such as pain or indigestion should be evaluated by a physician to determine the diagnosis. If necessary he can perform x-rays of the gastrointestinal tract.

Hemorrhoids

The veins of the rectum frequently become enlarged or tender, with sudden onset of brisk red bleeding. Called **hemorrhoids**, these annoyances are due primarily to our sedentary lifestyle, with the modern emphasis on refined foods containing little fiber. Sitting for prolonged periods or straining with bowel movements increases the venous pressure in the rectal area with the consequent development of these protruding veins.

External hemorrhoids are clusters of veins at the opening to the rectum (*anus*). They may develop a clot or *thrombosis*. These become excruciatingly painful and usually show an area of purplish or dark discoloration. Although gradual resolution will occur in 2-3 weeks with sitz baths, the most prompt relief is ob-

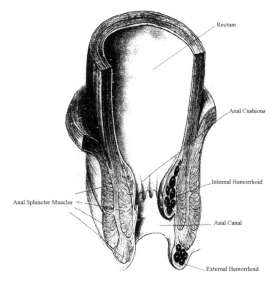

170

tained by the incision of the thrombosed hemorrhoid, removing the offending clots. This can be done with local anesthesia. Recurrence is uncommon.

Treatment of the **internal** hemorrhoid, which more commonly bleeds and ulcerates, is usually conservative. Hot and cold sitz baths are given, described in the chapter on **Hydrotherapy**. In combination with a high fiber diet, they will usually allow the condition to subside. At least two tablespoon of bran, with an abundance of fresh fruits and vegetables, are advisable to keep the stool soft. Aim at producing one or more substantial soft bowel movements daily.

Surgical treatment of refractory hemorrhoid disease was formerly a very painful and costly procedure. The development of the **band ligation** has changed this. A small rubber band is placed around the hemorrhoid high above the area of sensation, completely obliterating the hemorrhoid (*varicosity*). Two or three treatments in the office are necessary to complete this treatment. They are spaced at least three weeks apart to avoid excessive scarring. Rectal suppositories provide some relief from the pain of hemorrhoid disease, and may be purchased over-the-counter at most pharmacies. However, complications such as prolapse of the rectum or malignancy may present. The final decision on hemorrhoids is best handled by a physician.

Appendicitis

As in many above conditions, **appendicitis** has been linked to the consumption of refined foods. Quite rare in rural Africans, this acute situation is seen most commonly in individuals obtaining little dietary roughage. The pain of appendicitis usually comes on suddenly, and is associated with nausea and vomiting. A low grade fever develops, with rapid loss of appetite. The pain may at first be localized to the region of the stomach. It then migrates to the umbilicus, and finally localizes in the right lower quadrant of the abdomen. Deep pressure over the area will reveal a point of maximum tenderness. Stand the person on his or her toes, and ask the person to drop suddenly on the heels. This usually aggravates the pain **if** the appendix or a related internal organ is inflamed. Usually there is no bleeding or diarrhea.

Although some appendicitis cases can heal with simple measures, it is wise to obtain the counsel of a physician who can order the appropriate blood tests. If his pain does not subside promptly, surgery is necessary. **Rupture** of the appendix is a serious complication. Intestinal contents laden with germs may then contaminate the abdominal cavity, raising fever, increasing the pain, and becoming life threatening unless surgical drainage is accomplished promptly. Mortality is much lower for appendicitis than it was in previous years, but prompt diagnosis and treatment are still necessary to save lives.

Gallstones

The high fat diet of this "junk food" age has rapidly increased the incidence of stone formation in the **gallbladder**. Designed to be a reservoir of bile, the gallbladder has the capability of concentrating this liquid into a thick syrup. A diet rich in fats and cholesterol tends to overcharge the bile with bile salts and cholesterol, which readily crystallizes to form stones. Large single stones or many small stones may lie dormant for years, then produce a sudden crisis. In the area of the gallbladder, located just beneath the liver, pain develops, associated with vomiting, fever, or chills.

When a gall stone passes into the common bile duct, obstruction occurs, with jaundice, and even more excruciating pain. In such conditions surgery is mandatory to remove both the stones and diseased gallbladder. Nonsurgical treatment includes a low fat diet and strict avoidance of grease, oils, and other fatty foods. They may help the body to dissolve these stones. Contrast x-rays and **ultrasound** tests can easily be done to evaluate the gallbladder's progress. Check first to see if the patient is allergic to the iodine of the gallbladder dye. For best prevention I recommend steadfast control of obesity, and a lifetime adherence to natural foods. This will prevent most gall stones.

Peptic Ulcers

Usually **ulcers** involve the stomach or small intestine (*duodenum*) and can heal without surgery. The only conditions warranting surgery are severe gastrointestinal **hemorrhage**, or **perforation** of the ulcer with the spillage of stomach contents into the abdominal cavity. Also, the prolonged scarring of chronic ulcer disease can produce**obstruction** in the region of the stomach outlet (*pylorus*) or duodenum. When this occurs and prolonged vomiting ensues, the only recourse is to surgically bypass the obstruction and again provide a basis for adequate nutrition.

A fourth indication listed in many textbooks is **intractability**, meaning that the ulcer just won't heal and therefore surgery is necessary. In my opinion, this usually implies that the patient is "intractable." Often a refusal to quit smoking, eliminate coffee or alcohol, or change behavior patterns to a more peaceful, low stress mode lies at the root of the nonhealing ulcer.

In my medical and surgical experience, the best results in most types of ulcers are seen when the minimal amount of surgery is performed. Usually this means a *selective vagotomy*, in which the small nerves that influence only the acid forming portion of the stomach are cut. When necessary, an operation to enlarge the pylorus or to bypass scarring is done. As all surgeons know, tampering with normal stomach physiology in this manner is not without hazard. Iron deficiency anemia, the*dumping syndrome* (in which the ingestion of simple carbohydrates results in immediate diarrhea), abdominal cramps, and various types of malabsorption can occur.

For the typical ulcer patient whose pain occurs shortly after eating or is aggravated by stress or harmful beverages, the remedy is logical. Eliminate the offending substances—including spices, vinegar, tea, coffee, tobacco, alcohol, and fried foods. The recommended diet, although not entirely "bland," allows considerable variety of food intake. If these foods are thoroughly **masticated** good results can be seen.

Avocado is an excellent source of dietary fat to inhibit gastric secretion. With adequate intake of soft fruits, olives, or creamed foods, prompt relief of pain, as well as neutralization of the acid can occur. The intake of baking soda and use of aluminum containing antacids is discouraged, not only because of the cost, but also side effects elsewhere in the body. Hot packs over the abdomen and an abundance of cool water or diluted vegetable juices (carrot, cabbage, etc.) are also helpful in healing these common peptic conditions.

Varicose Veins

Tortuous dilation of surface veins in the lower extremities are also caused by our lifestyle. Prolonged standing and sitting allow an increase of venous pressure to develop in the lower extremities. Tight-fitting garments— such as girdles, belts and garters—will predispose to this degenerative condition. The increased venous pressure of late pregnancy often aggravates the situation. Elastic stockings are very helpful to prevent throbbing and progressive dilation of these large leg veins. Surgical treatment may be necessary, with the ligation and stripping of the veins, but this should be evaluated by an experienced surgeon competent to assess the indications—one who is inclined to avoid surgery whenever possible. Proper posture, daily exercise, deep breathing, and a diet that maintains good bowel action will all assist to keep the pressure low in the veins and thereby prevent unsightly legs, throbbing calves, or the ulcers that occasionally follow.

Tonsillectomy

Formerly the most common operation in the United States, **tonsillectomy** has fortunately declined in popularity. It is now known that our tonsils play a useful role in the formation of antibodies to respiratory infections. The incidence of poliomyelitis **and** cancer have been less in those fortunate individuals who were able to keep their tonsils. Infections in these organs will usually respond to prompt administration of simple remedies. Some of these will be discussed in Chapter Fifteen.

Indications for surgical removal of the tonsils are primarily limited to chronic recurring infections where the deep pockets (*crypts*) prevent adequate self-cleansing, and debris and infected material reside there. Recurring ear infections sometimes require the related lymph tissues in the nasal pharynx, called **adenoids**, to be removed. Both of these operations should be highly selective.

Coronary Bypass

Although the complexities of **coronary bypass surgery** are beyond the scope of this book, a few comments are in order. Briefly stated, this recent surgical advance is a procedure involving the removal of one or both of the major veins (*saphenous vein*) in the leg and its careful transplantation in the chest. After appropriate **cardiac catheterization** to determine the adequacy of the coronary circulation, the vein is placed between a hole made in the aorta as it leaves the heart and the more distant part of the coronary artery. With its 5-10% risk to life, the exorbitant cost ($30-50 thousand), and the lack of long-term statistics as to its effectiveness (at best 2 years), this operation should be regarded as a last resort.

Reconditioning programs are springing up around the country and offering a superior alternative to many bypass candidates. The combination of a low fat diet free of cholesterol and progressive exercise in a center with preventive capabilities will often minimize the necessity for cardiac drugs, while relieving chest pain and similar cardiac symptoms. Nevertheless, a few individuals with disease of all three coronary vessels or underlying impairment of the heart valves, may need and profit from this operation. In such cases, it is my recommendation that an medical center experienced in heart surgery be selected with much prayer and care.

Following the bypass operation, **cardiac rehabilitation** should begin in a lifestyle conditioning center where both diet and lectures are calculated to prevent recurrence. As rapidly as possible this will recondition the patient for a return to normal living. Otherwise, the temporary relief obtained by a revascularization procedure may be short-lived as the new vessels plug themselves with cholesterol once again. One can easily see how every aspect of coronary heart disease from the cradle to the rocking chair will benefit from preventive measures.

CHAPTER THIRTEEN

ACCIDENTS

AND

INJURIES

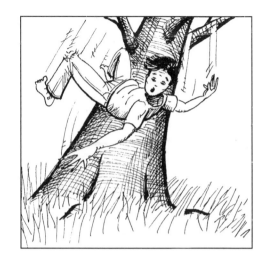

Unforeseen events occur in the lives of individuals every day. When these affect our health and cause bodily harm or injury, we usually call them **accidents**. Cases of extreme urgency, constituting a threat to life or limb, we term **emergencies**. Most hospitals are equipped with special facilities ranging from first aid stations to comprehensive trauma units. These *emergency rooms* are deluged with people having minor problems that have assumed the sense of urgency. However, many of these could well be taken care of at home. Some of the more common health hazards and problems will be outlined in this chapter.

It is well to remember the Boy Scout motto "**be prepared**" in obtaining necessary knowledge before the crisis. A calm, cool head combined with a knowledge of what to do in an emergency may prove the difference between life and death as crises erupt in the home. The words of Rudyard Kipling expressed it well, "If you can keep your head when all about you are losing theirs and blaming it on you . . . then you will be a man, my son." These poetic expressions apply to every nurse, homemaker, and lifesaver who can render first aid in an emergency, and *do the right thing, at the right time, in the right place, in the right way*. Such individuals are at a premium in our turbulent society.

Cuts and Bruises

Bruising results when the skin or underlying tissue has been traumatized. A kick, a blow, or a fall may not break the skin, yet result in trauma to the underlying blood vessels. When one of these vessels, small or large, is injured, bleeding occurs beneath the skin. The black and blue discoloration that often results from such injuries is called a bruise (*ecchymosis*). Applying ice packs immediately after such injury is helpful to reduce the bleeding, as well as relieve pain. Under NO circumstances should heat be applied to a bruise in the acute stage. Even in the healing phase, one should use heating measures with considerable caution.

Deep bruises in a muscle may produce swelling and considerable pain, but are located beneath the fascial planes and therefore show no visible discoloration. These also should be treated with ice. In the acute injury, some pressure is advisable to reduce the amount of bleeding.

When the skin surface is broken, several other reactions take place. First, there is a loss of blood, with the amount and rate of flow depending on the vessels that have been severed. Since the face and scalp are extremely rich in blood vessels, bleeding is often brisk. Yet because of its visible location, prompt pressure can reduce the blood loss.

A knowledge of appropriate *pressure points*, where arteries to the extremities come close to the surface, can prepare one to reduce blood flow in a very severe arterial injury. Pressure under the armpit, in the groin, or behind the knee may be life saving when a large artery has been ruptured. More commonly, however, the application of *direct* pressure over the wound will reduce the amount of blood flow. With the normal clotting mechanism inherent in body tissues, the bleeding will then stop, allowing coagulation or clot formation to secure the area.

The second problem that results when the skin is broken is that germs find entrance. Depending upon the amount of contamination, the wound may require thorough **cleansing** before any closure or bandaging is attempted. Thorough irrigation with water is the most effective, provided that the water is clean. Done early after an acute injury this constitutes the most important aspect of care, since infection is easier to prevent than to treat.

Contaminated wounds from the animal barn or farmyard should be exceptionally thoroughly washed. Unless the person has been adequately immunized against tetanus, a booster is recommended. In cases where no immunity exists the administration of *human tetanus antitoxin* will provide an additional safeguard. These injections would, of course, need to be obtained from a physician or emergency room.

Once the bleeding is controlled and the cut thoroughly cleansed or irrigated, appropriate closure can be attempted. Sometimes we use a *butterfly* bandage or adhesive tape to bring the opposing edges together. Often that is all that is necessary

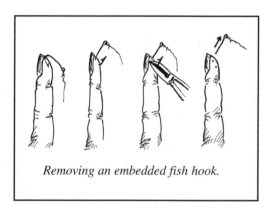

Removing an embedded fish hook.

to close the wound. Moreover, this simple closure, when free from infection, will produce the most rapid healing.

Sutures are necessary on occasion to close larger wounds, particularly those involving such delicate structures as the eyelid, lip, face, or hand. Deep wounds involving the hand must be carefully evaluated for possible injury to nerves or tendons. They should be repaired by a surgeon, whenever possible. For the best results in both healing time and preventing complication, lacerations should be repaired within a very few hours after their occurrence, the sooner the better. Cuts left open for longer than 8-12 hours nearly always have been contaminated with so many germs that suturing or other tight closure will increase the risk of infection. In such cases, open treatment and appropriate dressings are preferable.

Before proceeding with a description of suturing techniques, note two other types of wounds and their simple treatments. **Abrasions** are injuries made by rubbing or scraping. Some of these, called "floor burns" or "scuff burns," are very superficial injuries. They usually bleed briskly, and often can be very painful. Careful cleansing of these wounds is important to remove all sand, dirt, glass, or other foreign material that may have been ground into the skin. Porous dressings are advisable to allow the air-skin contact to form a crust or scab. Less commonly the extensive nature of an abrasion makes it advisable to apply an ointment, such as petroleum jelly with fine mesh gauze to prevent sticking.

Puncture wounds may also occur. Although these do not usually bleed as extensively, the risk of infection is high. A nail or tack may puncture or impale the skin. The most common place is the foot. Wear shoes or sandals and avoid playing in locations where rusty nails and broken glass abound. This will help to prevent most kinds of puncture injuries. Extreme care in the use of knives, scissors, power mowers, chain saws, razor blades, and firearms is likewise important to prevent penetrating wounds, particularly where small children live.

Techniques of Suturing

It is difficult to give a brief description of proper suturing technique to enable a person to acquire this art quickly. Several generalizations, however, will be discussed to help, remembering that practice makes perfect. As mentioned already, wounds that are over eight to twelve hours old are grossly contaminated and should **never** be sutured. Only when ligatures are necessary to control bleeding would sutures be indicated, or after careful surgical debridement and irrigation in an operating room. The placement of sutures to close a wound must take into consideration the location of the injury, the types of suture material available, the nature of the blood supply, the general body health, and the skill of the medic. Suturing around the more delicate parts of the body, such as the face, eyelids, genitalia, and hand should be reserved for surgeons who have proven skills.

Two-Hand Tie

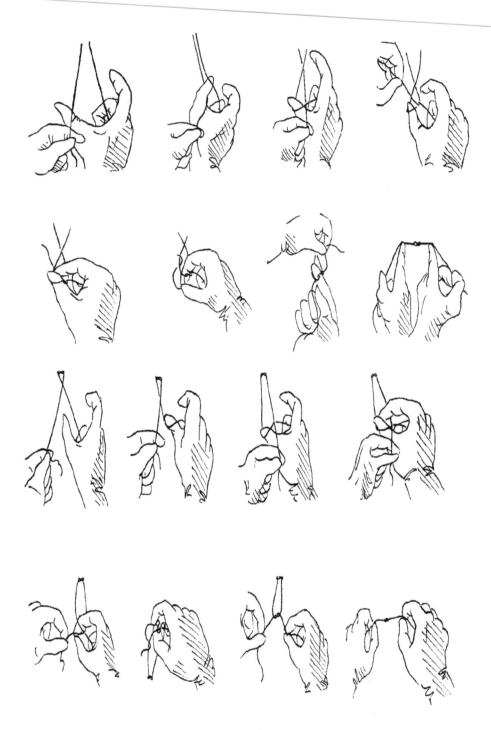

The *two-hand tie* for skin suturing. Practice this using a hook, chair rung, etc.

One-Hand Tie

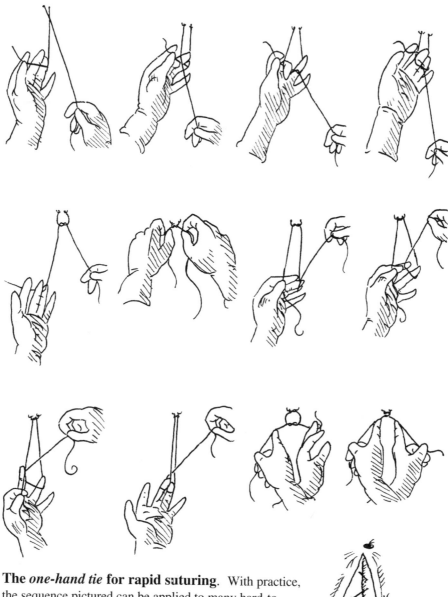

The *one-hand tie* for rapid suturing. With practice, the sequence pictured can be applied to many hard-to-reach places in surgery, as well as the speedy tying of knots when sewing simple lacerations.

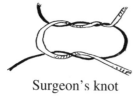

Surgeon's knot

Subcuticular running (continuous) suture

179

Instrument Tie Technique

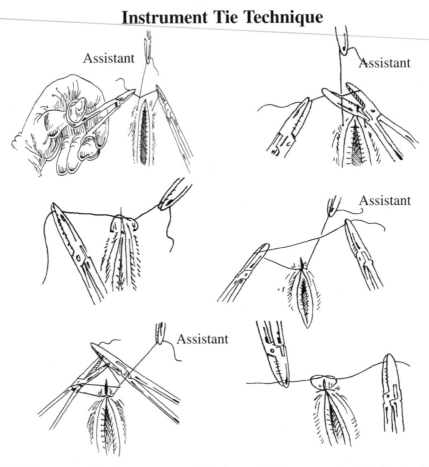

The Instrument Tie. This sequence shows the use of a *hemostat* or *needle holder* in tying knots. At least three knots should be used, one of them being the *surgeon's knot* to prevent unraveling. The ends are cut about ½" long to aid in suture removal later.

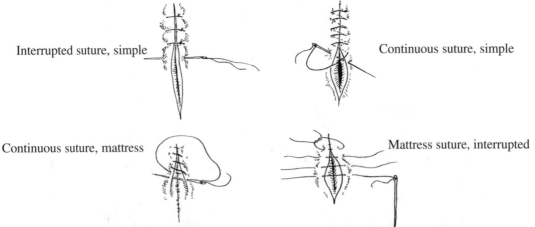

Common suturing techniques. The *continuous suture* laces the laceration in a way to conserve thread. *Vertical mattress* technique prevents the skin edges from turning inward, while adding the benefits of better *hemostasis*. *Subcuticular sutures* minimize scar formation.

To begin, let us consider the suturing of a simple laceration or incision on a flat area of the body with normal skin thickness and adequate blood supply. Sutures are usually placed 3/8 to 1/2 inch apart on an extremity, the trunk, or back. The distance between each suture should be more or less equal to the *span* of the suture itself. **Simple** sutures are used for skin edges that are not likely to turn under (invert), and are applicable to thicker areas of the body's surface. Around the face or in areas where unusual delicacy is required, very fine sutures of silk or nylon are placed 1/8 to 3/16 inches apart, and left in only three to five days. On larger areas of the body, the sutures are left in place approximately one week—for example, the upper extremities, chest, or abdomen. Leave sutures intact for ten days to two weeks in the lower extremities, back, or other areas where blood supply may be compromised. It is important **not** to tie the sutures too tight nor compress the skin edges so closely that free circulation is impaired. On the other hand, the suture should not be so loose to allow the skin edges to gape and thereby delay healing, as well as leaving open a route for infection.

During healing, sutures should be kept clean and dry. After three to four days showers are usually permitted, including shampooing of the hair after scalp injuries. Prolonged soaking, however, is inadvisable. Wet dressings should **never** be permitted to remain over sutures.

Silk and cotton sutures especially should be kept dry, as they may act as a "wick" to allow the entrance of germs resident on the skin surface. Nylon and *subcuticular* (buried) sutures are less likely to become infected. The latter type involves a special technique, comprising a back and forth sewing motion beneath the skin to "bury" the suture. This enables it to heal with scarring. Subcuticular sutures are particularly valuable in the perineum after childbirth, in the face to reduce scarring, and in children, where their removal several days later would be unduly traumatic.

Chromic,*Dexon*, or other absorbable material will provide a subcuticular closure with no necessity to remove sutures later. Properly done, this technique produces a very nice healed surface with minimal of scarring.

Nylon is not as suitable for subcuticular closure. When it or other nonabsorbable material is used, the ends must be left exposed outside the skin, and the suture removed after appropriate cleansing and at the proper time.

Skin edges that are prone to invert should be repaired using a *vertical mattress* technique. This enables the suture to encircle the deeper layers of the wound, as well as bring together (*approximate*) the skin edges. This is the usual method used to close abdominal incisions. Less often used in acute trauma, it is nevertheless appropriate in locations where careful attention to cosmetic results are indicated.

Removing the sutures is another skill that can easily be learned. It is often done at home. The dry, clean, healed incision is first disinfected with alcohol, merthiolate, povidone iodine (*Betadine*), or another suitable nontoxic germicide. These can all be secured at any pharmacy. When this cleansing is accomplished, one end of the suture is grasped with a hemostat or tissue forceps, while the end next to the skin is cut with **sterile** scissors. These instruments, if used at home, should first be boiled to sterilize them, before removing the sutures. Frequently, every other suture is removed as an incision has nearly healed. The alternate remaining sutures are removed when healing is complete.

When sterilized adhesive strips (*Steri-strips*) are employed to close the skin, they are removed after the same length of time as sutures. Lift the ends carefully, then pull them up on each side toward the center, avoiding undue traction at the laceration edge. After the incision has healed and sutures are removed, no further care should be required.

Care must be taken to avoid inadvertently leaving a segment of suture within the wound. This could form what we call a *sterile abscess*. A small area of the skin separates and the suture is seen in a small cyst-like area that drains fluid for a few days. Usually these pockets of fluid do not lead to further infection. Careful cleansing with *Merthiolate* or other household disinfectant will allow for complete healing in a few days.

Sprains

In contrast to pulled muscles (*strains*), **sprains** involve the tearing or traumatic injury of *ligaments*. These are strong, fibrous structures surrounding the many joints. Common areas where sprains occur are the knees, ankles, and wrists, though almost any joint can be affected. The typical "whiplash" injury of a rear-end automobile collision is also a ligamentous sprain. In reality, the entire spine is vulnerable to this type of injury.

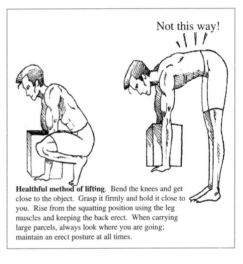

Not this way!

Healthful method of lifting. Bend the knees and get close to the object. Grasp it firmly and hold it close to you. Rise from the squatting position using the leg muscles and keeping the back erect. When carrying large parcels, always look where you are going; maintain an erect posture at all times.

The general characteristics of a sprain are as follows: there is acute pain, localized in the involved joint. Swelling follows, particularly if further ambulation or joint motion is continued, and the area is often held in a dependent position. When blood vessels are torn, bruising becomes apparent within hours, frequently turning the affected joint "black and blue."

There are several important first aid measures to be used in suspected sprains. These include the immediate **immobilization** of the extremity, its **elevation**, and the application of **ice packs**. All of these remedies reduce the amount of swelling and pain. They also help to control bleeding within the joint.

Pain in any joint is a message from "nature" to rest the injured member. For sprained ankles, wrists, or knees, elastic bandages, crutches, and occasionally plaster casting are used for immobilization during the healing phase. Hot and cold contrast treatments, used after the first 12 to 24 hours, aid in the resolution of these inflammatory changes. They also accelerate healing and reduce pain. Unusual persistence of pain in the involved area should alert one to the possibility of fracture, which is best diagnosed with an x-ray.

Simple Fractures

You may wonder why I would seem so bold to even suggest fracture treatment in a home-like setting. The reasons are twofold. First, many are completely unable to afford the expenses of emergency room care or the services of an orthopedist today. Second, many fractures occur in a remote rural setting in countries where medical services are not available. Therefore, it is advisable to know some of the basic principles of diagnosis and management, not only to alleviate acute suffering, but also to prevent residual deformity as the fractured bone heals.

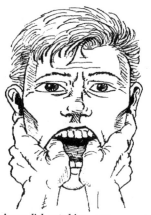

Reducing a *dislocated jaw*. With gauze or cloth to pad the thumbs, the hands are placed with the thumbs on the lower molars. The fingers underneath the jaw are used to elevate while the back of the jaw is depressed. With a rotational motion to depress the joint surface (*condyle*) the jaw can then be slipped down and back to relocate the joint and permit the mouth to close.

Fractures of the bones may be classified in several ways. The **greenstick fracture** is one in which only a portion of the bone is broken, leaving the major segment intact. This is more typically seen in children, since their bones are soft and still growing. Perfect diagnosis can only be obtained with x-ray. The **closed fracture**, formerly called *simple* fracture, is one in which the skin is not broken, and the bone is fractured in only one place. No other fragments are seen, and displacement is usually slight. A **comminuted fracture**, on the other hand, is one in which multiple fragments of the bone are present. It is usually caused by a more severe, shattering type of injury. **Open** (*compound*) **fractures** are those in which a sharp fragment of bone actually penetrates the skin, allowing contamination and a high risk of severe infection. **Osteomyelitis** of the bone is a common sequel of these extensive injuries.

The degree of *displacement* as well as the *kind* of fracture helps determine the appropriate treatment. Many traumatic injuries crack the bone either as a simple or greenstick fracture and leave no deformity at all. This can be seen particularly at the elbow with an *impacted* fracture of the radial head, or in the shoulder where fractures are caused by falling on an outstretched arm impacting the shoulder while fracturing the humerus.

The most common fracture seen in children involves the collar bone or clavicle. Usually some "overriding" (overlapping of fracture ends) is present. Prolonged fixation of the shoulders in a "figure of eight" splint is recommended, with manual evaluation or X-ray pictures determining the degree of shoulder-stretching required to keep the bones fairly well aligned.

Fractures of the **wrist** are the second most common type. They may be seen at any age. Often the deformity produced appears as a "silver fork." In order to avoid limitation of wrist motion afterward, with residual arthritis, careful setting of the bone is required. The easiest way to evalu-

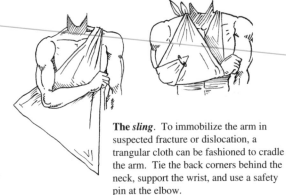

The *sling*. To immobilize the arm in suspected fracture or dislocation, a trangular cloth can be fashioned to cradle the arm. Tie the back corners behind the neck, support the wrist, and use a safety pin at the elbow.

ate an injured extremity for a suspected fracture is to feel with one finger along the involved bones. A fractured bone will usually be exquisitely tender right over the area of fracture. If the patient is seen before undue swelling has set in, the diagnosis can often be pinpointed.

Fractures about the **ankle** are also fairly common. However, X-rays are necessary to evaluate the extent of injury. Some can be treated with a compression type cast for 6-8 weeks, while others require the placement of pins or screws for accurate reduction. The goal is to restore complete weight bearing on the affected leg.

Unless obvious deformity exists, it is difficult to distinguish **skull fractures** from contusions or **concussions**. The presence or absence of unconsciousness is not always reliable in distinguishing skull fractures. Any fractures that cause slow bleeding into the space beneath the skull (*subdural*) are particularly dangerous. They may develop a symptomatic clot (*hematoma*) over a period of days to weeks, putting pressure on the brain.

Any prolonged impairment of consciousness or nerve function after a head injury should be evaluated by a physician, with the appropriate x-rays taken. Asymmetry of the eyes, double vision, an altered appearance of the facial bones, bleeding or clear discharge from the nose or ears should always alert one to the possibility of facial (*orbital*) fracture. Pain on biting or chewing, or altered position of the teeth may indicate a possibly fractured jaw. That also should be evaluated radiologically and appropriately stabilized.

Initial first-aid treatment of fractures is familiar to most emergency medical technicians and nursing instructors. The injured extremity should be put at **rest**, with appropriate splints. Boards, pillows, rolled newspaper, or the modern inflatable plastic splints should be used to immobilize completely the affected part. Ice packs should be applied to reduce pain and swelling during transportation. Ice may even permit appropriate manipulations for setting the bone, if the area has been rendered cold enough. No weight bearing should be put on an ankle, leg, or hip suspected of fracture, until appropriate examination and X-rays have established the *absence* of such injury.

When a fracture is well-aligned and stabilization is indicated, casts or splints can be manufactured. Bone setting, or the reduction of displaced fractures, is beyond my scope to teach here. Aluminum splints may be trimmed or cut, and shaped to conform to the injured part, making a suitable stabilizer to use with appropriate padding and an elastic bandage. **Cast materials** are available with plaster-impregnated gauze available in rolls or strips for the preparation of a cast. Usually a stockinette-type material or cotton padding about 1/8" thick is used to protect the skin, while the plaster on the outside provides stabilization. When the usual plaster rolls are used, wrinkles and excessive pressure over bony prominences must be avoided. Plaster casts are quite durable. Newer light cured epoxy materiels and fiberglass casts are light weight, but considerably more expensive.

Naturally, all plaster casts must be kept dry and free from weight bearing or pressure that exceeds the strength and thickness of the cast. When prepared plaster rolls are not available, an acceptable substitute may be prepared from roller gauze soaked in moist plaster of Paris. This is applied in the usual manner. Gauze strips may be laid **in** plaster and applied, gradually developing the cast. Be careful to avoid pressure over bony prominences. A general rule of fractured long bones is to immobilize the joints **above** and **below** the involved bone. Thus, a fractured forearm frequently requires casting above the elbow and down to the fingers. Exceptions to this are the ankle and wrist, both of which can frequently be stabilized with a shorter arm or leg cast.

The healing time of broken bones varies considerably, with babies' bones healing the fastest, children next, and adults more slowly. The aged take the longest. As a rule, a forearm in a child might heal well in 3–4 weeks, an adolescent or young adult in 6 weeks, and an elderly person 2–3 months. **Nonunion** is more common in the elderly, particularly in fractures of the leg bone (*tibia*), due to its less abundant blood supply.

The **removal of a cast** is quite easy. Without the usual equipment, such as cast saws and special scissors, a cast can be removed by soaking it in water until it softens. Another way of removal is with a knife or file. More commonly in a doctor's office, an oscillating *cast saw* is used, cutting the cast lengthwise on two sides, then taking it off in halves. After a cast is removed, begin using the extremity gradually. Hot and cold contrast baths or whirlpool baths are often helpful to improve circulation. Dependent areas, such as the leg and ankle, need to be wrapped for several weeks with an elastic bandage. Gradual weight bearing and ambulation will once again restore the normal venous and lymphatic return, preventing fluid collection or *edema* formation. With few exceptions, bones begin to heal from the time they are broken. After appropriate stabilization and care, a healed fracture can be as good as new within a short time.

Burns

Many thermal injuries can damage the skin. **Burns** include injuries caused by scalding, fire, radiation, caustic chemicals, and electricity. Although each type of burn requires individualized treatment, some generalizations are appropriate. **Classification** of burns is important to determine their severity, as well as to gauge the response to treatment. Traditionally, the extent is described by degrees. A **first degree** burn involves the superficial layers of the skin only, and manifests itself in reddening. The most common type is a *sunburn*. Prolonged use of heating pads or split-second exposure to a fire may also produce this self-limited, but occasionally painful type of burn.

Second degree or "partial thickness" burns also involve the skin surface or *epidermis*. This burn, however, transfers sufficient heat to the skin to produce blistering. These deeper types are more painful. Second degree burns of babies or small children are especially likely to become infected. If extensive, they may result in dehydration or shock.

The deepest burn, called **third degree** or "full thickness" involves both layers of skin, epidermis, and dermis. These may extend into the subcutaneous fat and muscle, destroying both blood vessels and nerves that supply the skin.

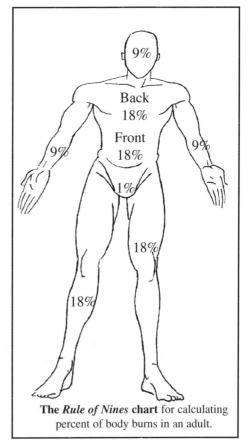

The *Rule of Nines* **chart** for calculating percent of body burns in an adult.

Small full thickness burns may be produced by electricity, although more commonly they are caused by fire or chemicals. Remember that a deep *partial* thickness burn may become badly infected, with extension of the burn to involve all the skin layers. In contrast to first and second degree burns which heal rapidly, the deeper full thickness variety is very slow to heal. The skin forms granulation tissue, with gradual progression to skin renewal, or grafting may be necessary.

Immediate first aid in the case of burns requires the application of *cold*. Often a potential third degree burn can be converted to a second degree or a second degree to a first degree burn by the immediate use of ice or other application of cold to counteract the thermal injury. This should be prolonged for thirty to sixty minutes, unless the burn is extensive enough to necessitate immediate emergency medical care.

A second way to classify burns is according to the **extent** of skin involvement. The "rule of nines" has commonly been used to approximate the burn area. The accompanying diagram helps illustrate how these burned areas can be calculated. Because of the ever present danger of contracture or scarring, burns involving the face or hands are especially serious.

Unless superficial, most burns can be treated like abrasions, with appropriate cleansing and protection against infection. Sterile dressings can be used to relieve pain and prevent the entrance of germs. Small burns are more amenable to the "open technique" than are extensive injuries. In this approach, the burn is cleansed and left open to the air to dry. Rapid formation of a **crust** seals off the burn, functioning like a scab to prevent infection while healing occurs beneath.

Many preparations have been advocated for the relief of pain from burns. And they may be used in a home setting. The mucilaginous gel from the *aloe vera* plant is immediately applied to burns in many countries. A portion of the plant is broken and the juice squeezed onto the affected skin. Pain is relieved, and the gel forms a soothing protective coating. **Vitamin E** oils may also be used. These seem to reduce the likelihood of scarring. The oil can be used directly over the burn and applied several times daily until the skin is healed.

Petroleum jelly (*Vaseline*) and fine mesh gauze can also be beneficial. They are quite easily applied to larger burned areas. A fluffy gauze dressing is used to cover the fine mesh. If no infection or drainage is present, this bandage can be left on several days until the burn is healed, at which time it will be dry and peeling. Daily dressing changes provide an opportunity to see the burn in the healing state. Whirlpool baths with disinfectants can be used when necessary for *debridement*. This term describes the peeling of dead skin or removal of crusts, thus allowing more freedom of motion around affected joints. The entrance of air exerts a drying effect. Treatment should always be continued until healing is complete.

Frostbite and Hypothermia

Two common cold injuries are **frostbite** and **hypothermia**. Taking precautions during winter weather can help you avoid them. First, never push yourself to exhaustion when exercising or working in cold weather. When you are worn out, you're more likely to fall or suffer injury. Take hourly breaks during long treks, skiing expeditions, or work that takes you outdoors for several hours.

Second, drink plenty of water when exercising in the cold, just as you would in warm weather. You can become dehydrated if you neglect to replace fluids, especially when sweating. This reduced blood flow to the skin, which could lead to cold injury.

Windchill Factor

Estimated Wind Speed (mph)	Equivalent Temperature on Exposed Skin When Thermometer Reads (°F):					
Calm	30	20	10	0	-10	-20
10	16	4	-9	-24	-33	-46
20	4	-10	-25	-39	-53	-67
30	-2	-18	-33	-48	-63	-78
40	-6	-21	-37	-53	-69	-86

Remember the **wind chill** factor when exercising outdoors on a cold windy day. Windchill means that a calm, subfreezing weather can do less damage to skin than a warmer, windy day. When exercising outside, head into the wind first, when you are fresh and dry. If you exercise awhile and become sweaty, the dampness will magnify the windchill factor. Rain, even a cool drizzle, causes greater heat loss when you skin stays wet. Snow, even though it has a special charm and beauty, can making walking or running hazardous. During a snowstorm your ability to see is limited. Driving visibility is reduced. Wear reflective clothing when walking.

Wear appropriate **clothing** for winter, but not too much. Exercise generates a lot of body heat. However, be sure your extremities are well covered. Heat can be rapidly lost via exposed skin. The smartest dress code is the layered look. Layers of clothing trap air to increase insulation and keep you warm. The inner layer should insulate and draw moisture to the outer layers where it can evaporate. Wool is good for the middle layer because it serves as a good insulator even when wet. The outer layer of clothing should be windproof, breathable, and water-repellent. Especially, cover your extremities, including fingers, toes, nose, and ears. These are the parts most vulnerable to frostbite. Because you can lose up to 40% body heat through your head, it's important to cover it. Wear a wool or fabric hat that covers your ears. Even a mask or scarf may be helpful in very cold weather.

Your body needs extra fuel when exercising in the cold. So eat **high-calorie foods** when on the trail. And, *NEVER drink alcohol.* It contributes to dehydration and widens (*dilates*) the blood vessels. This means more heat loss. Alcohol, moreover, impairs judgment and reduces sensitivity to cold.

If **frostbite** nips you or a friend, get indoors as soon as possible. Warm the affected area, using towels soaked in warm water. You may feel pain during rewarming. Never rub the affected area. Frostbite occurs when skin temperature (normally about 93° F.) drops below freezing. In very cold or windy weather, flesh can freeze in under a minute. Pay close attention to how your skin feels. Watch for burning sensations and whitening of skin. If you ignore these signs, you may get full-blown frostbite. Frostbitten areas may turn red, then blue, and blisters may form. Digits, both fingers and toes, have been lost through this type of thermal injury.

Exposure to cold also increases the risk of **hypothermia**. When your core body temperature drops to 95° F. from the usual 98.6° F., your life is in danger. If this loss of body temperature is not reversed, you may simply stop breathing and die. Furthermore, it may be difficult to tell that your body temperature is dropping. Heed symptoms like intense shivering, slurred speech, and disorientation.

Emergency treatment focuses on elevating body temperature. Provide warm (not hot) drinks, remove wet clothing, and warm your friends body as soon as possible. You can do this with blankets, your own body, or any other means possible. Get medical help as soon as possible. However, continue the warming efforts meanwhile. You may save a life.

Bites

Proper handling of injuries from animal or human bites requires experience and judgment. As a general rule, all bites that break the skin should be considered infected wounds. For this reason they should all be protected against tetanus with the appropriate **tetanus toxoid** booster inoculation. If previous vaccination has not been completed within the recommended period of time (usually 10 years), **human tetanus antitoxin** is also administered.

As soon as possible after an injury occurs, the wound should be washed thoroughly with water using the best available antiseptic soap. Careful irrigation and cleansing of the bite will remove most of the foreign substances that would otherwise produce complications or infection. When the laceration is severe or hemorrhage is present, ligatures to close the wound may be necessary. Smaller bites are best treated with the open technique, permitting them to heal by second intention (see section on wound care in Chapter 12).

Human bites are among the most likely to become infected, because of the abundant flora of germs resident in the mouth. The lysozyme content of a dog's saliva makes it less likely to contain virulent bacteria. But all animals, including cats, horses, dogs, and wild pets are likely to cause damage if they bite. Obviously, many of these injuries can be prevented by appropriate care in handling animals.

The bite of an animal infected with **rabies virus** is particularly serious. The animal usually exhibits strange behavior, and may be unsteady, foaming at the mouth, salivating, and unusually vicious. Rabies or *hydrophobia*, as it is sometimes called, is a viral infection of the central nervous system. Untreated, all known cases result in death. Proper rabies control requires vaccination of all pets, such as dogs and cats, with careful avoidance of untamed animals. **Never pet or attempt to fondle any strange animal!**

189

If an animal suspected of having rabies has bitten someone, the animal should be quarantined with the local health department or humane society. Within two weeks it usually becomes apparent whether rabies is present or not. If the bite is extensive or near the face, immediate inoculation of the patient with antirabies vaccine is begun. This therapy involves a series of daily injections for about two weeks. Although painful, they may be life saving. Most emergency rooms and health departments have information as to how the antirabies vaccine can be procured and administered. It is imperative to follow through with a full course of adequate protection to save the lives of such unfortunate victims.

Poisoning

Many die every year from accidental or intentional ingestion of toxic substances. Most cases of poisoning, however, are innocent and often occur in small children. Since infants are so prone to put unfamiliar substances in their mouth, careful surveillance by parents is necessary to prevent these incidents. The home should be inspected to be sure that cleaning fluids, medicines, insect poisons, and solvents are carefully secured beyond the reach of children. **Never put toxic substances into soft drink bottles or other containers that are normally used for food**. Particularly harmful preparations should be kept in a locked cabinet. As children are able, they should be instructed carefully concerning the danger of many household chemicals.

When accidental ingestion of a poisonous substance occurs, usually the first procedure is to **induce vomiting**. The sooner this is done after the ingestion of the poison, the better the results will be. Many substances are absorbed rapidly. If syrup of Ipecac is not available, give some lukewarm water or other liquid to dilute the poison. Then prepare at once to visit an emergency room.

Sticking the finger in the throat to induce gagging may be helpful when pills have been ingested, but should **never** be used in the case of swallowed lye, strong acids, gasoline, kerosene, or other hydrocarbons. Aspiration may result, producing a serious pneumonia. The caustic properties of lye make further corrosive burning of the esophagus a possibility. Even perforation may result if vomiting is instituted.

The most helpful remedy for poisoning is the early administration of **activated charcoal**. Every home should have a box of powdered charcoal on hand, as well as the "activated" capsules. Charcoal has phenomenal powers to adsorb poisonous chemicals. The usual dose of charcoal is thirty to sixty grams (2 to 4 tablespoons of the powder). It is mixed with water to make a "slurry." One must drink this water suspension as quickly as possible. The charcoal, administered early, can adsorb most drugs. Because of its insolubility, it is not absorbed into the bloodstream.

Many poisonous plant substances and mushrooms may be ingested. Botanical field guides are helpful to identify these substances. Some of the more common ones will be mentioned here. Every adult, especially every parent, should know how to identify the most common plants around their locality, and particularly be able to recognize the toxic species. Mushrooms are a most interesting class of plants. Some of them are nutritious and quite tasty, while others may be deadly when swallowed. The *Amanita* species are among the most toxic substances known to affect man. The recognition of this extremely poisonous mushroom should be thoroughly understood, so that no accidents will occur. Consult a field guide or first aid manual for any questions in identifying such toxic plants. The **poison control center** can be reached by telephone from most cities. Check your phone directory for the number.

Many *suicides* take place each year through the ingestion of harmful drugs. Overdoses of sedatives or tranquilizers are common. Most cases can be salvaged by early recognition and gastric lavage. All emergency rooms should be equipped with materials to wash out (*lavage*) an individual's stomach. However, the early induction of vomiting may make this unpleasant procedure unnecessary. **Activated charcoal** is usually administered to *adsorb* the drug and prevent its effect on the system. REMEMBER to take suicide notes, hints, and actual attempts *very* seriously!

Often the best response is a willingness to listen and sincerely attempt to understand the plight of the distressed individual. Tragic deaths or deliberate overdoses could be prevented by the exercise of love and mutual understanding when disturbances arise in the family. As in many other aspects of emergency medicine, your loving attention may reduce the toll that accidents are now taking in our turbulent society.

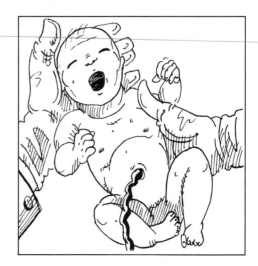

CHAPTER FOURTEEN

BIRTH

DEFECTS

Centuries ago in the land of Judea the disciples asked a question, *"Who did sin, this* [blind] *man, or his parents, that he was born blind?"* A prevailing idea at that time was that some transgression lay at the foundation of all congenital disease. It is true that conditions classed as birth defects may be related to parental transgression. Evidence implicating drugs (cocaine, crack, LSD, etc.) as the cause of many chromosome defects and genetically transmitted disease accumulates every year.

Some pharmaceutical drugs affect the growing embryo during key developmental phases. They may result in deformities of the cranium, limbs, heart, kidneys, or sense organs. Infectious diseases, such as syphilis, toxoplasmosis, and the cytomegalovirus can all produce serious damage to the unborn child. In order to understand genetic diseases, let us now consider some methods by which information is passed to our offspring.

In the *nucleus* of every cell lies specialized strands of nucleic acids called *chromosomes*. In human cells there are twenty-three pairs of these. Men and women differ only in the presence or absence of a **Y** chromosome (male – XY) or a pair of X chromosomes (female – XX). During the division of non-reproductive cells (*mitosis*) the chromosomes divide and duplicate themselves, forming identical nuclei in the "daughter" cells. When a reproductive cell divides, however, its chromosomes split and each resulting spermatozoa or ovum receives only one-half of each of the original twenty-three pairs, or **half** the complement of the fertilized ovum. This process (*meiosis*), then, results in cell division without duplication of original chromosome pairs and prepares the mature sex cell for fertilization.

In the chromosome lie a vast number of possible combinations (*genes*), each of which has the capability of governing growth, determining protein structure, and individuality. These **genes** make up the chromosomes. They are

192

able to start or stop protein synthesis, according to the need of the developing organism.

It is a marvel of genetic engineering to consider the possibilities. To produce a human being, while preserving perfect individuality and the near infinite variety of possibilities for facial appearance, height, bone structure, hair color, eye color, fingerprints is just amazing to our finite mind. In this chapter, however, I wish to consider some of the inherited tendencies and birth defects that cause great stress to parents and influence so profoundly the subsequent generation.

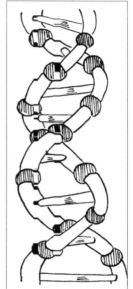

DNA. Located on each chromosome, the marvelous alpha-helix of *deoxyribonucleic acid* is the basis of our inheritance.

Behavior Problems

A whole new science of medical investigation has developed studying the influence of drugs and birth trauma on behavior. Many terms have been coined to describe these disorders of childhood, among them *minimal brain dysfunction* and *hyperactivity*. It is known that birth trauma—a difficult delivery, the traumatic use of forceps, or other conditions which result in oxygen deprivation—may produce long-term effects on behavior. Maternal use of drugs such as tranquilizers, cocaine, LSD, marijuana, and particularly alcohol (also numerous other substances) can induce changes that affect a person's learning ability for his lifetime. Many children of school age are unable to concentrate, sit still, or adhere to the discipline of a schoolroom. Multitudes develop patterns of truancy, then in adolescence become social problems or delinquents. The habits picked up tend to perpetuate the maladjustments. If pregnancy ensues, this antisocial pattern of behavior is reproduced. The science dealing with these problems is called **behavioral teratology**. Research in the field constitutes one of the most fascinating, yet ominous perspectives of medical investigation today.

Deformities

Many defects in the external physical appearance are related to chromosomal defects. The **Down's syndrome**, discussed below, is one of these in which characteristic facial appearance and retardation are evident. Many years ago a tranquilizer called *thalidomide* was administered to mothers during pregnancy. Complete or partial failure of development (*phocomelia*) of the hands, arms, or lower extremities resulted, creating thousands of permanently deformed babies from the simple taking of a nerve pill. Many drugs today have cautions against their use during pregnancy. But more drugs than we suspect may actually affect the unborn child. Pregnancy in women who are addicted to narcotics or the heavy use of alcohol runs a very high risk of developmental birth defects.

Infections in the early part or pregnancy, particularly the first trimester, may also produce deformities in the offspring. German measles or *rubella* may cause a wide range of birth defects, depending on when the infection occurred. Cleft palate, harelip, congenital heart disease, cataracts, and deafness are some of the afflictions that may stem from prenatal viral illnesses. A pregnant mother harboring *syphilis* germs may also cause deformities in her offspring with bowing of the legs, saddle nose, or characteristic chisel-like teeth. Nutritional deficiencies during pregnancy may result in congenital problems. Certain developing nations, because of their cultural taboos, prevent a mother from obtaining adequate sunlight, calcium, or milk. Congenital *rickets* can then develop, with failure to produce normal bones. Fractures, with life-long changes in the ribs, legs, or other growing bones are common. Conditions such as these are largely preventable.

Congenital Heart Disease

Many babies are born with defects of the heart, traced to chromosome defects, maternal infections, or the use of toxic agents. Two types of heart disease are seen. One is called *cyanotic*, because of the characteristic "blue baby" who has a dusky color to the lips, hands, or a general cyanosis. The most common of these is called the *Tetralogy of Fallot*, and includes four basic cardiac defects requiring specialized study for diagnosis. A number of surgical procedures have been devised to correct the congenital defects of the heart, reducing the mortality and extending the life of otherwise doomed children.

Noncyanotic heart disease such as ventricular or atrial *septal defects* and *stenosis* of the pulmonary valves describe defects in other parts of the heart. These conditions create an extra burden for the heart and if severe, may result in heart failure. *Patent ductus arteriosis* is another condition in which a normal shunting mechanism present in fetal life fails to close after birth. Surgical operations are being refined to deal with these problems and correct them early, to permit normal growth and activity in the young child.

Visual Defects

A number of eye problems are seen in the newborn. The most serious is **congenital blindness**, usually caused by *cataracts*. This is most frequently an aftermath of **German measles** in early (the first trimester) pregnancy. Avoiding exposure to this condition during the first three months of pregnancy or the inoculation of women who have not had *Rubella* prior to the childbearing years is preventive.

Less common today is blindness stemming from the use of high doses of oxygen for the newborn. **Retrolental fibroplasia** is a problem that was associated with the high concentration of oxygen used in treating an infant suffering from *hyaline membrane disease*. Modern pediatric care in a neonatal intensive care unit has greatly reduced the incidence of this serious, but usually preventable condition.

More commonly seen are a number of eye muscle imbalances present from birth. Some of the eye muscle shortening, called **strabismus** or "squint" may correct itself during the childhood years, as the eyes are alternately patched or treated with special glasses. The imbalance which results in double vision would eventually destroy the sight in one eye. It should be treated as early as possible with corrective surgery. This can be done successfully by most ophthalmologists and will preserve good binocular vision.

Hearing Impairment

Congenital deafness is very difficult to recognize in the newborn. A variety of causes are known, including heredity, drugs, and maternal infections. Deafness is a serious handicap which requires early recognition. Usually a mother notices that her child does not startle with the loud noises that arouse others. Vocal sounds fail to elicit appropriate smiles, and the child does not turn to face the sound of singing or other normal stimuli. Special hearing tests must be given to determine the type of deafness. Treatment may require hearing aids and special education. Early instruction in sign language, lip reading, and enrollment in special schools for the handicapped enable these children to compensate well for their lack of the marvelous gift of hearing.

Mental Retardation

Some of the most unfortunate types of congenital afflictions are those which affect the intellect. Untreated **hypothyroidism** (called *cretinism*) will inevitably result in retarded mental development, unless recognized early and treated with replacement doses of thyroid. A simple test using blood from the umbilical cord can detect this condition, which may be difficult to recognize clinically.

High levels of **jaundice** in the newborn period may produce a condition known as *kernicterus*. This may provoke seizures and retardation. However, if recognized early the appropriate use of light therapy or exchange transfusion may avert any brain damage and minimize the risk. **Anoxia** at birth may also trigger changes in the brain that result in retarded mental productivity. Safe obstetrical practices and the prompt treatment of newborn asphyxia can minimize these hazards.

195

Chromosome defects may cause retardation. The most common is called **Down's syndrome** or *Mongolism*. In such cases, a chromosome (number 21), is produced in a set of three instead of one pair. This is termed *Trisomy 21*. Other varieties occur where the chromosomes are broken or *translocated*. Changes in the palmar creases, a characteristic facial appearance with squinting eyes, an unusually round face, and an peculiar smile are all associated with mental retardation. Less commonly, cardiac or other internal organ defects are seen. Special education and an unusual degree of parental care are needed to train these handicapped children. Fortunately, most of them have very pleasant dispositions and can bring joy in unusual ways to parents who are willing to change their aspirations and accept the handicap of their offspring.

Cerebral Palsy

Also called *spastic diplegia*, **cerebral palsy** is a condition that usually results from oxygen deficiency during birth. The affected individual often has associated seizures and moderate to mild retardation. There may be a profound impairment in coordination, with inability to walk without "scissoring" in the lower extremities. Lack of hand coordination also may be evident. In the most severe cases normal development is completely impossible. "Patterning," the alternate repetitive movement of extremities in "crossed extensor" pattern (straightening out of one arm and the opposite leg) has been tried by devoted friends and family members to enable an affected individual to learn what otherwise would have come naturally. Some cases of cardiac arrest during childhood have resulted in cerebral palsy. With adjustment for the milder handicaps, many children can be educated to enjoy life with some useful skill.

Convulsive Disorders

Seizures can likewise stem from the lack of oxygen during birth. Infections in the newborn period or congenital *toxoplasmosis* can also produce convulsions. Usually in the newborn period, the seizures are of the *grand mal* type. The epileptic attack consists of characteristic violent jerking (*tonic* and *clonic*) convulsions, loss of sphincter control, and an aftermath of somnolence. During the seizure there is a tendency to bite the tongue or quit breathing for a brief period. **Fever** may aggravate the tendency to-

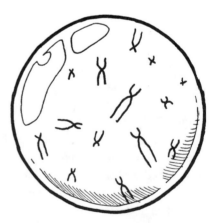

Chromosome analysis can often detect specific genetic diseases.

196

ward seizures. These should be distinguished from a true convulsive disorder. The *electroencephalogram* (EEG) can be very helpful in diagnosing the type of seizure and instituting a proper treatment. The next chapter will describe some of these problems, with a few suggestions for home management.

Fetal Alcohol Syndrome

Suspicion that **alcohol** could damage the unborn child has been in medical literature for many decades. Recently, however, convincing evidence has finally linked a mother's drinking of alcoholic beverages during pregnancy with a special set of problems visible in the newborn. A characteristic facial appearance with unusual-appearing eyes and nose is associated with the retardation of mental development and altered growth patterns. This has now been called the **fetal alcohol syndrome**. Some mothers have even been prosecuted for giving such a sad "birthright" to their babies.

The severity of this syndrome seems to be proportional to the consumption of alcohol by the mother. Reminiscent of the warning to Manoah's wife prior to the birth of Samson (read it in *Judges 13:13, 14*), this caution against alcohol drinking should strongly motivate modern mothers to take a non-drinking stand. When a baby has been born with the characteristic syndrome, it is destined to be handicapped, often for **life**. Although the mechanism of alcohol's toxic action on a developing fetus is not completely clear, the effects are nonetheless sure. Thus in considering the offspring from all angles—looks, intelligence (I.Q.), and general health, nondrinkers clearly have the advantage.

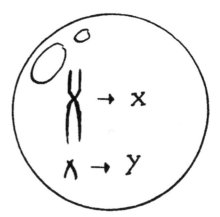

The **X** and **Y** chromosomes determine our gender

When Danger Threatens

With so many possible congenital deformities, many parents approach pregnancy with much worry and fear. Particularly when a mother has been exposed to **German measles** (*rubella*) in the early part of pregnancy or has a background of previous deformities, the thought of possibly terminating her pregnancy looms in her mind. Many of the **abortions** being done today are performed solely for convenience, relieving the unwed, the busy, and the unprepared from the stress of childbearing. A modern trend in genetic counseling, associated with the testing now available of chromosomes prior to birth (*amniocentesis*), advocates abortion in an attempt to prevent these possible deformities. Against the backdrop of the time-honored standards of medical ethics and the moral law given on Sinai, I wish to discuss some of the issues.

The currently accepted **definition** of abortion is a termination of pregnancy. Sometimes this occurs suddenly and spontaneously and may either be *complete* or *incomplete*. Most of the latter cases are treated with an emergency surgery called a *dilatation and curettage* (D & C) to prevent the risk of hemorrhage in a pregnancy that is already inevitably lost. **Therapeutic abortions**, however, are being performed in both the first and second trimesters of pregnancy *only* for the purpose of terminating the life of the unborn child. The major ethical consideration, in actuality, is just when does life begin? There is no reason to conclude other than this: LIFE BEGINS WITH CONCEPTION. Therefore, I believe that abortion at any stage involves the taking of life. The question then is, how can you sustain a life that will be obviously deformed?

It is well known that nearly two-thirds of pregnancies occurring in women who were infected with *Rubella* during their pregnancy will turn out **normal**. The other smaller group may have deformities ranging from cardiac defects to deafness. Most of these can be helped with remedial educational efforts or surgery. Certainly the handicapped person is difficult to raise. However, does the mere chance of having a deaf or blind child justify the sacrifice of his life before birth?

Because of documented experiences from other countries (Germany before World War II, China today) we need not await another generation to learn the long-term effects of this most unfortunate assault on the finer sensitivities and moral fiber of our people. Modern abortion practice notwithstanding, a truly dedicated physician or midwife **must** be true to his or her medical pledge and ethical traditions, kindly but firmly refusing abortion, while counseling toward alternatives.

An exceedingly rare case *may* exist where some mother's **life** could be so jeopardized by the continuation of pregnancy that therapeutic abortion might be considered necessary. Nevertheless, under such unlikely circumstances the multitude of counselors—including clergymen, physicians, and especially the Great Physician—should be able to provide wisdom. Most likely this instance would be so infrequent that many physicians could practice a lifetime without encountering it. Lives are so precious. Even the possibility of handicaps should not cause a mother, father, or medical advisor to compromise, thereby adding guilt to grief, regret to reality.

Coping With The Handicapped Child

The birth of a baby with congenital deformities adds a new challenge for devoted parents. The possibility of intellectual handicap is probably the most difficult to accept. Medical problems that can be managed or cured with appropriate surgery are not so hard to cope with. The possibility of having a disturbed child showing unusual behavior or a learning handicap tests the faith of a new mother or father to the utmost. Fortunately, there are many agencies prepared to assist with this adjustment.

Many physicians are versed in the medical needs of these children, and can give direction to agencies that provide learning skills, orthopedic evaluations, and special classes for the handicapped, deaf, or blind child. Although public health services, voluntary health agencies, and other governmental programs are usually available to give aid, the influence and assistance that a **church** may render should never be overlooked. Parents will need guidance and support, but should determine to accept the child as an *individual*, despite his or her limitations. This will not only set an excellent example for others in the community, but can also serve to bring out lasting desirable qualities in the siblings, if they are assured of their share of the parent's time and attention and interest.

Although institutional care is sponsored by most states to provide for the seriously involved child, home care wherever possible is without question the most beneficial. Especially during infancy and early childhood, a devoted mother or father can enable the handicapped child to develop maximally at every stage. Even severely disabled children can profit from tender loving care at home. *Mongoloid* (Down's syndrome) children, in particular, have a much greater potential if given good care in the average home than when placed in an institution from birth. With guidance, most families **can** handle their children's needs. The rewards to such parents are lasting, with character imprints that make it well worth every sacrifice.

Risk of Down's Syndrome Based on Age

Maternal age at birth	Risk of Down's in second trimester	Liveborn
25	1:1887	1:1250
32	1:563	1:794
35	1:274	1:386
39	1:100	1:141
45	1:20	1:39
49	NA	1:11

(from Creasy, RK, Resnik R: *Maternal-Fetal Medicine: Principles and Practice*, 2nd ed., Philadelphia, PA: W.B. Saunders, 1989.)

CHAPTER FIFTEEN

CHILDHOOD

AND

DEVELOPMENT

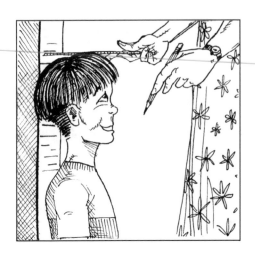

A home with small children is an exciting place to live. The activities of growing youngsters bring a never-ending series of delights. Yet life for these offspring is fraught with many perils. Although many of the infectious diseases that took the lives of babies and young children a generation ago have come under control with better public health and hygienic measures, certain infectious diseases and risks of accidents, are always threatening. The newborn period is especially a time when vigilance is needed.

EXAMINING THE BABY

From the time a new baby takes his first breath through the first few weeks of life, great care is needed to provide a protected environment of health. Assuming that anatomic development has taken place normally, that first vital breath is encouraged as mucus gets cleared from the nose, mouth, and throat. The rubber *suction bulb* is an indispensable device in the delivery suite, as well as the newborn nursery. Every parent should also have one of these suction devices in the home. It can be used to clear mucus, and is of considerable help during colds to maintain an unobstructed airway.

The newborn baby should usually **sleep** on his or her abdomen or be propped on one side, since for several weeks your baby is unable to turn himself or herself. Aspiration of regurgitated milk or other stomach contents can occur when he or she is on his or her back. **Temperature** stability is also important. A newborn entering the world is damp, and will immediately begin to lose heat. Therefore he or she must be dried, wrapped in a warm blanket, and either held close to the mother or in a special warming device.

In modern hospitals most nurses put a stocking cap over the baby's head to prevent rapid heat loss that otherwise occurs through a moist scalp, particularly those who have lots of hair. Avoid giving the newborn baby a bath too early, for this washes away the valuable cheese-like *vernix caseosa* that acts as a cosmetic cream to prevent drying and cracking of the baby's skin. Moreover, the greater necessity of warmth than cleanliness makes it advisable to delay the bath for several hours.

As one looks at the newborn baby, several **features** become apparent. In contrast to adults, whose head is about one-eighth the size of the body, a newborn baby is divided more equally with a larger proportionate head size. Charts are available to tell whether the circumference of the head is within normal limits. The height (about 20 inches) and the weight, which is usually 5.5 to 8 pounds (2500 to 4000 grams) also give a good estimate of the baby's maturity.

The newborn's **skin** is usually ruddy in complexion, particularly if the child has been left attached to the umbilical cord until pulsations cease. This extra blood that is "transfused" from the placenta can keep the baby's hemoglobin higher for several months, in spite of low iron intake. After his or her initial cry the infant may either continue with the same loud sounds or sleep quietly for an hour. A low level of excitement in the birth room and the absence of trauma during delivery will influence this reaction considerably. Usually the eyes are closed, but if they are open a light can be shined in to determine the presence of pupils with their "red reflex" off the retina. The ears are normally formed with well-developed cartilage, except in the premature, and the ear canals should be open (*patent*). The nose must be unobstructed to permit adequate breathing, as a newborn baby cannot breathe solely through its mouth. Obstruction in this area should call for urgent medical evaluation to save the child from asphyxia.

The **sucking reflex** is usually present from birth, as is the **rooting** reflex. To demonstrate the latter, the child turns his or her mouth and face toward the side of the cheek which is gently stroked. This sort of nuzzling prepares the way for breast feeding.

Small white dots on the nose (*milia*) and white "pearls" on the roof of the mouth (*hard palate*) are normal in a newborn. The neck turns from side to side, and the collar bone can be felt. Unusual lumps or masses in the head, neck, or large discolorations of the skin should be evaluated for associated birth defects.

The **heart** rate is still rapid in the newborn period, usually over 120 per minute. Gradually it slows to the childhood level within several days. Listening to the heart with a stethoscope, the examiner should detect normal first and second heart sounds with no unusual murmurs or rhythm irregularities. The lungs should expand equally without retractions between the ribs or any crowing, labored respiration.

The **abdomen** is usually protuberant. Although sometimes the edge of the liver or spleen can be felt on careful palpation, there should be no masses or hard tumors in the abdomen. The umbilical cord has three blood vessels—two arteries and a vein. These are best seen when the cord is clamped and cut before drying has occurred.

Careful examination of the genitalia to determine sex and, in case of males the presence of descended testes, is important. Usually there is no difficulty in urination. This spontaneously occurs within minutes to hours after birth. The need for **circumcision** in male babies remains a subject of controversy among pediatricians. However some decided benefits have been recently demonstrated, especially the lowered risk of urinary infection. Many parents still prefer this minor surgical procedure for hygienic reasons or for continuity of appearance among the male offspring. If so, this should be deferred for several days to allow the newborn to equilibrate from his birth experience and establish the pattern of breast feeding. The Biblical recommendation of circumcising a baby on the *eighth* day has value from a medical standpoint, in that the clotting ability of blood is usually restored to normal by that day, with the synthesis of **Vitamin K** in the intestinal tract. Most newborns by the eighth day will have little difficulty with hemorrhage. Aseptic surgical precautions are needed if a circumcision is performed, to prevent infection.

The examination of the extremities includes more than counting the fingers and toes. Creases in the thighs should be symmetrical, and leg length should be equal. The hips should be able to rotate outward and inward equally, without a "clicking" sound or obvious asymmetry. Some inward turning of the ankles may be seen, because of the intrauterine position. But any unusual club foot deformity should be brought to the attention of a physician.

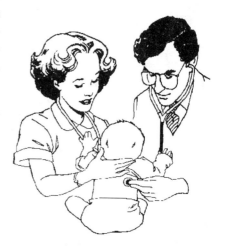

When the infant is dropped or jostled suddenly a *Moro's reflex* occurs. This involves a trembling of the hands with an outward grasping fashion. It is normal in newborns. The *Babinski reflex* is triggered by stroking the sole from the heel to the toe. It also is normal up to one year of age. It is positive when the great toe extends itself and the little toes flair. Unusual lethargy, a jittery appearance, the presence of seizures, or any failure to take liquids and suck normally should call for medical attention promptly.

FEEDING THE BABY

Nourishing the newborn is a precious privilege for a devoted mother. Modern scientific research has underscored the ancient belief that **mothers's milk** is unquestionably the best food for the baby. Its perfect balance of phosphorus, calcium, vitamins, and protein, as well as its ready availability in a prewarmed, sterile package makes it ideal for travel, as well as home. For the first few days sucklings brings forth a watery secretion called *colostrum*. This fluid contains valuable antibodies which will protect the infant for months against common infections and household germs. By the second or third day after delivery, the mother begins to notice engorgement in her breasts.

As her milk "comes in" a regular feeding pattern is started. Hospital routines of every four hours are not at all ideal for nourishing the newborn. Usually a system can be established with slightly more frequent feedings during the day and more sleep at night, awakening only once or twice to breast feed. The opposite policy of "demand" feedings should be discouraged, and the infant established on a *regular* pattern, according to his needs, as soon as possible. The nursing mother should be free from unusual physical strain, worry, or excessive work. Her fluid intake should be adequate to maintain a good milk supply, but she need not drink large amounts of milk in order to do this. Just as during pregnancy, a nursing mother should avoid taking drugs, many of which pass directly through to the milk and adversely affect the little one.

Many advantages can be listed for breast feeding the newborn. One of the most powerful reasons is the **bonding** that this develops between the mother and her new child. From the time of delivery on through the weaning process the physical contact between a mother and her nursing infant is an intimate one. The prophet Isaiah asked, "Can a woman forget her sucking child?" The obvious answer arises every few hours as engorgement of the breasts, as well as a hungry cry reminds the mother that feeding time is here.

The child will have less colic, and be more quiet and peaceful. With the natural limitation on work that nursing requires, breast feeding wins twice, for mother and child. A most ideal food is received through mother's milk. All attempts to develop formulas are merely fragmentary duplicates of the special product nature has designed in the mother's breast. Many dollars as well as hours are saved. The natural, prepackaged, prewarmed, sterilized, and readily available nutrients travel wherever mother goes.

There is another advantage, the physiologic spacing of pregnancy. Moreover, some degree of birth control is provided by breast feeding. During the first four months up to a year the full-time nursing mother may have no return of periods. Although exceptions exist, this physiologic "contraception" works well for many parents. Long-term benefits for the mother are also seen. There is a lowered risk of breast cancer. A breast fed baby has fewer gastrointestinal infections. Food allergies are more common with the early introduction of solid foods. Breast feeding affords impressive safeguard against allergic manifestations. The nutrients are so complete that solid foods are unnecessary.

When a baby's first teeth begin to erupt, at five to six months of age, it is time to contemplate introducing solid foods. Early feeding of table food should be discouraged for several reasons mentioned above. Ripe, mashed banana is an excellent food to commence with. Many others can be substituted, such as applesauce, peaches, and similar fruits low in sugar. Under normal circumstances, one new food should be introduced each week. Most children, when allowed to develop new tastes, one food at a time, will eventually have a wide variety of pleasurable eating experiences. This prevents the finicky food preferences of the traditionally "spoiled" youngster.

Cereal based foods should be introduced next, preferably those of whole grain composition. They can be "whizzed" in a blender or cooked for a very soft consistency, then ground through a food mill. Oatmeal, whole wheat, brown rice, and barley all form excellent cereals, always introduced one at a time. Use salt very sparingly, always less than mother's taste requires. The rest of the family should join in those well-planned breakfasts. Then the introduction of cereal foods can be a source of delight to parents and baby. Moreover, a little cereal will often quiet the fussy baby so he or she sleeps for several hours.

Gradually, after a variety of fruits and cereals have been introduced, the vegetables can be initiated. Soft foods like green beans, squash, creamed corn, and mashed peas are given. At first they should be pureed or strained. Later, as more teeth erupt and the child's chewing ability is established, more firm, chewy foods can be served.

Zwieback (twice-baked bread) and crackers constitute excellent foods for the child who has learned to grasp and chew. They are aids in teething, but should not be given as snacks. In fact, the more regular the child's feeding patterns are the better his or her disposition and health will be. Three meals a day of solid foods are quite adequate for infants, while older children and adults often fare even better with two substantial meals, breakfast and dinner.

DEVELOPMENTAL PATTERNS

It is fascinating for new parents to watch their child grow. The first smile of recognition is always reflected in the face of mother and dad. The infant's ability to grasp and mimic movements brings equal delight. Within the first few weeks after birth, most children learn to follow the mother's motion with their eyes. Particularly, if early bonding has taken place in a rooming-in experience, the child will feel more comfortable with the mother, and usually prefers being in the same room. Although the **grasp reflex** is present at birth, a child by two to three months of age will be strong enough to hold his head up and reach for objects that he or she can grasp and hold in his or her hand. It is important to take caution that objects within reach are safe, for most of them get sampled in the mouth.

Although most children are surprised when they roll over for the first time, this natural exploration of muscle power is seen by about three months. By five to six months of age the child usually crawls. Then the first one or two teeth erupt. By nine to ten months of age most children are able to pull themselves up, supporting their weight on both legs. Thus they develop the normal curvatures in the lower spine that an erect posture produces. By one year of age, we see the little one toddling around, taking his first steps. Parents should not become concerned if this is delayed a few months or be too elated when it comes early, for there is wide variation in normal development. During the second year of life excited parents hear their child's first words and phrases, then whole sentences. The child also develops increased coordination for running. These deeper emotional and physical expressions bring a never ending sequence of surprises and pleasures to the proud parents.

Discipline of the young child should never be neglected. Many parents have awakened with the realization that, unknown to them, their child has taken control of the home. Unless restrained, even a young child can manipulate each family member according to his whims, by temper tantrums, prolonged crying, and other demonstrations. Wise denial of food at improper eating times and firm insistence of obedience is essential to the development of a future adult, who will benefit society, bringing honor to the family name.

Parents need divine wisdom to guide their children properly. Never administer discipline in a harsh manner or when the parent is angry, exasperated, or upset. If something should be denied the child, firmness and consistency are needed. The mind soon learns to adapt to situations it is powerless to change. Yet, parents should be reasonable, mixing law with love and administering restraint with patience, praying for deeper understanding.

VACCINATIONS

If we lived in an ideal world where perfect heredity, perfect nutrition, and excellent health habits all combined to prevent disease, we would probably never need **vaccinations**. Nonetheless, it is a very real fact that germs exist and infections abound. Many illnesses are especially serious if contracted by a baby or young child. Others remain a threat throughout our life on planet earth. Some infections are more hazardous in tropical countries, while others inhabit specific areas, such as Asia or Africa. Here are a few guidelines to help parents select the program best suitable for their child.

In brief, vaccinations are inoculations of substances (antigenic proteins) which have been derived from an offending germ. There are two basic types of vaccines, one prepared from bacteria and the other from viruses. The viral vaccines are developed for human use by their repeated laboratory culture in cells of a fertilized egg. This *attenuation* of the virus makes it unable to produce disease, while retaining its surface proteins or antigens, which are necessary to stimulate antibody formation. This explains the basis for immunization to such diseases as polio and the common childhood illnesses, measles and mumps.

Smallpox germs, on the other hand, although a viral disease, were not used as the virus for vaccination. Instead the cowpox virus (vaccinia) was used as the agent. This produces only a mild illness in most people. Thankfully, the smallpox infection has been eradicated. For many years no infections have occurred, and the vaccination program has been discontinued worldwide.

The bacterial vaccines are prepared from the cell wall of killed bacteria. Many methods are used to prepare them. A commonly accepted vaccination program for babies and young children is as follows:

Oral **polio** vaccine (4 months, 5 months, 6 month, 18 months, 6 years).

Trivalent vaccine for **diphtheria, tetanus, and whooping cough** (DPT) (4 months, 5 months, 6 months, 18 months 6 years). Recent concern about the pertussis (whooping cough) component has led to developing **DT** vaccine—diphtheria and tetanus. In that case, the same schedule is followed. However, we are seeing more cases of pertussis. Public health concerns of possible future epidemics are understandable. It is better to be safe than sorry.

Viral vaccines—**measles** (*Rubeola*), **German measles** (*Rubella*), and **mumps** (*infectious parotitis*) are given at 12 to 16 months of age in one injection.

It is my belief that complete vaccinations against tetanus and also polio are extremely important for all children and adults. These diseases are fatal if contracted. Although not common today, both still pose a threat to numerous apparently healthy people. Whooping cough is much less common in this country now, but it is still dangerous in areas where hygiene and sanitation are less assured. Measles, mumps, and German measles are usually mild infections, although some children have developed encephalitis as a complication. It is especially important that a young woman who has not contracted German measles during childhood be vaccinated as a protection against the development of birth defects in her baby, should she later become pregnant.

Vaccination against **tuberculosis**, called the **BCG** (*Bacillus Calmette Guerin*) vaccine, has been used in many countries to protect against tuberculosis. TB experts in the United States believe that the risk of BCG does not justify its use, especially since the skin test converts to positive and becomes invalid for diagnosis or screening after the vaccination has been given. Other vaccinations for travelers to specific tropical countries are recommended just before departure, such as shots for typhoid, paratyphoid, yellow fever, or the temporary passive protection against infectious hepatitis afforded by gamma globulin.

COMMON CHILDHOOD ILLNESSES

Colds

Upper respiratory infections in the baby and young child are very common. Although few of these are caused by bacteria, such as the *Streptococcus* or *diphtheria* organisms, most sore throats are viral infections. More than one hundred different viruses can cause the same syndrome, so there is little likelihood that vaccinations will be developed as preventives. The principal measures that parents can use to prevent troublesome runny noses, sore throats, and similar congestions in their youngsters are the following:

1.   A diet low in refined sugar allows the body to defend itself better against invading germs. The white blood cells are better able to ingest bacteria (called *phagocytosis*) on a low sugar diet and recovery time will be hastened.

2.   A second factor is adequate clothing. In damp or rainy weather, the extremities should be clothes and the feet kept dry. The use of overshoes, raincoats, and umbrellas, although not fashionable with the younger set can definitely help to protect their health and prevent lost days from school for minor illness.

3.   Adequate fluid intake, plenty of rest at night, and some outdoor exercise on a daily basis will help to keep young bodies healthy and prevent colds.

4.   Baths should be terminated with a brief rub down. To improve circulation in the skin use the **cold mitten friction** (Chapter 17) for a minute or so in a cold shower, especially as the child gets older.

5.   A happy disposition also goes a long way toward improving the body's resistance to viral respiratory disease.

If one does take cold, the above measures will still prove healthful. A spare diet for a day with increased bed rest and an abundant supply of fluids aids the body toward a quick recovery. The use of a **vaporizer** by the bedside, usually of the hot steam variety, will increase the flow of mucus and relieve congestion. When bronchitis sets in and a hoarse, raspy cough develops, the vaporizer may make the difference between sleep or a fitful night of coughing with chest pain. Simple **COUGH SYRUPS** can be made at home with **honey**. To one cup of honey add 6 to 8 drops of **eucalyptus oil**, available at most pharmacies. Mix in a tablespoon or two of **lemon juice** for palatability. When this mixture is thoroughly stirred, the *honey-eucalyptus* cough syrup may be taken one teaspoonful at a time every four hours to relieve the discomfort.

A simple remedy for sore throat is the **heating compress** described in Chapter 17. Bacterial **cultures** of the throat should be taken if the fever is high or the soreness unduly prolonged. This is to be sure a *Strep.* infection or *infectious mononucleosis* has not developed. Most viral illnesses are self-limited and quickly cured by alert parents trained in the basics of home nursing.

Earaches

Many emergency room visits are caused by pain in the ear. Sometimes the only sign is a baby's persistent crying, associated with a fever, or the pulling of the ear, indicating that as a source of pain. **Earaches** are usually triggered by the buildup of pressure behind the eardrum. When the *Eustachian tube*, that connects the nose to the middle ear, becomes blocked with mucus, pressure builds up, producing pain, occasionally quite severe. Use a hot water bottle over the ear and the inhalation of steam to open the nasal passages. This can bring relief in the early stages. Several warmed drops of olive oil may be instilled into the ear canal carefully, and retained in place with a small tuft of cotton. Replace the ear drops every few hours. This also assists in relieving this uncomfortable symptom. Most earaches subside within hours to days. It is rare that a complicating bacterial infection or rupture of the drum makes surgical treatment necessary. Persistent high fever or increasing pain after several hours of intensive treatment should prompt a visit to the doctor.

Nosebleeds

At certain seasons of the year, children seem to be particularly prone to nosebleeds. This may occur after picking the nose or introducing a foreign body into one nostril. More commonly it is associated with allergies, in which the prolonged sneezing and irritated mucous membranes provoke one of the small veins to break. Pressure on the nostril, with the use of an ice pack will control most nosebleeds. If there is a bleeding disease, such as hemophilia, leukemia, or the blood pressure is abnormally high, sudden nosebleeds may be difficult to control.

If rest, pressure, and ice do not suffice to control the bleeding, the patient should be seen by a physician. An examination with improved lighting and suction available may be necessary to determine the source of the bleeding and allow the offending vessel to be cauterized. Local anesthetics and antibacterial precautions are valuable. It may even be necessary to pack the nose to control the more severe hemorrhages.

Swimmer's Ear

Infection of the outer ear canal typically results from participation in water sports. Although it may occur under other conditions, the main predisposing factor to *otitis externa* is residual moisture in the ear canal. In such case, pain is localized to the outer ear, and aggravated by pulling on the external portion. A watery or mucus-like drainage is seen in the canal, while the drum is seldom inflamed. Fortunately, hearing is unimpaired. The exudate material should be cleaned out thoroughly to allow the ear canal to dry. The use of **Burroughs' solution** (*sodium aluminum acetate*, available at any pharmacy) and specially made ear drops helps to kill or control any bacteria or fungi that are present.

Alternating hot and cold compresses are most helpful in reducing the swelling and pain associated with this condition. If it is necessary to visit a physician, he will usually take a culture and insert a cotton yarn "wick" with special medication to aid in the relief of pain. This procedure helps accelerate the healing process. To prevent swimmer's ear, after bathing in a public pool or lake, instill a few drops of *hydrogen peroxide* in each ear canal. If this is unavailable, a small quantity of warmed rubbing alcohol may be used. This aids in drying the ears that otherwise tend to retain moisture and thus prevent frequently recurring infections.

Bronchitis

A deep cough persisting in the chest may herald the onset of **bronchitis**. Inflammation of the bronchial tubes, if left untreated, may develop into **pneumonia**, a more serious pulmonary infection. Early treatment of bronchitis is important, with bed rest and the frequent application of fomentations to the chest. Chapter 17 describes the routine I have used successfully to alleviate the chest pain of bronchial irritation and quell the cough as quickly as possible. The *honey–eucalyptus* cough syrup, mentioned earlier in this chapter, may be helpful in reducing bronchial irritation. Try to avoid drying agents, such as antihistamines or decongestants. These drugs will make it difficult for the mucus to rise and be expectorated. A warm steam vaporizer by the bedside helps aid expectoration of the mucus. It should be kept going at all times until the cough has improved and the symptoms of fever or headache are alleviated.

Gastroenteritis

Nearly all viruses and bacterial toxins that cause intestinal upset are self-limited infections. However, in certain underdeveloped nations there are people who have a high infant mortality even yet from diarrhea infections of infancy. Two important principles must be remembered when a baby starts vomiting. First, provide an adequate fluid intake. Dehydration may develop quickly in a baby, unless fluid replacement is promptly administered. Many babies who develop diarrhea can still breast feed without difficulty. Some who are vomiting may be able to tolerate breast milk or an electrolyte mixture, while ordinary formula and solid foods are rejected. A simple **electrolyte mixture** in the home can be made with the following formula: Three tablespoons of *sugar*, 1/2 teaspoon of *salt*, 1/2 teaspoon of *potassium bicarbonate* (obtained from your pharmacy) and 1 quart of pure *water*. This or similar commercial electrolyte mixtures (*Pedialyte*) should be given as often as thirst requires to maintain hydration, while the stomach and intestinal upset gradually subsides.

Second, **Fever** always increases the fluid requirement, as does profound sweating. When diarrhea becomes more serious, as in *cholera* or *bacillary dysentery*, the drastic fluid needs may require the addition of intravenous fluids. Prolonged vomiting with dehydration or *diabetic ketoacidosis* may represent conditions where oral fluids cannot be tolerated. In such case a short hospital stay for intravenous therapy becomes necessary.

Later, it is frequently possible to add antidiarrheal mixtures, such as Kaopectate or the use of capsules of powdered **activated charcoal**, prepared in a *"slurry"* solution. This is accomplished by mixing about 2 tablespoons of charcoal powder in a glass of water and sipping the suspension or drinking it through a straw. The charcoal, in these diarrheas, *adsorbs* most toxins and reduces the inflammation along the mucous lining of the bowel. This is an excellent remedy for *tourista*, the diarrhea of international travelers. Muscle cramps in the abdomen can be relieved by applying hot moist compresses, a heating pad, or hot water bottle. Bed rest should be continued until the symptoms subside and recovery is complete.

Specific problems related to infectious bacteria and their unique clinical features are described in Chapter 3. The convalescence from diarrhea of an infectious nature, can be hastened by a wise, gradual transition to normal foods. Use diluted cereals, such as cream of wheat, oatmeal, rice water. Vegetable broth, applesauce, milk toast, and other bland foods may also hasten the recovery and avoid irritating the intestinal tract until it is healed. Sometimes a temporary *lactose intolerance* results from the gastrointestinal infection, making it advisable to avoid any cow's milk except yogurt for a time. Fried or greasy foods and spices, carbonated or caffeine beverages, and concentrated sweets should be eliminated for the most rapid healing to occur.

Worms

Children typically put their fingers in the mouth. Close contact in schoolrooms and families, as well as sharing dishes and towels, also encourage the development of parasitic infections. In the United States the commonest type of infestation is *pinworms*. This causes itching around the anus, and may lead to considerable irritation and scratching, even during sleep. In actuality, the female pinworm customarily migrates through the intestinal tract to irritate the anal opening during sleep.

Pinworm eggs can be obtained with a piece of *Scotch tape* applied to the anus (sticky side down) early in the morning, before defecation or bathing has occurred. The tape is then placed on a glass slide, which is examined through the microscope, revealing the characteristic appearance of the pinworm eggs. Most other parasitic infestations either produce no symptoms at all in the early stages or exhibit vague ache and pains, failure to grow, anemia, or general lassitude, headache, and weight loss.

An **examination** of the stool under the microscope can detect each type of parasite eggs. Their recognition provides specific guidelines for proper therapy. Specific infestations and their treatment are described in Chapter 3. There are obvious preventive measures such as hygienic food preparation, hand washing, the wearing of shoes, and purification of drinking water. Many parasites respond to purgatives that completely cleanse the intestinal tract, associated with deworming medication. Garlic in high doses, such as six capsules or three cloves a day, may work well. However, resistant cases should be evaluated by a physician and appropriately treated to prevent family spread and chronic illness.

Urinary Infections

Usually it is little girls who develop infections of the urinary tract. The closeness of the urethra to the anus is the principal reason for this. Mothers should early teach their little daughters how to cleanse themselves after going to the toilet. Wiping the perineum should be done from front to back in order to avoid contaminating the urethra and vagina with germs present from the stool. Careful hygiene may require special washing with soap and water after a movement. Drink an abundance of fresh soft water. It also helps to keep the kidneys cleansed. If a relaxed atmosphere surrounds the **toilet training** process and copious water drinking is encouraged, your child will have a healthful preventive to infections which otherwise could damage the kidneys for life.

The usual symptoms of urinary tract infection are burning or irritation with urination. These may be associated with vaginal discharge, fever, or back pain over the kidneys. You can find in most pharmacies a urine testing dipstick to analyze the specimen for infection. Urine examinations with the microscope can demonstrate the presence of bacteria and pus. The urine culture provides further guide to appropriate treatment. Make the urine acidic with *cranberry juice* or supplemental *Vitamin C* (500 mg. four times a day). This will help to eliminate bladder germs by inhibiting their multiplication in the bladder. The *hippuric acid* in **cranberries** also helps to decrease bacterial adhesiveness to the bladder wall. Hot and cold sitz baths, hot half baths or moist heating packs (as described in Chapter 17) over the kidney areas help to increase urine flow and white blood cell defenses in the area.

Constipation

Occasionally, the pediatrician will see a child who simply refuses to move his or her bowels. Usually this is a psychological problem. **Obstipation**, as it is called, could accompany a difficult toilet training process, in which punitive measures or ridicule were used to reinforce the parent's desires. A carefully performed rectal exam with the little finger will help to rule out the presence of a congenital obstruction. Further examination with a *sigmoidoscope* or a *barium enema* x-ray may be needed to exclude a congenital deformity or acute disease. Proper **toilet training** may then begin in a relaxed way. Rarely, stool softeners are necessary to increase the ease of elimination. Psyllium seed, flax seed, and bran, all provide a natural lubrication and softening. Most of these items are available at a pharmacy or supermarket.

Regularity of bowel function is very important. After a meal, such as breakfast or dinner, the urge is often present and should be responded to promptly. The toilet training atmosphere must be relaxed and private, with punitive measures studiously avoided. Difficult cases may require medical counsel. The earlier this problem can be solved the healthier teen and later years will be, for the bowel habits of childhood tend to perpetuate themselves into adult life.

Miscellaneous Conditions

The reader is referred to Chapter 9 for discussion of common skin rashes present in babies and children. The **Appendix** contains several formulas for treating common skin conditions. It should be helpful to every parent dealing with these problems. Allergic diseases of children are discussed in Chapter 10. Sections there include the common childhood problems of asthma, food allergies, and various types of eczema.

Headache is a symptom common to school-age children. Although not a disease itself, this symptom warrants investigation and, when possible, removing all known causes. Most headache in childhood are related to **tension**, often reflecting pressures at school, interpersonal conflicts at home, or deep inner security and its need for expression. A warm sympathetic attitude on the part of parents is important to win the confidence of children. When security is lacking in the home, youth usually turn to peer groups, whose advice is often unreliable.

De-emphasize the "miracle drug" approach to pain relief before your children. Parents themselves can set the example, analyzing rationally and treating physiologically their own health annoyances as they occur. Extra water intake, hot tub baths, and "early to bed and early to rise" are habits that can quickly remove the headache. The pain is then soon forgotten. The *hot foot bath* is helpful. More importantly, a firm trust in God through a personal experience in prayer can prepare the child for the "vicissitudes of life," developing in him or her a headache-resistant personality.

Since vision is critical for normal learning in the child, any pain in the eyes demands immediate attention. **Eyestrain** is a common cause for headache. It has been increasingly associated with the early exposure of a child to reading when his constitution is not yet ready for the challenge. Many children who wear glasses can trace their nearsightedness back to the early reading classes that should have been postponed until age 8 or 10. Contemporary urgency to send *Johnny* off to school at age 4 or 5 for a "head start" program, followed by kindergarten, then the competition of the first grades only invite problems of emotional adjustment, premature eyestrain, and physical symptoms. Most can be avoided by delayed entrance into school.

Infections of the eye are not uncommon in childhood. Some newborns have a discharge from their eyes. It is traced to injury or rubbing of the eyes, and the introduction of antibiotics or silver nitrate drops required by the public health departments to prevent newborn *gonorrhea*. This material can be removed from the eyes with a warm soft washcloth. If excessive, hot saline compresses several times a day will clear the condition quickly. Make them using one half teaspoon of table salt in an eight ounce glass of hot water. Zinc sulfate (0.2%) drops, although innocuous to the baby's eyes, will help to clear this *conjunctivitis* when it is resistant to the above measures.

Pink eye in childhood is quite contagious. It is usually caused by a *Hemophilus* organism (See Chapter 3). The childhood conjunctivitis can be spread from one eye to the other, and to other children by rubbing the irritated part with the hands. Careful hand washing, combined with frequent hot saline compresses, or the use of a *charcoal poultice* placed over the eyes (See Chapter 17) will clear the infection in its early stages without requiring antibiotics. Avoid undue irritation in order for these simple remedies to do their best job.

Finally, let us consider the **foot problems** of children. Many infants are born with a tendency for the toes to point in or out. Sometimes this appears as an inward curving of the foot itself (called *metatarsus valgus*). This usually requires corrective shoes. Some infant's feet can straighten with normal growth, while the parents reverse the left and right shoes on the feet, doing this each day for several months.

The *night splint*, which maintains the child's feet in shoes at a prescribed angle, can be used to correct unusual **outward** pointing of the feet. This must be worn for several months in order to be effective. Pigeon-toed children are usually treated with a *Thomas heel*, which provides a slight inner wedge to direct the foot outward, placed on the shoe when walking begins. From one to two years of age, this special orthopedic heel can help to straighten the gait and enable running to develop smoothly later on. "Bow legs" and "knock knees" in children are usually self-correcting and only rarely require orthopedic evaluation.

The most serious foot deformity is the **clubfoot** (called *talipes equinovarus*). It usually requires a series of corrective casts or surgical procedures to straighten the feet and enable gait training to proceed normally. An orthopedist should be consulted.

213

THE CHILD IN THE HOSPITAL

A baby in the hospital feels keenly the mother's absence. The unfamiliar surroundings, combined with procedures that may be painful, create constant fear and apprehension. The taking of blood samples, preparation for surgery, dressing changes, or confinement in cribs or mist tents all elicit emotional responses hard to define. It is not unusual for a child, hospitalized the first time, to regress in his or her toilet habits, eating preferences, and dependencies. If possible, it is best for a parent, usually the mother, to stay with her child during the period of hospitalization. When a rooming-in arrangement can be secured, the hospital stay can be made as pleasant as possible with stories, puzzles, games, and most important, the presence of someone who loves him or her most.

Surgery presents another challenge to the child. Lacking complete understanding of the exact reasons for and techniques of the contemplated procedure, a child often develops fantasies and fears that are difficult to understand. Drawings or dolls can be used to illustrate the anticipated surgery, providing support and understanding to lessen the child's fear. Spiritual resources available to parents and children at times like this help also to allay any fear of disfigurement, pain, or death that often accompanies entrance into the hospital. A frank discussion by the physician or surgeon, as well as the nursing team, is of great significance to inspire trust and confidence.

Postoperative convalescence can be hastened with the presence of parents and familiar objects from home. Stuffed animals, favorite toys, or pictures can be brought to make the hospital room seem as much as possible like the child's household domain. Unless contraindicated by the nature of the illness, some catering in regard to favorite foods will assist the rapid return of appetite. Do everything possible to facilitate the cheerful adjustment to the strangeness of hospital routine. As much as possible rest at night should be undisturbed. Too many visitors and flowers should be discouraged. As soon as feasible, resume normal activities with return to school. It will likely bring the transient emotional changes to an end, as health is restored.

Any child with a terminal illness presents the greatest challenge. Youngsters with leukemia, malignant cancers, or advanced cardiac disease often "understand" better than their parents. Many become willing to discuss the approach of a fatal outcome. At such times, it is exceptionally important to discuss the future in a candid, yet sympathetic way. Spiritual support and a strong trust in God, with continued presence of devoted parents, will ease the approaching pain of separation, while clasping to a hope of future reunion should final "farewells" be required.

CHILDHOOD HABITS

It is well said that "**thoughts lead to actions; actions repeated form habits; and habits determine character**." Many actions are repeated during childhood, some good, others detrimental. Some of the more common habits creating concern in parents will be discussed here.

Thumb sucking is one of the commonest habits of early infancy. It is thought to be normal by some psychologists. This habit often indicates a need for oral gratification and contact with something human. In the early months of life it does no harm, if the hands are clean. Thumb sucking prolonged into later childhood and school years is a source of embarrassment, as the peer group makes fun of any child so habituated. Dental development is additionally affected, with the tendency toward protrusion of the incisors (*buck teeth*). Security gained in other ways, with a gentle education away from the habit is generally able to "wean" the reasonable child.

Bed wetting or *enuresis* is another distressing problem, particularly to school-age children. When this habit is prolonged after age three it deserves gentle but corrective measures. Usually there is no anatomic problem in the urinary tract. Stress factors and psychic tensions appear to be the commonest underlying cause. Inner security combined with an avoidance of undue attention will bring help to most of those affected. The use of antidepressant drugs or stimulants should be positively avoided.

Restrict fluids at bedtime, with rewards such as stars on a calendar for dry nights, may provide the motivation for mild cases. Avoid shaming the child or drawing undue attention to his or her failures by corporal punishment. Electrical devices are available for some difficult cases, but are not universally successful. Usually the problem subsides spontaneously. Some children have found that sleeping on a very hard bed or even on the floor aids in the bed-wetting situation when excessively deep sleep is a factor. If persevering efforts are unsuccessful by age six to eight, a physician should be consulted to thoroughly test for anatomic disease.

Stammering or **stuttering** is very common in the school-age child. Occasionally this results from starting the child to school too early. It may be eliminated by keeping the youngster at home another year or two. The pressure and tensions of the schoolroom may be an inciting factor. Usually thought to be a nervous habit, stuttering is amenable to speech correction when the therapist is a calm, supportive, understanding person. Patience on the part of parents and gently nonpunitive correction of the speech disorder will usually succeed in retraining the speech.

Genital exploration is not uncommon among small children. The attempt to understand their anatomy should be of no concern to parents when it is seen casually in very young children. Boys and girls early in life notice the difference between themselves. Sexual identity should be established at an early age. The wearing of different clothes for boys and girls—such as, pants vs.

215

dresses, helps to establish this identity and aids the development of male or female personality in a healthful direction.

Persistence in the manipulation of the genital organs or habitual stimulation is defined as *masturbation*. Sometimes called *self abuse*, this habit has been linked by many health writers to long-term health problems. Just as all violations of natural law have their penalties, the unnatural habit of masturbation will affect greatly the developing personality. Promoting sexual desire, including in some the tendency toward homosexuality, the effects of this practice are pernicious. Those who continue the practice during adolescence often develop a habit pattern, which is almost impossible to break.

The most current explanation of these health hazards involves **zinc** metabolism. Of all body fluids, semen is the richest in zinc. The prostate gland secretes a fluid which is high in this trace mineral. With frequent sexual stimulation, whether masturbation or another sensual activity, there is rapid loss of body zinc stores, approximately what can be absorbed from the intestines in one day! When the dietary zinc is marginal, and true zinc deficiency results, many health problems develop, including impotence. Dr. Carl C. Pfeiffer Ph.D., M.D. went even farther to state in his book *Zinc and Other Micro-Nutrients*, "We hate to say it, but in a zinc-deficient adolescent, sexual excitement and excessive masturbation might precipitate insanity."

It is this author's clinical impression that adolescents, who have continued with frequent habitual self abuse, may set the stage for diseases later in life. The immune system is especially impaired. Infections of the liver and lungs, neuralgia, rheumatism, diseased kidneys, and even cancerous conditions can possibly be traced back to the unconquered habit of masturbation. Mental depression and complete breakdowns are not uncommonly seen in these patients.

For the child caught in the grip of this self indulgence there is still a ray of hope. Hard physical labor and closer contact with parents is a substantial aid to the child struggling to conquer the habit of self abuse. A nonstimulating diet, avoiding spices, caffeinated beverages, a high intake of sugar, and even meat and eggs will aid the child in recovery. He must shun all fantasy on lustful themes portrayed in popular magazines, television, and theater to help in developing a pure mind that is invaluable to health of the body. Cold sitz baths and the avoidance of much time in the hot showers may also help. Perineal hygiene is essential. Spiritual counseling should not be neglected.

ADOLESCENCE AND PUBERTY

The teenage years are often turbulent ones. Changes that begin in the preteen find full-blown expression in the adolescent. Girls develop earlier than boys. They begin at age 11 or 12 with *budding* of the breasts. The development of hair growth in the pubic and axillary region is next. This is followed by other secondary sex characteristics. The growth in height, as well as a developing feminine body are precursors to the actual time of **menarche**. This date marks the beginning of menstruation. It has been arriving earlier in girls in Western cultures. In comparison with many Orientals, who begin menstruating at age 15 or 16, the average American girl menstruates at 12 years. I believe this to be related to the increased protein (especially meat, containing steroid hormones) in the Western diet, as well as the general acceleration of maturity that popular education and entertainment seems to foster.

Associated with these changes, a growing preoccupation with "the boys" often transpires. Wise parents will seek as long as possible to preserve the simple loyalties of childhood in their young teenagers and foster **family** activities, parental togetherness, and close supervision of sports and recreation. Interest in studies and home duties are a great safeguard against the moral depravity and unhealthful practices creeping into high schools, colleges, and universities—even Christian ones.

Young men mature a year or two later than their feminine counterparts. The growth spurt usually begins around 13 to 15 years of age, but occasionally comes even later. Sometimes a young boy will grow 2 to 4 inches in one year! The voice changes with a humorous (to others) break of pitch (called *falsetto*) right during mid sentence. It becomes quite embarrassing to the awkward earliteen.

Muscular development, strength and athletic ability, as well as other secondary sexual characteristics (whiskers and beard) are a frequent source of pride, tempting many youth to "show off." Tendencies to hazardous driving practices, risky athletics, daredevil stunts, and excessive play should be discouraged by serious parents, who really want their bright star to shine some day. A part-time job, household chores, and encouragement in study and spiritual growth can be fostered in a close-knit family setting.

If it becomes necessary for young boys or girls to leave home and live in a school dormitory, their roommates and close associates should be chosen with care. With drug abuse and sexual permissiveness becoming increasingly common, any serious devoted parents should spare no pains to bring their young people up in the *"nurture and admonition of the Lord."* The rewards to youth, as well as to society are compelling indeed.

CHAPTER SIXTEEN

DISEASES

OF

DIGESTION

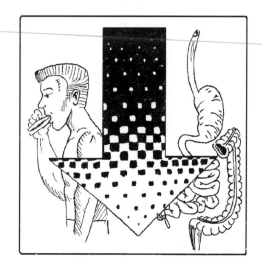

The system of the body dealing with digestion of foods includes all of the related structures in the mouth, such as the **teeth**, **salivary glands**, and **taste buds**. It extends down through the **esophagus**, the **stomach**, the small and large **intestines**, and includes three *accessory* but equally essential organs, the **pancreas**, the **liver**, and the **gallbladder**. A great many infectious, degenerative, and malignant disorders can develop in these highly specialized, yet diversified organs.

Congenital problems involving the intestinal tract or trauma may affect the digestive system. The more common problems, however, are related to our lifestyle, particularly the diet. In some people, the digestive system constitutes the target organ for stress, reacting to built-up tension with pain, vomiting, or diarrhea. Most of the proprietary medications available at any pharmacy are marketed for disorders of digestion, including antacids, laxatives, and dental aids. I plan to look at some of the problems that afflict this most interesting body system, in a way that can be both preventive and therapeutic.

Dental Caries

The **teeth** are valuable for nutrition as well as appearance, being normally absent only in newborn babies. Heralding the interest and need for solid foods, tooth eruption begins at five to six months of age. This continues until the "baby teeth" or *decidual* set, with a complement of twenty, are all in place. Five or six years later the incisors begin to loosen and are gradually replaced over the next six years with the *permanent* set of teeth. A complete ᵊntal set in the adult would have thirty–two teeth, paired "uppers and lowers" as follows: four incisors, two canine teeth, four premolars, and six molars. The third molars, which come in last are sometimes called "wisdom teeth." In many modern Americans the crowded jaw conditions which resulted from poor nutrition require their removal. Because 30% of Americans "outlive" their teeth, the cost of dental care is tremendous. Tooth decay is a problem to be studied by everyone concerned with the prevention of disease.

The tooth is not dead, as many think, but is actually a live structure requiring a constant blood supply. It has many delicately sensitive nerves. In fact, you can easily detect a small grain of sand between your teeth. Sad to say, **dental decay** (called *caries*) often begins in childhood. Drinking cola beverages and other soft drinks, with the free use of candy and between-meal snacks sets the stage for the development of dental decay, beginning in the preschool years.

Bacteria present in the mouth normally cause little damage, unless there is a high intake of sugar. Bacterial *fermentation* of sugar produces an acid which erodes the sensitive enamel of the tooth surface. As a pocket or **cavity** is formed, bacterial action further destroys the tooth until invasion of the pulp produces acute pain, and an abscess develops. Research in the past two decades has also shown the protective benefit of *fluoride* in the diet as well as drinking water. As little as one part per million in the water supply, will enhance the resistance to dental caries, even when the diet is not good. Over three parts per million of fluoride, however, causes *mottling* of the enamel. So the tolerances are small. Although I commend the efforts of public health authorities to improve the dental situation, there is no question that diet is the major factor in a promotion of dental health.

Proper **brushing and flossing** of the teeth is also valuable to remove food particles and prevent the build-up of *plaque*. At least every twenty-four hours the teeth should be brushed, preferably with soft bristles, in order to remove a small film that forms after eating. If it is not removed, the base of each tooth will gradually harden and calcify (forming what we call *plaque*). Plaque formation is one of the major causes of **pyorrhea** (or *periodontitis*) that eventually, if untreated, will loosen the tooth and infect the surrounding tissues.

Flossing the teeth involves cleaning between them with a special type of string or tape. If done properly, this will remove small particles of food that lodge there and aid in the fight against decay. Regular checkups by a dentist and prompt treatment of cavities is important to prevent tooth loss. When dental destruction is complete, it requires the more expensive and troublesome *dentures*. So for dollar savings, looks, and especially function, it is well worth preserving our permanent teeth.

Swallowing Problems

Difficulty in swallowing is not common but is very troublesome. At all ages this may occur. A newborn baby who experiences difficulty in swallowing should be carefully evaluated for a possible **congenital** deformity. An abnormal connection called a *tracheoesophageal fistula*, between the esophagus and the windpipe may lead to *aspiration pneumonia* or even death. Congenital *webs* in the esophagus may obstruct swallowing. Some babies are even born with failure of esophageal development (*atresia*). Correction of this disorder requires surgery.

Children who accidentally or intentionally swallow *caustic* materials, such as hydrocarbons, lye, or strong acids may develop **stricture** of the esophagus. This narrowing and scarring usually occurs where the esophagus joins the stomach, but may produce symptoms higher in the chest or neck, including a feeling of fullness or frequent regurgitation. Fluoroscopic observation of a *barium swallow* is essential to establish the diagnosis. It is necessary to dilate a strictured esophagus with the passage of mercury-filled tubes (*bougies*) for several weeks to prevent further scarring or complete obstruction.

Swallowing difficulties in middle to later years of life may be caused by a problem in muscular peristalsis (*motility*). This may produce the characteristic painful spasm in the chest that occurs when a large chunk of food is accidentally swallowed. At all ages it is extremely important to **masticate** the food well to aid digestion, especially the smooth passage of food from mouth to stomach. Large amounts of liquids should not be taken with the meals. Rather, thorough chewing mingles saliva with the food, allowing it to slide smoothly down the esophagus. Food should not be washed down. Moreover, it is important to avoid "greasing the chute" with overusage of fats or margarine.

Excessive gastric acid and its stimulation caused by caffeine drinks tends to relax the sphincter muscle at the lower end of the esophagus, allowing regurgitation of stomach contents to occur. Symptoms of **heartburn** are then noted. If hydrochloric acid is allowed to remain within the lower esophagus, it sets up an irritation (*esophagitis*) that may even lead to permanent scarring. In an older individual any persistent difficulty in swallowing, especially associated with weight loss, should prompt a careful search to discover the cause. **Cancer** may develop in the lower esophagus, which all too often is inoperable, almost 95% fatal by the time it is discovered. The avoidance of tobacco, alcohol, and irritating foods is preventive for this serious malignancy.

Gastritis

Inflammation of the stomach, or **gastritis**, is quite common. Symptoms of acute gastritis, especially nausea and vomiting, may appear suddenly. They are usually caused by toxins produced by infectious organisms. **Staphylococcal food poisoning** is one type that runs its course within a few hours. Chronic forms of gastritis are seen in alcohol users, where the toxic effect of beverage alcohol produces a gradual thinning and drying of the gastric mucus membrane. Associated with this, not infrequently, is the high level of acid secretion indicative of **peptic ulcer**. Certain *atrophic* forms of gastritis may produce the opposite effect, namely the absence of gastric acid and *intrinsic factor*. It is responsible for the absorption of **Vitamin B$_{12}$** by the small intestine. *Pernicious anemia* will develop, with its characteristic blood picture and neurologic signs.

Treatment usually requires the lifelong administration of monthly vitamin **B$_{12}$** injections to replace this essential vitamin. Although some doctors advocate a *bland* diet for the treatment of gastritis, it is really only necessary to avoid irritating substances. Tobacco, alcohol, coffee, cola drinks, spices, condiments, and corrosive drugs should be eliminated, giving the stomach an optimum chance to heal itself and restore normal levels of enzymes essential for the digestion of protein. Moist heat applications over the stomach area can relieve pain and spasm. Avoiding extremely hot or cold drinks will allow the stomach, with its marvelous regenerating powers, to heal, often within days.

Hiatus Hernia

Discussed already in Chapter 12, **hiatus hernia** is an increasing problem in western civilization. A widespread American habit is the consumption of very large quantities of food, especially near bedtime, and drinking several cups of liquid with each meal. This chronic over-distention of the stomach weakens the sphincter at its upper end and tends toward *acid reflux*. Regurgitation of this sour and slightly irritating material is aggravated by obesity, tight belts, girdles, and stooping, bending or lying down immediately after a full meal. X-rays of the upper intestinal tract help to confirm the diagnosis, Corrective dietary measures must avoid the above "causes." Occasionally the use of elevating blocks at the head of the bed, will control nighttime heartburn for most people.

Peptic Ulcer

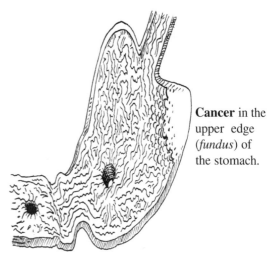

Ulcers in the stomach and duodenum are quite common in alcoholics, slow to heal in smokers, and occasionally are caused by aspirin and similar irritating drugs. However, it is my belief that most cases of peptic ulcer have their root in the **stress** mechanism. It is generally established that ulcers do not form in the absence of gastric acid. On the other hand, even spicy stimulating diets may not be associated with ulcer formation. Profiles of the so-called "ulcer-prone personality" characterizes him or her

Cancer in the upper edge (*fundus*) of the stomach.

Ulcers of the *duodenum* and *stomach*.

as intense, competitive, easily upset, and one who internalizes many pent–up emotions. Gastric analysis often shows high levels of acid secretion.

Factors that damage the protective mucous membrane that safeguards the stomach lining are spices, such as *eugenol* in cloves, *cinnamic aldehyde* in cinnamon, and *piperadine*, the primary irritant in black pepper. Repeatedly coupled with borderline vitamin deficiency, an irritating highly spiced diet will frequently produce an irritable person. Thus, the stage is set for peptic ulcer. In evaluating the cause of this unhappy problem, you should never overlook the influence of drugs. Some of the most common medications that produce ulcers are aspirin, cortisone and its synthetic derivatives (methylprednisolone, prednisone, Medrol, etc.); indomethacin (Indocin), phenylbutazone (Butazolidine); and related classes of non-steroidal anti-inflammatory— NSAID—preparations (ibuprofen, Advil, Motrin, Voltarin, etc.), all used in the treatment of arthritis. Nearly any drug, however, can irritate the stomach, and these should be suspected whenever there is pain.

The **symptoms** of peptic ulcer can be confusing. Usually the burning pain is located over the stomach, slightly to the right of the midline. Pressure in this area aggravates the pain. Symptoms are relieved by food, and usually by antacid preparations. After coating the ulcer, and providing temporary relief, the pain returns. Large ulcers may be painful, persistent, and disabling. Complications, such as obstruction, perforation, and hemorrhage are infrequent, but normally require surgery as described in Chapter 12. Most cases, however, can be handled by strict attention to dietary wisdom and more effective stress coping mechanisms.

Many physicians refuse to treat a person with peptic ulcer who continues to use cigarettes. It is essential to abstain from all tobacco and alcohol. Alcohol stimulates acid secretion, while tobacco interferes with acid neutralization. Coffee and other forms of caffeine also increase acid production, aggravating the tendency to ulcer disease. Spices and condiments gradually erode the mucous protective lining of the stomach and increase the susceptibility to damage by the acid and pepsin present in the gastric glands. Emotional tension must be relieved with periods of meditation, exercise, adequate rest, and the cultivation of a tranquil, accepting personality. Spiritual renewal and prayer are all essentials in achieving this state of peaceful digestion essential to health.

Antacids, although popularly used, do not possess curative powers. Neutralization of the acid can be done in alternate more physiologic ways. Small amounts of food, particularly those high in fat content, such as avocados and olives, are helpful to the digestion. They retard acid production, as well as gastric emptying. High protein diets and acid fruits are usually avoided in the acute stages. Vegetable juices are preferable. Liquids on the cool side tend to reduce gastric secretions more than do hot drinks. On the other hand, because of reflex connection to the autonomic nervous system, moist hot packs over the stomach can reduce acid secretion, as well as give a splendid pain relief. These should not be prolonged, but may be used frequently through the day. Within a few weeks, in all but the complicated cases, symptoms will subside. Healing is usually complete.

Malabsorption

Selectivity in absorbing nutrients is one of the most important characteristics of the human intestine. A newborn baby has the ability to absorb many large protein molecules. This is one of the reasons why antibody protection is secured from the mother's *colostrum*, the early form of milk. For this reason, the early introduction of solid foods should be discouraged. Absorption of too many complex proteins can set the stage for food allergies that last a lifetime.

Once digestive integrity has been established in infancy the intestinal absorption is quite specific. Proteins must be broken down to amino acids, fats to fatty acids, and carbohydrates to the simple six-carbon sugars—glucose, fructose, and galactose. Absorption of these end-products of digestion requires adequate amounts of specific enzymes. Please refer to Chapter 23 for a review of this digestive physiology, essential to understanding the problems that may result in malabsorption.

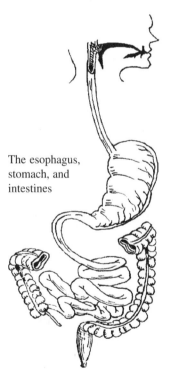

The esophagus, stomach, and intestines

One common defect in the absorption of carbohydrate is a deficiency in the enzyme *lactase*. Other *disaccharides*, less commonly, acquire deficiencies of their final splitting enzyme. In typical **disaccharidase deficiency** there is a failure to split lactose into its simpler sugars, galactose and glucose. Lactic acid accumulates, and bacterial fermentation rapidly follows. This produces cramps, bloating, or diarrhea. It is reported, in fact, that 60 to 90% of the Black and Oriental races have *lactase* deficiency. This is likewise present in Caucasians, but to a lesser extent. For this reason many people avoid milk in adult life and get along very well. Others follow popular customs or childhood patterns and do not realize that their increased flatulence and diarrhea are due to a hereditary problem. An accurate diagnosis, followed by elimination of milk from the diet relieves symptoms completely.

Sprue is another type of malabsorption. The *nontropical* variety, in recent years, has been identified as a hypersensitivity to wheat, hence is called *gluten enteropathy*. It is characterized by foul smelling stools, nutritional deficiencies, and diarrhea. Fortunately, the condition entirely clears when wheat is eliminated from the diet. Intestinal biopsies are sometimes used to confirm the diagnosis, but diet therapy is "curative."

Temporary malabsorptive states are seen after bouts with gastrointestinal infection. Certain antibiotics, most notably *Clindamycin* have been associated with the development of malabsorption. The *fish tapeworm* can induce malabsorption, with the development of B$_{12}$ deficiency. Certain similar states may occur after partial removal of the stomach, and some other intestinal operations. Less common causes of malabsorption must be diagnosed with *intestinal biopsies*, with special diets prescribed to improve the patient's nutrition.

Regional Enteritis

Crohn's disease, or *regional enteritis*, affects primarily young adults. Characterized clinically by episodes of diarrhea, cramps, and occasional intestinal bleeding, this problem resists most attempts with natural therapy. The cause is unknown. A granuloma formation gradually develops in the small intestine, occasionally producing obstruction. Numerous operations may be required to relieve the obstruction and remove involved portions of the small intestine. A relationship to stress and emotional tension has been seen in many of these patients.

I have observed beneficial results on numerous occasions with the prolonged use of hydrotherapy treatments, using hot and cold contrast over the abdomen. Careful elimination diets select out any foods to which the individual is sensitive. Persistence in adhering to a strict pattern of eating, eliminating allergenic foods, spices, and undesirable foreign chemicals may arrest the progress, or at least control the symptoms.

Colitis

A more common inflammation of the bowel is **ulcerative colitis**. Affecting children, as well as adults, this inflammatory change involves the colon, with gradual development of shallow ulcers and episodes of cramping pain, diarrhea, and rectal bleeding. As in gastric ulcer, association with stress has been prominent, and the disease termed a *psychosomatic* one. We do not know whether use of antibiotics, other drugs or chemicals are involved in the production of colitis, though this is often suggested. The disease tends to run a chronic recurring course with diarrhea predominating. A change of occupation may become necessary. Modern drug therapy for this condition is rarely curative. Cortisone steroids in particular tend to borrow upon the body's reserves elsewhere to control the symptoms. Specific causative factors should always be investigated and dietary measures strictly followed to control this disease.

Treatment requires a tranquil, peaceful lifestyle in order to effectuate a complete cure. Adequate dietary fiber should be encouraged, with the avoidance of irritating foods such as spices and seeds which might be sharp or erosive. Avoid any food to which the individual shows sensitivity. Thoroughly chew the food, and use fruits at one meal and vegetables at the next. Cultivate a tendency toward simplicity in the diet. It will usually prove most rewarding.

Hydrotherapeutic measures are indispensable to control the pain. Prolonging the colitis beyond eight or ten years has been shown to increase the risk of cancer in the colon. Preventive care may rarely require a *colectomy*. For this and other reasons, medical consultation should be periodically sought during the chronic bout with colitis.

Irritated Colon Syndrome

A much more common and often confused condition is the **irritable colon syndrome** or *spastic colitis*. I prefer the term "irritated" colon for reasons described below. The symptoms usually occur in episodes. Watery diarrhea alternates with periods of painful constipation. There is extreme spasm in the colon, most often on the left side. The colon may become tender, but fever and inflammation are not striking. Excessive mucous production may produce an alteration in the color of the stool. Most typically the irritated colon syndrome is seen in individuals who are always "on the go," tense, anxious, and often too hurried to regularly move their bowels. The diet in such patients is frequently refined, with inadequate fiber to give good intestinal tone.

One most important measure in treating the irritated colon is reassurance concerning its benign nature. *Sigmoidoscopic* examination and a *barium enema* x-ray are needed to be sure that there is no cancer or other disease. Negative diagnostic findings and a typical history makes the diagnosis likely. The diet should be high in fiber, with the addition of one or two tablespoons of bran daily. An abundant use of fruit and vegetables will improve the bowel habits and normalize the transit time, reducing the frequency of both diarrhea and constipation. Adequate fluid intake and a more relaxed attitude toward life are quite beneficial. Hot packs over the abdomen should be used to relieve spasm. Stimulants and condiments should be avoided. Drugs that alter the intestinal tone, tranquilizers, and laxatives should also be eliminated, as they tend to perpetuate the situation. Usually, with appropriate remedial measures, this condition can be stabilized. It is compatible with a normal life span.

Hemorrhoids

Although I discussed the treatment of **hemorrhoids** in Chapter 12, additional comments are appropriate here. This painful condition is common in our "constipated" Western culture. Millions of dollars spent on laxatives hardly substitute for a natural diet that could nearly eliminate the problem. The total vegetarian diet has plenty of *fiber*. It is likewise helpful in reducing irritation

225

from hemorrhoids. Your intestinal transit times move more quickly, keeping the entire body in better health.

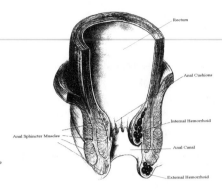

Regular bowel habits are important. Thorough cleansing of the anal area using warm soapy water after each bowel movement aids in the elimination of offending bacteria. This extra hygienic measure is important to allow the rectal area to heal. Various over-the-counter *suppositories* can be used to relieve itching, but are not routinely needed.

The most helpful simple treatment for hemorrhoids is the hot and cold contrast **sitz bath** (see Chapter 17). Take the treatment three times daily. It will both improve the circulation and bring relief of pain. Physical activity, with the avoidance of prolonged sitting, will improve the abdominal circulation, avoiding congestion in the sensitive region. Prolonged or more serious cases may need the rubber band ligation or surgical procedures described in Chapter 12.

Many people erroneously conclude that all bright red rectal bleeding is due to hemorrhoids. **Every** person with rectal bleeding should be investigated to exclude cancer or ulcerative conditions. Rectal pain can also be caused by disorders other than inflamed hemorrhoids. **Anal fissures** are particularly painful, usually aggravated by the passage of stool. Infections and abscesses may also develop in the anal region and should be excluded by a careful examination.

Cancer

Malignancies of the digestive tract have already been described in Chapter 6. **Stomach cancers**, common in Oriental nations, are fortunately decreasing in frequency in the United States. Difficult to diagnose and cure, this particular malignancy requires careful observation of the people at risk with periodic screening tests to detect early signs or risk factors. A diet free of extremely hot foods, spices, or fermented soy preparations (commonly used in Korea and Japan) will help to reduce the incidence of this dreaded condition.

Far more common in this country is **cancer of the colon**. Eighty percent of these lesions are within sight of the sigmoidoscope for early diagnosis. This simple procedure, *sigmoidoscopy*, is recommended for individuals above the age of 40, every other year or so, at the physical examination. Any rectal bleeding should be investigated with appropriate studies to exclude malignancy. Screening tests with the *stool guiac* or *Hemoccult* paper may detect trace amounts of occult bleeding. Keep in mind, however, that a meat diet can produce small amounts of blood in the stool, not related to any disorder in the body itself.

The presence of black tarry stools in the absence of charcoal or iron ingestion should alert one to the possibility of gastrointestinal hemorrhage. This may be caused by ulcers, diverticulitis, and other conditions, including cancer. In the event of severe hemorrhage prompt medical diagnosis is imperative to determine the cause.

The recognition of cancer in the colon in its early stages mandates prompt **surgery**. After appropriate preparation, the tumor should be completely removed, if possible. When this is done early the colon is usually reconnected (called *anastomosis*), permitting bowel function to restore normally.

Extensive lesions or obstruction may require a temporary or permanent *colostomy*. This is an opening in the abdominal wall that permits the fecal waste to empty into a bag. After removal of the obstructing tumor, the bowel may be reunited. In cases of *abdominal-perineal resection* for cancers low in the rectum, the colostomy remains the permanent site for evacuation of feces. When this unfortunate procedure is necessary, a positive outlook is exceedingly important to recover the confidence to function normally, and care for the appliance at home. Descriptive brochures with instructions are available from most colostomy equipment manufacturers.

As we look at most of the gastrointestinal problems mentioned above, it becomes apparent that true preventive answers lie principally in proper diet. The lifestyle, including daily exercise, relaxation, adequate fiber, thorough mastication and regularity in elimination can prevent many troublesome conditions that affect the digestive system. Frank discussion with your family physician will help uncover symptoms previously unrecognized, while in unusual situations the medical practitioner can do additional tests, finally arriving at the proper diagnosis.

FIBER FACTS

Breads	*serving size*	*grams of dietary fiber*
Bran muffin	1 medium	3
Whole wheat bread	1 slice	2
Pumpernickel bread	1 slice	1
Rye bread	1 slice	1
Raisin bread	1 slice	<1
White bread	1 slice	<1
Saltine crackers	4 squares	0

Cereals and Pasta	*serving size*	*grams of dietary fiber*
General Mills Fiber One	1 ounce	13
Kellogg's All-Bran	1 ounce	9
whole wheat pasta	1 cup	5
Kellogg's Complete Bran Flakes	1 ounce	5
Post Fruit & Fibre	1.25 ounces	5
Kellogg's Raisin Bran	1.4 ounces	5
Nabisco Shredded Wheat	1 ounce	3
General Mills Total	1 ounce	2.5

Fiber Facts, continued

General Mills Wheaties	1 ounce	3
General Mills Cheerios	1 ounce	2
Post Grape-Nuts	1 ounce	3
oatmeal	1 cup	2
popcorn	3 cups	2
Kellogg's Corn Flakes	1 ounce	1

Cooked Legumes	*serving size*	*grams of dietary fiber*
kidney beans	1/2 cup	10
baked beans	1/2 cup	7
navy beans	1/2 cup	10
pinto beans	1/2 cup	10
lentils	1/2 cup	2

Vegetables	*serving size*	*grams of dietary fiber*
cooked frozen peas	1/2 cup	5
baked potato (with skin)	1 medium	4
cooked broccoli tops	1/2 cup	3
cooked young carrots	1/2 cup	3
cooked corn	1/2 cup	3
fresh avocado	1/2 medium	3
cooked green beans	1/2 cup	1
Brussels sprouts	1/2 cup	3
cooked eggplant	1/2 cup	2
cooked sweet potato	1/2 medium	2
raw cabbage	1/2 cup	2
raw lettuce	1/2 cup	0
raw celery	1 stalk	0

Fruits and Nuts	*serving size*	*grams of dietary fiber*
almonds	1/4 cup	5
dried prunes	3	4
apple (with skin)	1 medium	3
banana	1 medium	3
blackberries	1/2 cup	3
dried dates	5	3
nectarine	1 medium	3
peach (with skin)	1 medium	3
roasted peanuts	1/4 cup	3
strawberries	1 cup	3
cantaloupe	1 quarter	1
olives	10 medium	2
orange	1 medium	2
creamy peanut butter	2 Tbsp.	2
tangerine	1 medium	2
walnuts	1/4 cup	2

CONDIMENTS

These herbs are currently considered SAFE TO USE:

Bay leaf
Caraway seed
Cardamom
Celery seed
Chives
Coriander
Dill seed
Fennel
Garlic
Italian seasoning
Marjoram
Mint
Onion

Oregano
Paprika (Spanish type)
Parsley
Peppermint
Saffron
Sage
Savory
Spearmint
Sweet basil
Thyme
Turmeric
Wintergreen

These herbs are known to be HARMFUL:

Allspice
Cassia
Cayenne pepper
Chili powder
Chicken seasoning (some)
Cinnamon
Cloves
Curry

Ginger
Horse-radish
Mace
Mustard
Nutmeg
Paprika (Hungarian)
Pepper (black and white)

CHAPTER SEVENTEEN

HYDROTHERAPY

AT

HOME

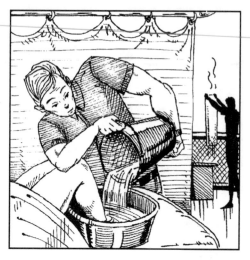

It was only natural that water became the mainstay for simple treatments of disease. It is absolutely essential for the survival of mankind, and consequently must be universally available wherever people live. Thus, water early found its place in the therapeutic approach to illness. Anciently, **hydrotherapy** came into common usage among the Egyptians, then the Jews, the Greeks, and the Romans. There is good reason why water's therapeutic applications are so comprehensive. But I often wonder why modern hospitals have largely turned to other quicker and more remunerative measures.

Considering all the divisions of physical therapy, hydrotherapy is most *versatile*. Water is abundant around the world, hence is almost always *available* for application in therapy. It is one of the most *economical* substances known. Taken internally, water is not irritating, and can also be used in contact with the skin freely, within the limits of body tolerance for certain temperatures. Water is a physiological *solvent*, dissolving most inorganic and many organic substances. It gives off and absorbs large quantities of heat and has a high *specific heat*. Its heat-absorbing capacity, for example, is thirty times that of mercury! In fact, the specific heat of water is higher than that of any other substance, making it the standard of comparison! At useful temperatures for therapeutic application water exists in three *states*—solid, liquid, and gas—making it extremely versatile.

Most people are acquainted with the **thermometer**. This device measures the *intensity* of heat. The *Fahrenheit* scale places the freezing of pure distilled water at sea level at 32° and the boiling point at 212°. A gradual tendency to utilize the *Celsius* (Centigrade) scale is developing. On the *Centigrade* thermometer the freezing point is 0 degrees and the boiling point 100 degrees.

Definitions that apply to hydrotherapy temperatures range as follows (using *Fahrenheit* scale):

Very hot	over 104° F.
Hot	100° to 104° F.
Warm	92° to 100° F.
Neutral	94° to 97° F.
Tepid	80° to 92° F.
Cool	70° to 80° F.
Cold	55° to 70° F.
Very cold	32° to 55° F.

Another property of water that makes it excellent for hydrotherapy is its **latent heat** of freezing and vaporization. Latent heat is the quantity of heat necessary to convert a substance into another physical state without changing its temperature. It requires nearly eighty times as much heat for ice to melt without change of temperature, as it does to warm it one degree above freezing. The latent heat is usually defined in *calories*. This is the amount of heat a gram of water absorbs or gives off in changing its temperature 1 degree (Centigrade).

Thus, one gram of ice in melting absorbs enough heat to raise a gram of water from zero degrees to 79.2° Centigrade. This is called the *latent heat of freezing* and for water it is 79.2 calories.

In converting 1 gram of boiling water to steam, a much greater amount of heat is released. The *latent heat of vaporization* for water has been found to be 537 calories. Thus, when steam condenses it gives off an immense amount of heat. This explains the intense heating effect of a Russian steam bath, also the value of steaming fomentations. Moreover, the intensity of burns produced by steam is easily understood, as well as the cooling and soothing effects of an evaporating wet sheet pack.

In order for water or any other substance to communicate heat to another body, it must remain some time in contact. The impression of heat or cold is perceived immediately when a substance comes in contact with our skin. This sensation transmits nerve impulses to the brain, which interpret the feeling. We sense heat when the substance is warmer than the body, or cold when it is cooler than the skin. Thus, the temperature of the skin is the starting point or zero of the temperature sensing mechanism. This awareness varies in different areas of the body. However, it explains why a neutral bath 94° to 97° F. produces the least thermic impression.

Since water stores so much heat and gives it off so readily, it often seems hotter or colder than other substances. For example, the temperature–conducting capacity of water is 27 times that of air! One may appreciate this fact more naturally by stepping from an atmosphere of 75° F. into a tub of water at the same temperature. The latter always feels cool. For these reasons a thermometer should usually be consulted when using water baths or treatments involving immersion to give with safety the desired reaction to the body.

Mechanical friction can be employed to enhance the effect of water treatments. The application of cold, combined with friction, can act cooperatively to produce a much greater influence than either alone. The same is true of water douches and sprays. The percussive effect of a water stream adds greatly to the reaction produced, partly because of the perfect *fluidity* of water as a solvent.

As a cleansing agent, water is used in shampoos, the enema, and the douche. The benefits from drinking *pure soft water* are partially due to dissolving and washing out poisons from the system, and the beneficial cleansing effect on kidneys and bowels. Some waste products in our bodies require a great deal of water to dissolve them. Furthermore, constant hydration of the tissues must always be maintained. For these and countless other reasons, water is a great blessing to mankind.

How The Skin Works

As indicated in Chapter 9, the largest organ of the body is the skin. Some writers have called it "keyboard of the hydrotherapist." Through the numerous blood vessels and nerves of our skin, and their reflex connections with the internal organs, practically every organ of the body can be influenced by applications of heat or cold to the skin surface. Small muscle bundles are found in the *dermis*, connected with the hair follicles. Contraction of these *arrectores pilorum* muscles cause the hair to stand erect, producing a peculiar roughness of the skin known as "goose flesh." Applications of cold or sensations of chilliness can bring this condition. With cold, the skin also becomes blanched, as blood squeezes out of the vessels by this muscular contraction. An enormous network of lymphatic vessels, veins, and capillaries is present. These tiny tubes that constantly convey fluid back to the heart contain thousands of valves and nerve fibers. This gives them the ability to shift blood flow from one area to another.

Several times a minute, changes occur in the diameter of our blood vessels. As they *contract* and become smaller, blood is forced onward. During the relaxing or *dilating* phase, they fill with blood. This "pumping" action is another powerful factor in the circulation of these vital fluids. It is sometimes called the "peripheral heart." Circulation slows when the nerve control of these vessels is interfered with, and the extremity becomes dusky in color and cold. Paralysis succeeding a stroke, infectious diseases, and even emotional problems can alter the flow of blood in the skin. This adds to the burden on our heart, making it work under a disadvantage. Contrasting temperatures of hydrotherapy treatments produce powerful circulatory reactions, which enhance these rhythmic changes and alternating contractions in the blood vessels of the skin.

Massage also aids the return of lymph to the heart, and briefly empties the veins when it is done properly. Movement of a limb by active **exercise** likewise enhances the circulation. Since the body weight is 1/13 blood and about

1/4 lymph (*interstitial fluid*), a large amount of fluid can be affected when hydrotherapy applications are given. Results are seen in the body as a whole.

Sweat glands are found throughout the entire skin, but are especially numerous in the underarms (*axillae*), the palms, and the soles. It is estimated that 1 square cm. of skin on the palm may have about 3,000 of these tiny "mouths." Estimating the total surface of their ducts at 11,000 square feet, it appears obvious that this secretory function is of considerable importance.

Sweat is about 98% water, but contains small traces of impurities which are thrown off from the skin. It also contains assorted salts, such as sodium chloride. About twice as much water is excreted by the skin as the lungs give off each day! When the excretory function of the kidneys is diseased, the sweat becomes loaded with toxins. Unfortunately, the sweat glands may also be diseased when kidney afflictions are of long duration. To encourage free perspiration during a hydrotherapy treatment, it is appropriate to drink water before and during the applications. Hot drinks are very helpful. An environment that is warm, comfortable, quiet, and free of stress is likewise beneficial.

Certain diseases produce such alteration in the ability of sweat glands to eliminate heat, that extreme precautions must be made in giving these treatments. Extensive **burns** may destroy the skin nerves and abolish normal reflexes that occur in response to temperature. **Alcohol** intoxication may obliterate the response to heat, making heat stroke a distinct possibility if appropriate precautions are not taken. Reflex effects on distant organs are also influenced by damage to nerve endings in the skin. The perception of heat and cold, our control of circulation, and the beneficial effect derived from hydrotherapy treatments may be compromised in numerous diseases. Careful observation and study are essential, along with medical consultation where indicated.

Effects Of Heat and Cold

The application of heat to skin produces local **dilation** of the blood vessels with an increase in the rapidity of flow. Localized hot applications additionally increase the capillary pressure, causing an increased flow of fluid into the lymph spaces, then back to the heart through those channels. Local heat also increases perspiration. When treatments are prolonged, the sweating becomes generalized. One outstanding effect of all forms of heat is the relief of pain. Relaxation of muscle spasm may account for some of this benefit. Inflammatory congestions are also relieved.

Prolonged applications of heat tend to produce greater **relaxation** or dilation, ending in a slowed circulation. Venous blood predominates in these relaxed vessels, making the skin appear more reddened and congested. Heat penetration is quite limited, since a healthy circulation distributes warmth rapidly to other parts of the body. Internal parts are still affected, however, by **reflex effects** discussed below.

When cold water contacts the skin for a short time, it becomes reddened with an increase of blood. This is especially evident when the cold stimulus is accompanied by friction. Nerves in the blood vessels are stimulated, and a type of "vascular gymnastics" follows. The blood vessels pump vigorously with alternating dilation and contraction. Extra amounts of oxygen are delivered to the skin during these maneuvers.

When intense **cold** is applied for a prolonged period, the vasoconstriction tends to be preserved. This "suppressed reaction" occurs whenever an ice bag, for example, is applied for 15 to 30 minutes. Immersion baths in cool salt water, particularly when it is charged with carbon dioxide gas (the European *Nauheim bath*), are powerful stimulants of the blood vessels. The heart rate decreases and high blood pressure goes down during these particular treatments.

When fomentation treatments with heat or cold are followed by mechanical stimulation, as in a *percussive shower*, the metabolic effects frequently double. This clarifies the stimulating effects of cold sprays to the spine, cold mitten frictions (Chapter 17), and the therapeutic spray, compared to more mild treatment using similar temperatures.

Blood pressure is affected by hydrotherapy. It increases after a hot bath over 104°F. Blood pressure usually oscillates during thermic applications above skin temperature. Prolonged heat overrides this reaction, and the blood pressure falls. Neutral baths relax blood vessels, and help lower the blood pressure. Frictions, massage, and additional mechanical stimuli are sometimes combined with cold treatments to raise blood pressure in asthenic or frail individuals.

Blood distribution is quite uneven in states of physical inactivity. The liver, spleen, and other solid internal organs tend to collect blood during bed rest or sedentary activity. Moderate exercise helps to equalize blood flow, so that more cells are found in the circulation. Cold water therapies, associated with mechanical stimulation, increase the number of red and white blood cells circulating vigorously in both arms and legs. Red blood cell counts increase slightly along with a transient surge in hemoglobin.

The principal advantage, however, comes from the **white blood cells**, which swarm into the blood stream after a hot and cold contrast treatment. They have defensive maneuvers to perform, fighting infection and safeguarding the body from germs. Contraction of the spleen after a treatment forces its millions of sequestered blood elements into the whole body. With prolonged applications of heat, circulating blood volume increases. Both hot and cold baths, moreover, trigger an increase in the white blood cells. It is not known exactly how this occurs, but the benefits are wholesome.

Most people have experienced the **relief from muscular fatigue** that comes after a warm bath. Normal rest and restoring sleep is promoted by this relaxing and quieting influence. On the other hand, if a warm tub bath is followed by vigorous cold applications—such as a cold shower, ice water pour, or cold mitten friction—the body acquires new energy. The brain is more alert, the extremities are warm, and more work can be accomplished without the injurious after effects from drug poisons such as caffeine.

A very opposite effect is produced by hot baths. The muscles become more fatigued, and are able to do less work. Mechanically stimulating your muscles with a hot spray douche will give a transient increased working capacity, but this is slightly less than with cold treatment. Maximal stimulation occurs when the alternating hot and cold **percussion douche** is used. While the hot spray should be of a brief duration, it must be sufficiently prolonged to prepare the body for the cold.

Remember, however, these general treatments affect the entire body, including the nervous system, the liver, and the body chemistry, as well as the muscles. The conversion of lactic acid, from fatigued muscles, back into useful sources of energy is enhanced. Oxygen delivery is also improved, to enable the muscles once again to work effectively. In contrast to many chemical stimulants, hydrotherapy gives no *false* sense of energy. Treatments such as the warm baths are conducive to a perfect relaxation that normal rest and sleep require for recuperating powers of the body.

Prolonged contact with cold substances chills the body and depresses its vital functions. In contrast, the application of moderate heat stimulates the pulse and respiration, quickening the circulation. Digestion is enhanced, the muscles "come alive," and sensation from the skin is more accurately perceived.

If, however, the body remains in contact with cold water for a brief time, its activities are heightened instead of slowed. These "**thermic impressions**" are not related to the transfer of heat, but react by way of the nerves.

The response of the body toward any disturbing agent, in this case cold, consists of several phases. The **thermic reaction** involves an increase of heat production within the body. As exposed skin becomes reddened with increased blood flow, a circulatory *reaction* takes place. The nerves tingle with new life and in this "nervous reaction" there is a feeling of renewed energy for work. Any therapist administering hydrotherapeutic procedures must be aware of this phenomenon.

Occasionally, there is an **incomplete reaction**, with duskiness of the skin, "goose flesh," shivering, cold feet and hands, and a feeling of congestion in the head. In this complication, treatment has failed to produce adequately vigorous surface circulation. Measures must be taken immediately to warm up the patient. On occasion, it may be desirable to suppress the reaction. Usually, local cold, such as an ice bag is applied and prolonged. In other circumstances, a short application of heat is given immediately after the cold to suppress the thermic response. Repeated reactions, however, are usually beneficial to secure maximum results. They occur with all effective alternating hot and cold applications. However, the power to react is subject to fatigue. So after two or three successive fomentation changes, each reaction is less complete. Percussion or cold mitten friction can be added to intensify this response.

The ability to *react* is limited in the extremes of life. Neither infants or aged persons bear cold treatments well. Certain disease states also produce a profound weakness. Anemia and emaciation, as well as some nervous conditions require the modification of cold contrast. It may be better to apply heat alone, by means of sunshine, electric heating pads, or the light bath, to secure a mild stimulating effect.

Exercise warms the body sufficiently to promote reaction. It quickens the circulation and brings blood to the surface. Body heat is increased, so that surface blood vessels become dilated. This helps to increase heat reaction. In cases of extreme exhaustion, no cold treatment at all should be given, since the reactive powers have been taxed to their utmost.

When the patient is warm, reaction occurs promptly. The internal temperature of body organs may be ever so great, yet reaction is impossible if the skin is cold and clammy, pale, or manifests goose flesh. The skin should be warm, even ruddy, before cold applications are used. If it is not, some sort of hot treatment should first be used to draw blood to the skin. The room temperature where the patient is treated should be warm. A hot drink may be offered to warm the person. Warm feet are especially important. As a rule, if the feet are cold, they should be warmed with a hot foot bath before giving any other treatment. This may even be beneficial as preparation for an enema, to prevent chilling and weakness afterwards.

After finishing the treatment, a short period of rest with additional covers or blanket, will help secure a prompt and complete reaction. A little carelessness may undo much of the benefit which otherwise would occur from these hydrotherapeutic procedures.

Reflex Effects

The body is whole, and all its organs are interrelated. In addition to exquisite control exercised by the ductless *endocrine* glands and the vital nutrients supplied from food, nerves exercise a continual influence, regulating the activities of numerous internal organs and body structures. Reflex reactions can be accelerated, retarded, and changed in various ways by electrical impulses traveling through delicate nerves. This especially is true of the blood vessels, since change in their diameter affects blood flow so profoundly. An easy experiment to demonstrate this uses the hands. Apply ice to one hand, and the blood flow decreases in the opposite hand. The reverse is true with heat application. Thus, through nerve connections and reflexes in the spinal cord, a distant effect is the same as the local effect of heat, cold, as well as some other stimuli.

While strong stimulation of any nerve in the body changes flow rate in most blood vessels, these variations in size are most pronounced in certain parts that have a close nerve connection with the part stimulated. For example, an ice bag applied over the stomach may cause a brief change in the size of the blood vessels in the brain, but the most lasting changes are produced in blood vessels within the stomach. Actually, for each internal organ there is an area on the skin, which when stimulated, causes a profound shift in the circulation to that organ. In most instances this area of reflex nerve connection is the skin surface overlying that organ.

These interesting nerve impulses traverse definite pathways. The stimulus produced by heat, cold, electricity, or pressure travels to the spinal cord by sensory (*afferent*) nerves. In the spinal cord incoming impulses circulate to various levels upward or downward. Sensitive nerve endings start other impulses over outgoing (*efferent*) nerves. Impulses that are destined to influence internal organs pass to nerves in the **sympathetic nervous system**. These connect with blood vessels from internal organs, as well as muscles and glands. When an application to the skin interacts with another part of the body through some nerve pathway, it is said to produce a "**reflex effect**." Let's now consider a few reflexes and their applications in home therapy.

Reflex or *consensual* effects may be classified under three headings, (1) circulatory, (2) muscular, and (3) glandular. All of these effects are illustrated in the abdominal organs. A fomentation (as described in Chapter 17) applied to the skin of the abdomen causes diminished intestinal activity, decreased intestinal blood flow, and decreased gastric acid secretion. When an ice bag is applied over the heart, its rate is slowed, and the force of each contraction increases. Cold applied to the epigastric area over the stomach induces diminished tone in the stomach muscles, with complete quieting of the stomach's outlet (*pylorus*). These are obvious reflex actions since the warming or cooling of the stomach directly by drinking a hot liquid or ice water will increase or decrease respectively the peristalsis and acid secretion. It is just the opposite of what would be expected from a direct temperature effect on the stomach.

We therefore find it possible to influence intestinal and internal organ function with applications of hot or cold to the skin area *reflexly related* to these organs. A few remote skin locations relate to some organs at a distance, and their nerve pathway is more difficult to trace. The accompanying outline will illustrate some distant reflex relationships which have been documented with medical research.

Here are the more important reflex areas employed in water treatments.

(1) The skin areas of the face, scalp, and back of the neck are reflexly related to the brain.

(2) The back of the neck is reflexly related to the mucous membrane of the nose.

(3) The skin of the neck is reflexly related to the throat and larynx.

(4) The skin of the chest on front, back, and sides are reflexly related to the lungs.

(5) A close reflex relation exists between the area over the heart (called the *precordial region*) and the cardiac accelerator nerves.

(6)   The skin over the lower right chest is related to the liver.

(7)   The skin over the left chest is related to the spleen.

(8)   The skin of the lower back and lumbar spine are reflexly related to the kidneys.

(9)   The skin of the central abdomen is related to the kidneys and ureters.

(10)   The skin of the lower lumbar and sacral spine is related to the pelvic organs.

(11)   The skin over the epigastrium is related to the stomach.

(12)   The skin of the entire abdomen is reflexly related to the intestines.

(13)   The skin of the lower abdomen, including the groin and upper inner surface of the thighs is reflexly related to the pelvic organs.

(14)   The saddle shaped area covered by a sitz bath is in reflex relation to the prostate and seminal vesicles in men and to the pelvic organs in women.

(15)   The skin of the feet and legs is related to the pelvic organs.

(16)   The skin of the breasts is reflexly related to the pelvic organs.

Two general classes of effects are produced by thermal and mechanical applications. The first is **stimulating** and **tonic**; the second, **depressant** and **sedative**. A stimulating effect is greater than a tonic effect, but both increase the vital activity. The intensity of the effect will be proportionate to the intensity of the application. On the other hand, depressant and sedative effects are both due to a decrease of activity. They differ in the *extent* of the decrease.

Whatever the *degree* of reflex effect be, it is similar to the *direct effect* on the skin area treated. Four principal changes occur in the skin and the internal organs related to it. Try to remember them when treatments are given:

(1)   The blood vessels are contracted and remain so, as long as the application is in place, sometimes longer.

(2)   The nerve sensibility is decreased.

(3)   Glandular activity is decreased.

(4)   The muscles contract firmly.

In healthy organs the vascular changes may not be excessively marked, but in congested or inflamed organs, these changes are often profound.

Special reflex effects are seen with prolonged cold and differ from those caused by short applications of cold. Similarly, there are special effects from prolonged hot applications that differ somewhat from those of short duration. These are summarized in standard books on hydrotherapy. But before studying about the treatments and their indications, I will review some reflex principles involving generalized heat.

All applications produce reflex effects. But applications of heat to a very large area **dilate** so many surface blood vessels that blood is withdrawn from internal or distant parts. Therefore, the reflex dilation of the blood vessels in this distant part is overcome, wiped out by the mechanical or *hydrostatic* effect. This is called **derivation**.

Conversely, when cold is applied to a large area or the surface of the body is chilled, blood is driven from the outer parts. Then the internal blood vessels are filled and become dilated. Internal organ congestion results, called **retrostasis**. The above outline shows these different effects. Heat draws blood to the surface—*derivation*. Cold produces local vasoconstriction, driving blood to the interior—*retrostasis*. Then a secondary effect of cold draws blood to the surface again—*derivation*.

Furthermore, blood distribution is altered by other external heating and cooling measures. Normally, the human body maintains its temperature at a fairly constant level. The main factor in *thermostatic* regulation is the skin with its connections, especially the brain. About 78% of our body's heat loss is eliminated through the skin. At ordinary environmental temperatures, 73% is lost by **radiation** and 14% by **evaporation** of moisture from the skin surface. As the temperature rises, more and more heat loss occurs by evaporation, until this becomes more important than radiation, as a means of temperature control.

So efficient is this cooling mechanism, that it is difficult to produce significant rises in body temperature by applying heat in a dry atmosphere. Both radiation and evaporation require dilation of skin blood vessels to eliminate the heat. These changes in vascular diameter, the caliber of the vessels, are under the control of heat-regulating centers in the central nervous system. These centers, in turn, are controlled by the autonomic nervous system.

When heat is applied to the body surface, our heat regulating mechanism goes into action, and the skin vessels dilate to eliminate heat. First, this occurs in the upper extremities. The lower ones follow shortly thereafter. Although maximum dilation occurs in the area heated, in actuality it is more or less a general cutaneous dilation.

In contrast, when the surface of our body is chilled, even in a small area, there is general constriction of the skin vessels. This is produced by the nervous system temperature control mechanism in an endeavor to prevent heat loss. If cold is applied for a short time only, *reaction* occurs within a few minutes, and the skin vessels dilate, provided the patient is able to react. If the cold application is prolonged, this vascular constriction is also prolonged.

Chilling of the surface causes dilation internally in those areas which are constricted by peripheral heat. This makes it clear that these so-called *hydrostatic* effects are closely bound up with temperature regulation. They are mediated through the "thermostat" center of the brain together with the autonomic nerve supply to the skin.

In health, a warm application to the skin surface draws blood almost equally from all parts of the body, chiefly from the interior. Where there are congested organs, a hot application will draw proportionately more blood from the congested organ than from other parts of the body. This decreasing of congestion is known as **depletion**. The means of producing it is called **derivation**. Internal organs having the most practical use for these hydrostatic effects are specifically the brain, the lungs, and the pelvic organs.

With lung congestion—such as in colds, influenza, and the early stages of pneumonia—a hot foot bath with fomentations to the chest is most useful. It is also beneficial to take hot beverages, and use blanket coverings to produce sweating. Tonic treatments, such as the cold mitten friction should finish the therapy session to prevent recongestion. Congestive headaches find relief with the hot foot bath, applying cold compresses or ice bags to the head and neck.

Acute inflammatory diseases in the pelvic organs requires most vigorous derivation. A hot hip and leg pack, combined with ice bags to the bladder (*suprapubic*) area is often effective. If preceded by a hot vaginal irrigation, the relief of pain usually comes within ten minutes. This treatment should likewise be finished with a cold mitten friction.

TECHNIQUES OF LOCAL HEATING PROCEDURES

Fomentations

A **fomentation** consists of local application using moist heat to the body's surface. The fomentation cloth is typically made of blanket material—50% wool to retain heat, and 50% cotton to retain moisture. The combination gives greater durability. A fomentation **tank** can be constructed to employ boiling water or steam. A kettle of boiling water, such as that used for home canning is quite sufficient. At least four fomentation cloths should be assembled, with a few Turkish (terry cloth) towels. A basin for ice water and the foot tub completes the setup.

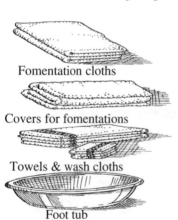

Fomentation cloths

Covers for fomentations

Towels & wash cloths

Foot tub

Preparation for Home Treatments

During the procedure, keep the room warm and free of drafts to prevent chilling. Avoid bright lights shining in the patient's eyes. Protect the furniture, bedding, and carpets from moisture, especially when giving a room treatment. Do not be very talkative. Avoid discussing the patient's ailment, and keep all conversation positive, uplifting, and cheerful. Make every move count for something, conserving energy and economizing on time.

First, start the water boiling. Fold a fomentation cloth in about three thicknesses. Grasp the ends and partially twist the cloth. Then submerge all but the ends in the boiling water until thoroughly soaked. Stretch or pull the fomentation to wring it as dry as possible. Untwist the "fomie" quickly and wrap it in a **dry** fomentation cloth.

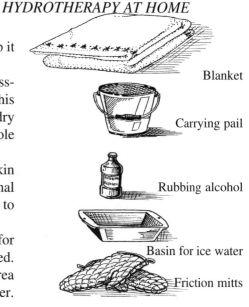

Blanket

Carrying pail

Rubbing alcohol

Basin for ice water

Friction mitts

Materials for simple remedies

Next, fold the fomentation double cross-wise. Roll it together to hold the heat. Unfold this then at the bedside and place the inner side on a dry towel on the area to be treated. Cover the whole application with a towel.

If the fomentation is very hot, rub the skin underneath until the heat is tolerable. An additional towel may be placed under the fomentation to prevent burning and to absorb moisture.

Each fomentation should be left in place for 3-5 minutes. Three applications are usually used. When the last fomentation is removed, cool the area with a wash cloth wrung out from cold water. Finally, dry the skin thoroughly. All fomentation changes should be made quickly. The part treated should **never** be left exposed. During the treatment, it is usually advisable to apply a cold cloth to the forehead or neck in order to keep the head cool. This helps prevent headache. Preheating the patient with a hot foot bath aids in the derivative effect mentioned above.

Fomentations are very useful to relieve congestion from chest colds, coughs, bronchitis, and influenza. Fomentations can relieve pain in neuralgia, arthritis, and other inflammations. They may *stimulate*, when alternated with cold, or *sedate* in nervous conditions. For sedation, apply them to the spine, not too hot, but quite prolonged. Elimination of toxins is enhanced by sweating, especially when the fomentations are applied properly. Take great care to avoid burning the patient, particularly when there is paralysis, anesthesia, atherosclerosis, diabetes, edema, or recent surgery.

Protect the prominent bony areas specifically, lifting the fomentation frequently to allow steam to escape. You may also pad them with an additional wash cloth or towel. When fomentations are used in heart disease an **ice bag** should be placed over the heart. This can keep the pulse slow. It also helps avoid apprehension. Fomentations should *not* be used in cases of acute abdominal pain, heart failure, suspected heart attack, or gastrointestinal hemorrhages, such as from peptic ulcer. Nor should they be applied to the chest in pulmonary tuberculosis. Caution should be used in severely hypertensive patients also. Check the blood pressure frequently.

A special type of fomentation, called **revulsive compress** is used in infectious states. The fomentation is applied and allowed to remain a few minutes, then followed with a hand towel wrung lightly out from ice water. This contrast spreads out over the surface after the fomentation is removed. Then, after drying the skin, another fomentation is applied. **Alternating hot and cold** is similar, except that instead of the cold compress, the therapist rubs a piece of ice back and forth over the skin between the fomentations.

241

This produces a vigorous **stimulant** or *tonic* treatment, greatly enhancing the circulation, increasing the muscle tone. It usually produces a beneficial reaction.

Hot Foot Bath

As you would expect from the name, a **hot foot bath** involves the immersion of both feet and ankles in water at a temperature ranging from 100° to 115° F. This increases blood flow, locally and reflexly, through the feet and entire skin surface. As a *derivative effect*, the hot foot bath produces decongestion in the internal pelvic organs as well as the brain. For this reason, it is often applied to relieve congestion in the head and chest, and as a treatment for headache. Pelvic congestion frequently responds. Even a nosebleed can be stopped by this simple treatment, combined with ice packs over the face.

A second use for the hot foot bath is in conjunction with fomentations to warm up the body generally, preparing for the application of heat. **Tonic procedures**, such as the salt glow, cold mitten friction, and the percussion shower douche can likewise be enhanced when preceded by a hot foot bath. If prolonged, the hot foot bath will induce sweating. It often helps to prevent or abort a common cold. Relaxation and comfort are encouraged. Of course, any local inflammation of the feet receives relief with this simple measure.

Find a metal foot tub or plastic container, large and deep enough to contain the feet and ankles. Even a five gallon can or plastic wastebasket will do. If a thermometer is not available, test the water temperature with your elbow or hand. Protect the bed or floor from spilled water. Combine any prolonged treatment to the feet with a cold compress to the forehead to facilitate the derivative effect and avoid head congestion, producing headache.

Hot foot bath with **cold compress** to the head. This sitting position is used, with a blanket wrapped around to encourage sweating.

After testing accurately the water temperature, introduce both feet carefully to avoid burning. Vascular disease in the extremities and complications of diabetes, in which the sensation is reduced, are **contraindications** to this treatment or require moderation of the temperature. *Frostbite* may be treated in a warm foot bath, but very hot applications should not be used. Except for some vascular diseases mentioned above, the water temperature is usually started at about 103° F. Add hot water from time to time, increasing the temperature to tolerance. The treatment is continued for 10 to 15 minutes, changing the cold head compress frequently. When finished, lift the feet out of the water, pour cold water over them, remove them from the tub, and dry them thoroughly. For general perspiration, give an alcohol rub or a cold mitten friction, then dry the skin thoroughly.

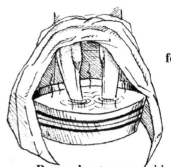

The **hot foot bath** may be given in bed or in a chair.

Remember to use a cold compress on the forehead to prevent congestion or headache.

Cold Mitten Friction

One of the finest hydrotherapy measures for stimulating blood flow in the skin is the **cold mitten friction** (CMF). Enhanced circulation benefits the entire body. As a tonic, the skillfully performed CMF is better than anything found in a bottle. After fomentations, a CMF treatment is excellent to close the pores and tone up the skin. It heightens nerve and muscle tone, and skin sensibility. Heat production is increased, as well as tissue oxidation. Reflex effects in the internal organs induce stimulation of muscular, glandular, and metabolic activities. Helping to fight infections and fevers, the CMF increases antibody production and *phagocytosis* (where white blood cells destroy and "eat" harmful germs). Thus, it builds up general body resistance and is helpful for those suffering from frequent colds. For individuals sensing a lack of energy, particularly when the habits of coffee or tobacco are being eliminated, this treatment is invaluable.

A wash cloth can be used to deliver the cold mitten friction. However, it is more effective to sew a thick hand towel into the form of a mitten. This mitten is dipped into ice water, wrung out lightly, and rubbed **briskly** on the skin, up and down two or three times. The upper extremities are treated first, beginning with the fingers and rubbing alternately up to the shoulders. Each extremity is dried and covered before the next portion gets treated. The chest and abdomen are rubbed briskly with the friction mitts, then dried and covered. The lower extremities are treated similarly, finishing with the back.

The friction is given as vigorously as the patient can tolerate it, repeated until the skin is nice and pink. This so-called "vascular gymnastics" is one of the finest physiologic tonics known. A CMF is so simple that one can do it to himself or herself after the shower each morning for a quick "jump start."

Sitz Bath

One of the oldest hydrotherapy procedures is the **sitz** or sitting bath. Many abdominal and pelvic conditions were treated thus by the Austrian practitioner Priessnitz, who used water as a curative remedy.

The modern sitz tub is made of metal or porcelain and fashioned in such a size and shape that the patient may sit in it comfortably. The feet extend outside, positioned comfortably in a foot bath. A wash tub or plastic basin may serve the purpose at home, slightly tipped and made stationary with blocks of wood. A smaller tub or basin may be employed to give the foot bath. It should be considered part of the sitz treatment. An ordinary bathtub may also be used for a hot sitz bath. The patient sits in the tub, drawing up the knees so that only the feet and pelvic areas are submerged. Alternatively, one can take a **hot half bath** in which the water depth is deep enough to reach the navel.

Water temperature varies, depending upon the effect desired. As used in this text, the following Fahrenheit temperatures will correspond to these relative hydrotherapy terms:

cold: 55° to 75° F.
neutral: 92° to 97° F.
hot: 105° to 110° F.
very hot: 110° to 115° F.

Cold sitz baths are useful treatments for constipation and chronic pelvic inflammation. **Hot sitz baths** are used to treat pelvic pain during the menstrual cycle and in acute pelvic inflammatory conditions. They are also helpful to assist patients who are unable to urinate. Alternating hot and cold sitz baths are valuable for the treatment of hemorrhoids and prostate trouble, and after surgery of the perineum or rectum.

The patient should be protected from contact with the tub by placing towels behind his back and under his knees. Cover him or her with a blanket. Sufficient water should be used to cover the hips and reach the abdomen. The temperature of the foot bath should be several degrees hotter than the temperature in the sitz tub. Friction may be used with the cold sitz bath, if a person feels chilly, or when it is desirable to intensify the effects of the bath. Finish hot sitz baths by cooling the water to neutral for one or two minutes, or by pouring cold water over the hips and thighs. A cold sitz may be concluded by rubbing the hips and thighs with warm alcohol. Cold compresses to the head and neck should be used with some of the hot sitz baths. The patient should be observed closely for fainting.

If one avoids drafts or chilling the benefits will be great. After these and most other hydrotherapy treatments, the patient should rest for 20 to 30 minutes. As a reliever of pelvic pain and an improver of the circulation, the hot sitz bath or a contrasting one works well for treatment in the home.

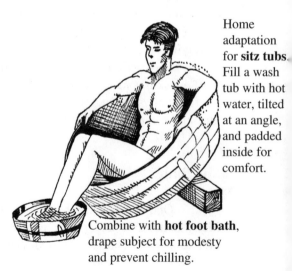

Home adaptation for **sitz tubs**. Fill a wash tub with hot water, tilted at an angle, and padded inside for comfort.

Combine with **hot foot bath**, drape subject for modesty and prevent chilling.

Centripetal Peripheral Rub

The **centripetal peripheral rub**, usually called CPR, consists principally of stroking (*effleurage*) movements toward the center of the body. It is a type of light massage designed to expedite the circulation, particularly in the superficial veins. The CPR is a most relaxing treatment when used to finish a *general hydro* treatment, particularly one designed to relax spastic muscles and give a general feeling of well-being. Mild applications of CPR can hasten the absorption of edema fluid from either lower extremities or the hands.

The technique is as follows: Apply a lubricant such as body lotion or light oil to the extremities, one at a time. The first motion lubricates the extremity. In the arm, go from the fingers to the shoulder, returning with rotary sweeps. Stroking is done first to the back of the hand, the palm, the forearm, the elbow, then the upper arm and shoulder with free sweeping motions in each area. A knowledge of muscle configuration is helpful to make this most effective.

In the CPR, stroking is always done **toward** the heart, emptying the veins, and at the same time kneading the muscles lightly. Brief percussion is given the extremity with a "clapping" (palms cupped) up and down, then quick light "hacking" (using edge of hand), finally finishing with a very light stroking motion again. This percussion maneuver is avoided over the chest and abdomen, but it is very effective on the back and large muscles.

When rubbing the back, the first lubrication motion is followed by a stroking type of *effleurage* down the spine and out the lateral muscles. From the neck and shoulders down to the buttocks, the muscles are symmetrically massaged with firm pressure and gentle stroking. Kneading motions are typically alternated with the stroking. Finally after a brief percussion, called *tapotement*, a light effleurage completes the treatment. This most basic type of massage is very helpful to tone a sluggish circulation, relaxing the person for rest or sleep.

Contrast Baths

As the name implies, a **contrast bath** consists in the alternate application of hot and cold water to any part of the body. The alternate contraction and dilation of the blood vessels which results, improves the circulation and rapid removal of waste products from the area. By repeated changes this effect is heightened, resulting in a greatly increased blood flow through the area.

Oxygen and nutrient elements, necessary for nature's healing processes are provided, as well as white blood cells, which help the body defend itself against infection.

To begin a contrast bath, secure two containers, large enough to allow the water to cover the extremities. Basins, plastic or metal garbage pails, or a double sink in the kitchen will work fine. Consult a thermometer for proper temperature, since it is important to have the heated water at the correct temperature.

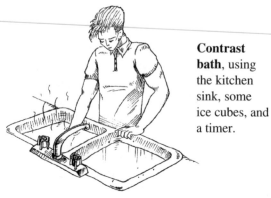

Contrast bath, using the kitchen sink, some ice cubes, and a timer.

The affected limbs are placed in hot water, at 105° to 110° F., for three or four minutes, then immersed in cold tap water or ice water for 30 to 60 seconds. Begin with the hot water and end with the cold water, changing back and forth, from three to six times. After each treatment, the extremity is dried carefully and kept warm.

Contrast baths are useful in several conditions. Poor circulation caused by many blood vessel diseases can be improved, although in such situations temperatures above 105° are usually contraindicated. The cold water should be used for only about 30 seconds, and a treatment should be finished in neutral to hot water, instead of cold. **Arthritis** improves with contrast baths. Begin with temperatures of about 110° F., and change to tap water on a four and one minute cycle. After four to six changes, end with **hot** water. The treatment should be repeated at least twice daily.

Infections of the upper or lower extremities lend themselves well to these easy-to-perform contrast baths. The extremes of hot and cold temperature should be as great as can be comfortably tolerated. The more hardy person can start with ice water, changing five to six times, and finishing with the ice water. A powerful release of white blood cells into the circulation helps the body to combat infections such as cellulitis. Obvious improvement in the redness and relief of pain occurs after each treatment.

After initial *first–aid* application of ice packs (see Chapter 13) for sprained ankles or wrists, the hot and cold contrast bath is used to promote healing and take away pain. Swelling decreases more rapidly, and a return to full use of the injured joint is accelerated.

Heating Compresses

A **heating compress** is in actuality a cold compress, so covered as to prevent the circulation of air. This causes a rapid accumulation of body heat, warming the treated area for several hours. Most commonly these heating compresses are used around the throat. They are also effective over a joint, such as the knee or elbow. Using a larger cloth and wrapping, one can treat the chest or abdomen, giving great relief in certain conditions.

Use a strip of cotton cloth or muslin, long enough to encircle the area twice and wide enough to cover the area being treated. This cloth is immersed in cold tap water and wrung "dry." After wrapping the moist cloth around the treatment area, a strip of wool flannel is then used to cover snugly. Pin the outer wrap in place with safety pins. Leave the compress on overnight, removing it in the morning. Finally, rub the skin briskly with cold water before drying.

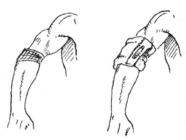

The heating compress used on the throat measures about three inches wide and thirty inches long. The wool flannel covering is about four by thirty-four inches, allowing it to completely encircle the other cloth. This remedy is effective in cases of sore throat, laryngitis, tonsillitis, and similar illnesses.

Heating compress to the upper arm. Apply a wet cotton strip or gauze, then cover with wool flannel. Hold it in place with a safety pin.

A **heating chest pack** may be made in the same way. Apply it to the chest, rolling a broad cloth, about ten inches wide and seventy-two inches long, around the chest and over the shoulders diagonally, after first wringing it out in cold tap water. Secure it snugly at all points, but not so tight as to restrict respiration. After covering the moist cloth with a wool flannel one, secure the chest pack with safety pins. Leave it on overnight, then finish with a brief alcohol rub in the morning. A sweater or firm knit pajamas may be worn over this to aid in the heating effect. Chest packs are useful in treating pneumonia, bronchitis, pleurisy, and whooping cough. Materials for a heating compress to the chest should be kept available in every home.

A similar cloth is used over the abdomen as a **moist abdominal binder** for the treatment of indigestion, constipation, and other digestive problems.

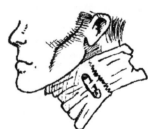

Heating compress to the neck. Put on at bedtime and remove in the morning.

When a heating compress is applied to a joint, such as the knee, it is likewise left on overnight, followed in the morning by a brief massage. Medications can be applied to the skin, such as diluted *oil of wintergreen* to aid the heating effect and relief of joint pain. You can purchase it at a pharmacy of health food store. The acutely painful joints of rheumatic fever, as well as chronic inflammations respond to these simple measures.

Paraffin Bath

Water in its various forms is a versatile medium to convey or withdraw heat from the body. Water's high *heat conduction* property explains its value for this. **Paraffin**, however, has a low heat conduction. It therefore can be used as a vehicle to apply heat to a local area for a longer period of time. Paraffin adheres to the skin and does not allow evaporation or heat elimination to take place. Therefore, local skin temperatures can be elevated more than would be tolerated by water alone.

The **paraffin bath** is used in arthritis cases involving joints of the hands or of the feet. Circulation to these joints is increased. Even the small blood vessels are dilated.

The paraffin (purchased from any super market) is prepared in a double boiler, using one pint of Mineral Oil to five pounds of paraffin. A thermometer capable of registering up to 150° F. should be employed. Usually a temperature of 120° to 130° is used for the immersion. To sterilize paraffin in a tank, heat the temperature to 180° to 200° F. When the paraffin cools and a film forms over the top, dip the hand or body part six to twelve times, allowing several seconds for cooling after each dip. After repeatedly dipping the hand (or foot) to form a wax glove, hold the extremity still to avoid cracking the paraffin. Then wrap it in plastic, and cover with a towel, preserving the heat for another 15–20 minutes. If both hands are to be treated, dip one hand first, then remove and wrap it in plastic while the other hand is being done.

After the treatment, remove your paraffin glove and place the wax in a basin. The "glove" may be used for finger exercise (squeezing and kneading), or it may be cleaned and replaced in the tank. **Remember that paraffin is flammable. DO NOT SPILL IT ON THE STOVE.**

Treated daily, arthritic hands and feet soften and joints improve their function when these simple baths are used. Never use paraffin, however, when there is an open lesion, an unhealed scar, or a skin infection. Also, use great care in treating old, weak, debilitated individuals. Peripheral vascular diseases, where circulation is compromised, constitutes another contraindication for the use of paraffin.

For cases of sciatica or bursitis, spread the paraffin with a brush, using 10 to 12 coats. Then cover the part with oiled silk or wax paper. Apply a towel or flannel. A heat lamp will help to keep the paraffin warm for another 10 to 30 minutes. Consult a physician if questions arise regarding indications or if results seem unsatisfactory.

Medicated Steam Inhalation

Colds, coughs, and influenza are particularly common during the colder seasons of each year. Significantly, a definite relationship has been found between a person's resistance to colds and the temperature of his skin, especially the upper chest and back. If your skin does not warm up rapidly after being chilled, the temperature of mucous membranes in the respiratory tract is also lowered. When this occurs, the resistance of these membranes to nose and throat infection is diminished. Congestion follows, and there is a feeling of stuffiness and excessive drainage. In cases of bronchitis or pneumonia, there follows a harsh cough, which becomes deep and raspy, as the sputum loosens.

The **steam inhalation** is an excellent agent to supply warm, moist air over the congested mucous membranes. A **vaporizer** which heats water electrically can generate steam most effectively. Care must be taken not to burn the sick person with such a device. However, it most effectively increases the humidity. Water may also be boiled in the kitchen, on a hot plate or a wood stove, to increase the ambient humidity. This is especially important in northern winters, when central heating dries out the air, drying out the skin and also the mucous membranes. When a vaporizer is used, *oil of eucalyptus* or *tincture of benzoin* (from a pharmacy) may be added to increase the potency of steam on mucous membranes.

A simple tent can be constructed, using an umbrella over the bed, with a sheet to cover it. Steam may be directed into this tent, increasing its effectiveness.

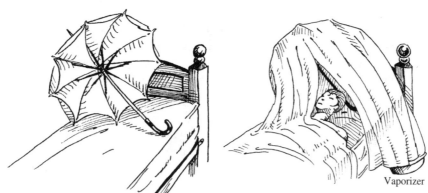

Home adaptation for the **steam tent**. Use it to treat bronchitis and other respiratory conditions.

Vaporizer

Precautions must be taken to avoid ALL risk of burning. Drafts in the sick room should also be avoided. Particular care must be given in treating children, so that accidents are prevented.

The steam inhalation or vaporizer effectively relieves cough and inflammation of the mucous membranes in the nose, throat, and larynx. It helps as well in throat irritation and draining sinuses.

People who suffer from acute asthma usually do better using a **cool mist humidifier**. This device delivers a fine spray into the room, thereby increasing the humidity. It is not used with medication, as a rule, but helps in cases of wheezing or severe allergies. Newer types employ *ultrasonic* principles (sound waves) to create a fine mist. They are helpful devices, but need careful adjustment to prevent such excessive humidity that will literally take off the wallpaper. Clean these appliances carefully between use to prevent mold or mildew accumulation. Many asthmatic patients are allergic to the spores.

Wet Sheet Packs

Fevers involving babies and small children respond particularly well to the **wet sheet pack**. Use it early in the course of an infection before high fever, chest congestion, or vomiting develops. This simple remedy may avoid the necessity for many emergency medical consultations and antibiotic prescriptions.

Before giving the wet sheet pack, however, it is often well to assure complete elimination with an **enema**. As a preheating measure, give a **full hot bath** to draw blood to the skin and lessen congestion. Immediately after the hot bath, your child may be placed in the wet sheet pack and wrapped up quickly. This is comfortable and well tolerated, even with a small child.

Several stages of response occur as time progresses. The *first stage* is one of cooling. To enhance this effect, before the sheet has been warmed to body temperature, the blanket may be folded back and cold water sprinkled on the patient over the sheet. He or she may be fanned then to hasten evaporation and thereby lower the temperature.

The *second* or *neutral stage* begins when the temperature of the pack reaches or slightly exceeds that of the skin (about 94° F.). This stage may be prolonged by removing some of the dry coverings after the warming has well begun. The neutral stage has a marked sedative effect, inducing relaxation and sleep. It is especially helpful for those in danger of convulsions or excited and nervous patients.

The *third stage* of heating begins when the skin temperature rises slightly, and ends with the beginning of a general perspiration. Tonic and heating effects may be prolonged by applying cold water to the head and neck continuously. This helps to check excessive sweating. For a tonic effect, this stage should be continued about twenty minutes.

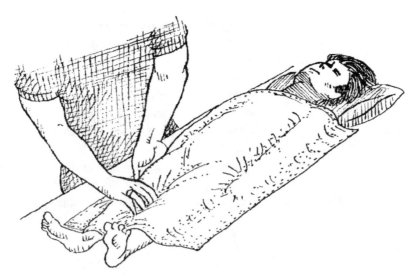

Wet sheet pack **for childhood fevers.**

A *fourth stage*, of sweating, develops as the pores open and the body attempts to cool itself. Sweating may be increased by applying hot water bottles or fomentations within the folds of the dry blanket. Drinking hot sugar–free lemonade or hot water can promote your elimination of impurities through opening skin pores. Cold compresses on the forehead should **not** be very cold or renewed too frequently. This eliminating stage is salutary for delirious fevers, alcoholism, infantile convulsions, and many other common ailments. When the subject falls asleep, the pack gradually returns to a neutral stage, going through other stages as it cools.

In giving a **wet sheet pack** properly, it is important that the wet sheet come in close contact with the skin at all points. A dry blanket applied over the patient must prevent entrance of air or chilling may result. Warming up begins immediately. During the entire treatment the feet should be kept warm. Administer only water—or clear fluids if pack extends through mealtime. The attendance of a sympathetic, interested therapist helps to allay fear and secure cooperation. With these few suggestions, a wet sheet pack will find increasing use in the treatment of infectious illnesses of obscure origin.

Ice Packs

It was Priessnitz of Austria who first advocated the use of cold compresses after injury. Applications of cold are now given not only to relieve minor injuries but also for anesthesia. In proper situations, applications of cold can be just as appropriate as the use of heat.

For a sprained wrist or ankle, ice packs, snow, or cold water should be applied at the earliest possible moment. Combined with elevation of the injured extremity, the application of cold will prevent swelling and lessen the black and blue discoloration which occurs when blood vessels are injured. Cold contracts these blood vessels and keeps blood from oozing into the torn tissues. If the injured extremity is kept elevated and bandaged with an elastic support, healing will usually take place rapidly.

Applications of heat should be avoided for the first day or two in sprains or bruises. If more blood is drawn to the part by heating, tissue swelling increases. Cold packs should be applied in this type of injury to slow down the circulation and overcome the reaction of the body. Cold also relieves pain. Any application of ice or snow, however, should be removed periodically, so that the body can maintain its ability to react to temperature changes.

Cold is employed by immersing the sprained ankle in ice water or cold tap water for 30 minutes out of every two hours. Do this for at least four to six treatments. If it is difficult to put the sprained limb into cold water an ice bag or **ice pack** may be applied while the limb is kept elevated. Since an ice bag cannot cover the joint entirely, try preparing the pack as follows:

First, protect the bed or furniture with a piece of rubber sheeting or oiled silk. Then lay down a piece of plastic, such as a section of shower curtain, large enough to wrap the joint. Cover this with a one inch layer of thick towels. Then wrap the joint in a light flannel strip or bandage. Finely crushed ice or snow is then packed around the joint, not directly contacting the skin. A layer of toweling is then wrapped around the joint and pinned into place, finally surrounded with the plastic. This application can be removed after 30 minutes and reapplied every two hours, until the pain and swelling has abated. Between treatments it is helpful to give support by elastic bandaging. Avoid weight bearing. It may be painful.

Movement of the affected joint should begin as early as possible to prevent stiffness. Similar ice packs may also be used in cases of acute joint inflammation, in gout, in rheumatoid arthritis, and in acute bursitis. **Burns** of the skin should always be treated by immediate cooling with ice or cold water. Often, the extent of a burn can be reduced by this emergency first-aid measure.

Cleansing Enema

Four principal channels for the elimination of waste products are the lungs, the skin, the urinary tract, and the colon. In illness the elimination of toxic waste products is of primary importance to the healing process. In home care it is sometimes necessary to give an enema for colon cleansing or to stimulate bowel activity.

An **enema** can be given in several positions. For an extremely weak or sick person, it is best given in bed, with the patient lying on his left side. A salt solution is usually used with 1 teaspoon of salt to 1 pint of water. Tap water can also be effective, but soap suds solutions should be avoided, because of their irritation. In cases of colitis or unusual chronic inflammations of the bowel, a *charcoal slurry* solution can be made by stirring powdered activated charcoal into water. Then use only the cloudy solution which results after the liquid has set for a couple of hours. This "slurry enema" will reduce inflammation locally, giving considerable relief.

After inserting the enema tube carefully into the rectum, using a lubricant to aid passage, the container is elevated and the solution allowed to run in slowly. By slowly distending the colon, a normal stimulus to defecation is induced. The height of the can above the bed and the degree of pinching of the tubing regulates the rate of the flow. If

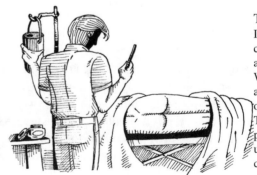

The **enema**
Insert the tub[e] carefully, usi[ng] adequate lub[ricant.] Water shoul[d run in] as the patien[t lies] on the left si[de.] The knee ch[est] position can [be] used for hig[h colon] cleansing.

a person complains of a desire to expel the enema, stop the flow for a few seconds by clamping the tubing. A small volume of solution repeated is better than a large amount, because an over distended bowel loses the tone necessary for vigorous contraction.

The individual should then be placed on a bed pan or assisted to the commode. If your patient is very ill, he or she should be continually attended to until the evacuation is completed and he or she is comfortable again.

Hot Water Bottles

Someone has said, *"If a procedure is capable of doing good, it is also capable of doing harm."* The **hot water bottle** is generally considered a simple home remedy, but precautions are necessary to make it safe and effective.

Patients who are paralyzed or unconscious have an impaired sense of temperature and cannot tell if a hot water bottle is too hot. Those who have cold extremities may likewise have some impairment to the circulation. Burns may result if caution is not exercised in the use of hot water.

Water at 115° to 125° F. can be poured into the hot water bottle making it 1/3 to 1/2 full. Air should be expelled by placing the bottle on one side, until the water reaches the neck. The top is then closed securely and the device checked for leaks. A flannel cover or towel is used to cover the hot water bottle. It should NEVER be used without some protective covering. Avoid placing heating devices in contact with patients who are unconscious or paralyzed, who have poor circulation or advanced diabetes. If used properly, hot water bottles can relieve pain, relax and warm a bedfast patient, and even prolong the effect of fomentations. Congestion is relieved and sleep assisted by the use of this simple home remedy.

Sprays and Douches

The **sprays** apply water from multiple "needle" spray heads striking the entire body surface, except the head and the feet. They are used, not only for cleansing, but as a tonic measure, with or without previous application of heat. Women should wear a shower cap. Ambulatory patients may prefer to wear thong sandals.

After the individual washes himself or herself with soap and rinses well, the therapist adjusts the spray from a sedative temperature to hot and then to cold. The most sedative effects are seen with a *neutral spray*, while hot and cold contrast can be used as a vigorous tonic. The latter has a definite fatigue-relieving effect and can be employed as a progressive program in vascular exercise.

Tub Baths

A **neutral tub bath** with a temperature of 94° to 98° F. is a valuable sedative. Effective in exhaustion of the central nervous system, insomnia, and nervous irritability, it becomes one of nature's finest tranquilizers, as well as an inducer of restful sleep. The tub should be filled with water at the above temperature to *cover* the individual up to the neck.

The room should be quiet, with subdued light, and a pillow or folded towel placed under the head. When the individual lies quietly and relaxes in the water, the tub should be covered with a sheet to preserve the water temperature, as well as for privacy. The skin should be dried by gentle blotting, without friction or unnecessary rubbing, and at least thirty minutes of undisturbed rest should be allowed after this treatment.

Other types of baths can be used with medication. **Dry starch** may be added to a tub of water at neutral temperature to relieve skin irritation. *Aveeno* or finely pulverized oatmeal (sold at most pharmacies) may also be used, adding two cupfuls to a full tub of water for the relief of skin irritation. An **Aveeno bath** is not as drying as a starch bath. Lumping may be avoided by placing the Aveeno in a coarse muslin bag and soaking it in a towel of hot water first. Since these substances may make the bottom of the tub slippery, care should be taken to prevent falling. For itching of the skin a water dispersible oil such as *Alpha Keri*, or *oil of juniper* (Almay Tar) may be used. A **pine oil bath**, using one-half ounce of *balpine oil* to a tub of water, is a pleasant, refreshing sedative and produces slight redness of the skin. Look in health food stores for these oils.

Steam Baths

A full-body **steam bath** may be taken either reclining or sitting. The *Turkish bath* is done in a cabinet with the individual seated and the head exposed.

A full-body steam bath with the patient reclining is called a *Russian bath*. These are used to produce sweating and for mild fever therapy. The body temperature is increased in this environment of 100% humidity, preventing heat loss. There is usually an increase in pulse rate, blood pressure, and metabolism. Alcoholism and other addictions, rheumatoid arthritis, obesity, and certain cases of influenza respond well to the steam bath.

Home style **steam treatment**. On a hot plate place a tea kettle or pan of boiling water. Place this under a wooden stool, on which the patient sits. A shower curtain or some waterproof material is placed around the patient, with a hole for the head. **Be careful to avoid burns!**

Since this is a more vigorous treatment than other heating measures, certain considerations should be regarded. A generalized steam treatment is contraindicated in hypertension, diabetes, and cardiac impairment. An individual should have had a bowel movement within 24 hours previous to the treatment time and should void before taking the treatment. Adequate fluid intake should be encouraged during and preceding the treatment, as any increased perspiration helps eliminate some wastes.

Preheating the body with a hot foot bath or using a fomentation to the spine is helpful. In the home, a hot plate with a kettle of water may be placed under a wooden stool or chair, on which the patient is seated. The feet are placed in a hot foot bath. A shower curtain with a hole cut out for the head may be wrapped around, much as in the barber chair or at the hairdresser's. With complete covering in this way, the steam filling the area will cause a rapid onset of sweating. It may be necessary to apply a cold compress to the head, changing it frequently. Finish the treatment with a graduated spray. Patients should be adequately cooled after every steam treatment and rest for 1/2 to 1 hour.

With aromatic medications, such as *tincture of benzoin, camphor gum, menthol,* or *eucalyptus oil,* the steam bath can be therapeutic in relieving the inflammation of mucous membranes, common colds, sinusitis, and bronchitis. Other chronic conditions of the respiratory tract improve when these inhalant mixtures are used in conjunction with the steam.

Ultraviolet Therapy

Natural sunlight (*heliotherapy*), of course, is the best source for ultra-violet light. Most people today get too little sunlight, except in short doses during the summertime. A source of *ultraviolet radiation* which approaches natural sunlight is the **sunlamp** bulb. It may be used on any household AC current and screwed into a standard reading lamp. Privacy should be secured and the eyes protected, covering them with a black cloth, or using dark glasses. Special precautions should be taken to avoid the burns that result from direct rays of the sunlamp. For average people the maximum time for first exposure should be about six minutes, with a distance from the lamp of thirty inches. For greater safety, a greater distance can be employed, with exposure time proportionately increased, depending upon the lamp manufacturer's directions. One minute daily may be added to the exposure, up to fifteen minutes maximum. The eyes should always be protected. Gradual skin tanning will usually occur.

Ultraviolet rays aid the body in producing **Vitamin D**. This helps us absorb calcium, thus building strong bones and teeth. Infections in the skin are improved and a general tone of the body results from the regular use of sunlight or ultraviolet. Many other physiologic effects are being discovered, but the benefits can be had only by those who *use* this valuable remedial agent.

These are only a sample of many forms of hydrotherapy useful in home treatments. More complicated procedures can be given in sanitariums and hospitals where this therapy is emphasized. Water treatments do take time. So, remember that nature, if assisted, will do her work wisely and well. Hydro-therapy, massage, and physical medicine will continue to find their place in homes and hospitals where diseases are treated physiologically and where the body's *needs* are truly regarded in your recovery from illness.

255

CHAPTER EIGHTEEN

MEDICAL

BOTANY

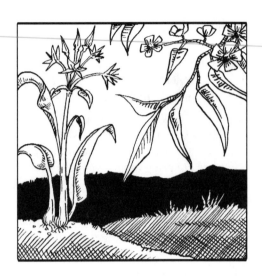

Nature study of all types can be most fascinating. The infinite variety displayed in the plant kingdom, and particularly the array of colors, aromas, and designs seen, delights the serious student of botany. Among the various grasses, trees, wild flowers, and other herbs, there exist a great many healing properties. The study of these medicinal agents and their use in the treatment of simple illnesses is called **medical botany**.

In studying healing properties found in plants the student and health practitioner alike must always remember that *"what is new is not necessarily true and what is true in not necessarily new."* Furthermore, this sage advice by Alexander Pope is still applicable: *"Be not the first by whom the new is tried, nor the last to lay the old aside."* As we consider the various medicinal plants and their usefulness in health and disease, let us also look at the many years of change that have either amalgamated or mutated these plants, causing some of them to be poisonous.

Closely parallel and an equally fascinating field is the use of wild plants for food. Nearly everyone is familiar with the appearance of tomatoes on the vine, potatoes in the ground, and various fruits on the trees. Few people, however, realize the vast food resources in the wilderness, by the roadsides, and upon majestic mountains where wild flowers, roots, trees, and grasses proliferate. They supply food in abundance, not only for animals, but for man. A knowledge of *edible wild plants* is valuable in preparing for survival when future economic pressures or crop failures may make such simple nutrition mandatory. In the scope of this volume, however, only a few select plants can be covered, thus whetting the "appetite" to pursue similar studies in growing numbers of references that guide more detailed research in botanical lines.

MEDICINAL PLANTS

Let us look now at several healing herbs that come widely recommended to relieve symptoms and treat common diseases. This list is selected, and far from comprehensive, since among more than 40,000 plant species, many *hundreds* have been used by Indian herbalists and herbal practitioners of other nations. Some herbs can be cultivated and grown in greenhouses, in ornamental garden patios, even window ledges. Others are found among the wild grasses or flowers of forest and meadow, challenging nature lovers to take a walk now and then, to gather, to classify, and dry these medicinal botanicals for use at a future occasion.

Aloe Vera

Easily grown and very decorative, the **aloe** plant provides a quick and certain relief for many minor burns. At the barbecue or a kitchen stove, any first or second degree burn can be soothed with pain rapidly relieved by the juice expressed from the *aloe vera* leaf. Usually a simple house plant, the aloe grows in warm humid climates, and is cultivated beside the outdoor barbecue of most Hawaiian residences. Every home should have one or two of these valuable plants.

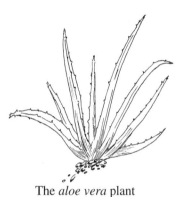

The *aloe vera* plant

Buchu

Known by its botanical name *Rutacae*, this low shrub has small leaves and angular branches. Flowers range from pink to white in color. Dried leaves are used for medicine, prepared as a tea. A usual standard remedy consists of 1 teaspoon of the dried powdered leaves steeped in a cup of hot water. Take it in small doses. A preparation of **buchu** stimulates the appetite, increases the flow of perspiration, and acts as a natural diuretic. This is a valuable tea for chronic disease of the urinary tract—such as cystitis, urethritis, and prostatitis. It may have value in cases involving stones in the urinary passage, and historically has also been useful in cases of vaginal discharge (*leucorrhea*).

Camphor

Steam is passed through the chipped wood of large trees in Taiwan to obtain the **camphor** distillate. The preparation is then heated until evaporation to obtain the oil. It is frequently used as an inhalant in vaporizers. Internal usage should be strictly limited, although some have claimed it beneficial in intestinal worms, various types of rheumatism, and respiratory infections.

Cascara Sagrada

Of the tree family *Rhamnaceae*, the medicinal preparation comes from the bark. **Cascara** acts as a gastrointestinal irritant. The fresh bark should be stored for at least a year, because of its powerful properties. As a laxative, the bark is usually steeped, 1 teaspoon to a cup of boiling water. It should not be used regularly, as even herbal laxatives may weaken the body's normal intestinal reflexes.

Castor Oil

This well-known cathartic and purgative obtained from the castor bean plant has a mild action to evacuate the bowel. One to four teaspoons may be taken to produce very complete elimination. Usually the castor oil is blended with cracked ice and orange juice, or taken in fresh or warm milk to disguise the oily taste. Castor oil may also be applied externally to relieve joint pain or itching of the skin.

Catnip

This herb from the *mint* family is available in capsules in many health food stores. But **catnip** is typically taken as a tea. Its effect helps to calm the nerves, but catnip also aids in removing gas from the intestinal tract. And it induces perspiration. The dried leaves are boiled. Like most mints, catnip is easy to grow around the house.

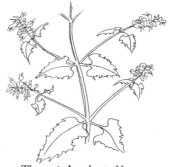

The **catnip** plant, *Nepeta cataria*, has square stems, true of all *mints*.

Chamomile

Chamomile is a humble roadside herb is well known as a simple remedy for nervous problems. The flowers and leaves are dried and powdered, then they are steeped in boiling water to prepare a tea. Pain has been relieved with poultices prepared from the chamomile flowers.

Comfrey

Known by several other names, such as *Gum plant* and *healing herb*, this perennial beautifies many a planting box or garden. The leaves are large and hairy, usually dark green with pointed ends. A fair amount of sunshine is needed, with good soil and plenty of water, to produce prolific growth. Although **comfrey** is probably used for more different purposes than any other herb, I list but a few that have shown favorable results. A tea made from comfrey is prepared with hot water, into which is stirred an ounce of the powdered root or leaves. This may be taken several times a day. It is a rich source of calcium.

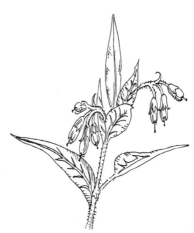

Comfrey, *Symphytum officinale* showing leaves and flowers.

Various irritations of the stomach, even diarrhea, have responded to the soothing effects of this cleansing agent. Mucous membrane irritations improve. Hot compresses or poultices may be made from the comfrey plant, using the moistened powdered herb or crushed green leaves. Prompt scab formation will follow the direct application, with considerable acceleration of healing to a cut or wound.

Comfrey is a nutritive food. Often the fresh leaves are blended in a base of unsweetened pineapple juice, to which mints or parsley has been added to make a healthful "green drink." Give it a try in your herb garden.

Charcoal

Although not strictly an "herb" in itself, **charcoal** is derived from the incomplete combustion of many plant products. Usually obtained from a hard wood, charcoal is produced by slow combustion in a relative absence of oxygen. Although most hard woods can be utilized in the manufacture of medicinal charcoal, *eucalyptus* wood seems to be one of the best. In a home-like setting, charcoal can be scraped or chipped from the charred hardwood. After being

259

moistened with water, it is forced through a food grinder. Commercial sources of charcoal are also available, principally obtained from *coconut shells.*

Treatment with superheated steam, or another industrial method, can produce "activated" charcoal, which is capable of much improved absorptive effect. The use of medicinal charcoal goes back to ancient Egypt, and was found in an Egyptian papyrus dated around 1550 B.C. In the time of Hippocrates *wood chars* were used to treat various ailments.

Charcoal's adsorptive property is due to a myriad of micropores, the walls of which have surface areas that range from 400 to over 1800 square meters per gram! Thus, the surface area of powdered charcoal is phenomenal. Finely ground charcoal particles are so small that it takes about 50 million to make one pound! One should not confuse the properties of activated charcoal with burnt toast or charcoal briquettes.

Many poisons can be *adsorbed* by charcoal, although the properties are quite selective. DDT, dieldrin, strychnine, malathion, and parathion are some industrial toxins that become inactivated by this "miracle" substance. Many drugs are likewise adsorbed by charcoal. Several more common ones include aspirin, barbiturates, cocaine, opium, nicotine, morphine, penicillin, and sulfas. Inorganic substances are adsorbed, such as mercury, phosphorus, chlorine, iron, lead, and silver. For this reason, **charcoal should be an important constituent of the emergency kit in every household**. Better than the *universal antidote* in case of acute poisoning, a rescue worker has merely to induce vomiting, followed with a large dose of activated charcoal to render most substances harmless. Usually 30 to 60 grams, about ¼ cup, is needed, suspended in water and taken as soon as possible after the injection of any toxin.

Charcoal may be employed to reduce or eliminate distress from intestinal gas. Its adsorbing and deodorizing properties are welcome in skin ulcers. For colostomies, place a tablet in the bag with each cleansing. Charcoal can act as an air purifier in a sickroom, in the refrigerator, or where recycling of air is necessary, as is common in a submarine.

Although a charcoal filter in cigarettes may remove three times as much of the toxic vapor as ordinary filters do, the carbon monoxide and nitric acid present in the smoke are **not** efficiently adsorbed. Charcoal has furthermore been used in the filtering of blood for the victims of kidney disease who must undergo repetitive dialysis. Depressed individuals who have taken an overdose of drug medication may additionally be saved with a specially designed charcoal filter that will revitalize the blood, while removing impurities.

Newborn babies who experience **jaundice** will usually be improved with activated charcoal. Bile secretion from the liver into the intestines is usually followed by an efficient reabsorption process. Charcoal binds this bile and carries the pigment out, reducing risks from jaundice. Charcoal can be mingled with the baby's formula, or for breast milk expressed into a bottle, may be mixed with the mother's milk and given for several days until the neonatal jaundice clears. The need for exchange transfusions and hospitalization has been reduced considerably with this simple measure.

Charcoal is moreover a valuable remedy for **diarrhea**. Two table-spoons of activated charcoal powder in a glass of cold water, is taken every 4 to 8 hours until the diarrhea is under control. Charcoal capsules should be in the **travel kit** of any one going to countries where the danger of *Tourista*, traveler's diarrhea, exists. If unusual intestinal irritation occurs, so that vomiting is a problem, the charcoal can be allowed to stand and settle, then one drinks the clear looking *slurry* water on top. Millions of charcoal particles are present in this "clear" liquid, as can be demonstrated by shining a light from the side. It reveals a cloudiness, called the *Tyndall phenomenon*. Even a baby will get considerable relief from this charcoal water.

Skin infections can respond to charcoal mixed with water, and applied as a poultice. Water and activated charcoal are stirred until the consistency is that of a thick cream. The mixture can be "geled" with boiled *flax seed*, *aloe vera* gel, or *agar*, then poured onto a piece of cotton flannel. This pack is placed directly over the area of inflammation, covered with a piece of plastic, and finally secured with tape. You should change the poultice every 6 to 8 hours or when it becomes dry. This natural adsorbing agent will reduce pain and inflammation in cases of cellulitis, bruises, and superficial burns. When properly used such a simple, inexpensive, and harmless medicine will save many lives.

Eucalyptus

Eucalyptus (also known as *blue gum*) leaves have many beneficial effects. Distilled as an oil, eucalyptus may be inhaled freely for sore throats and infections of the bronchial tubes or lungs. It helps to reduce swelling of the mucous membranes in asthma and can be used with most vaporizers. A **cough syrup** may be prepared from the eucalyptus oil with three to ten drops stirred into a cup of honey. A small amount of lemon juice may be added for flavoring. One teaspoon of honey–eucalyptus "cough syrup" may be taken every few hours to relieve a sore throat or cough associated with many common respiratory illnesses.

Figs

A common fruit tree in subtropical climates, the **fig** is not only delicious to eat, but medicinal in several aspects. Dating back to Biblical times (See Isaiah 38:21), the fig has been used for various skin afflictions. For painful **boils**, the ripe, fresh fruit should be split open and laid over the lesion. Its powerful proteolytic enzyme *ficin* helps to liquefy and dissolve necrotic tissue. The osmotic effect and high sugar content help to draw poisons from the wound, as well as inhibit the multiplication of disease-producing bacteria. Other sores may similarly respond. A fig tree finds its place around the patio of most southern homes, if for no other reason than for the delicious fruit it bears.

Garlic

Garlic belongs to the same family as the onion. This powerful plant has great medicinal value, in spite of the offensive breath it produces. There is considerable evidence that it may reduce high blood pressure. As an expectorant, garlic tends to remove mucus from the throat. It is a natural antibiotic, inhibitory to yeast organisms as well. Most easily taken in capsules or "pearls," garlic drops may particularly aid the expulsion of intestinal worms. More experimentation is needed to determine just which parasites respond most promptly to this common bulb.

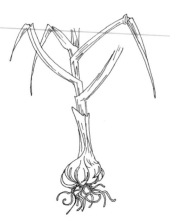

Garlic, *Allium sativum*. Good for what ails you.

Golden Seal

This herb grows plentifully in virgin forests of the United States. However, **golden seal** is becoming more scarce as a wild plant, and if cultivated, should be planted in well-fertilized soil. Abundant shade and good drainage will aid in its cultivation. Golden seal generally has a vasoconstrictive effect on the body. Blood vessels are tightened, improving conditions in which running secretions or catarrh are seen. In combination with bicarbonate of soda, golden seal may serve as a mouth wash for the relief of sores in the oral cavity, especially the gums. It may also have a styptic effect in certain cases of nosebleeds.

Jewel Weed

A beautiful late summer wild flower in the southern United States, **jewel weed**, or **spotted touch-me-not**, is a favorite habitat for hummingbirds. The fresh stem and leaves may be boiled in shortening to form an ointment for hemorrhoids. Weeping eruptions, such as poison ivy, may also respond to the plant juices rubbed on the affected skin at frequent intervals.

Hops

Dried leaves of the **hops** plant may be taken in capsule form or steeped for an herb tea. The alkaloid *lupulon*, present in the hops plant, is a sedative. In some scientific studies it has been shown to slow brain wave patterns. Hops tea is therefore valued when a person needs assistance to induce sleep. Chronic insomniacs may need several capsules. The strong hops flavor may be modified with a small amount of lemon or honey to make the tea more palatable.

Honey

Delicious as a food, **honey** is useful also in medicine. The high sugar concentration of pure liquid honey completely inhibits bacterial multiplication. Thus, honey is usually free of contamination by micro-organisms, more than most natural substances.

Honey may be used with other agents to prepare a natural cough syrup. It also is valued as a covering balm over skin infections. With its osmotic drawing power and bacterial inhibition honey may rapidly aid in wound healing. Particularly, honey is helpful as a flavor enhancer and sweetener for many herb teas that otherwise would be difficult to take because of their strong flavor.

Kelp

This seaweed is found along coasts and bordered inlets of the north Atlantic and north Pacific oceans. Being without a true root, stem, or leaf, **kelp** grows near the surface of sea water, attached to rocks. The high *iodine* content of this plant makes it a valuable supplement in cases where iodine deficiency has produced thyroid disease. Other trace minerals are present that may help in blood formation. Some vitamins are also found.

Lemon

The juice of the **lemon**, a citrus fruit, may be used as a disinfectant for minor infections, Rich in *Vitamin C*, lemon has become a popular remedy for coughs and colds. It may be mixed with honey to make a healthful syrup. Some reported beneficial effects of lemon in cases of arthritis or other chronic diseases may be due to its Vitamin C content, rather than other special herbal properties.

Oats

Cultivated extensively in the temperate zones, the common **oats** thrive best in wet soil. Oatmeal and rolled oats are prepared by removing the husks: the kernels are then rolled or ground. So-called "quick oats" are kernels, first partially cooked before rolling. This lessens the time required in preparing the product for food. Oats may be used for many conditions. The fiber of this healthful grain makes it a value in cases of indigestion and constipation. Oat bran also helps to lower cholesterol. Itching skin may respond to *poultices* of oatmeal. A bath taken in oatmeal water (*Aveno* is a common brand) will be therapeutic in many allergic conditions of the skin.

Olive

This often used remedy for constipation is a popular laxative for children. As eaten *in* the **olive**, natural olive oil is healing to an inflamed stomach. It also may be of value in chronic infections, such as tuberculosis. Olives are good for kidney infections and nephritis. Used externally, pure olive oil may be applied as an ointment for bruises, burns, scalds, and other skin conditions. A drop of warm olive oil may be placed in the ear to relieve the pain of mild earache.

Onion

Commonly used in flavoring and valuable as a source of Vitamin C, **onions** can additionally be made into a poultice for tumors or ulcers, especially where there is pus formation. Pain may be relieved in a short time, particularly with the use of the milder onion varieties.

Plantain

The leaves of the common **plantain**, a green wild flower, have a pleasant, cooling effect upon the body. The juice helps stop bleeding from minor wounds. Fresh plantain leaves may be rubbed directly on parts of the body stung by insects, or on the skin rash produced by the stinging nettle.

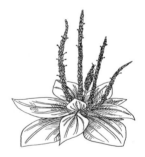

The **common plantain,**
Plantago major.

Pine

The aromatic properties of **pine** needles are highly valued in respiratory afflictions. Boiled in water or used in vaporizer, the *balsam* of the pine, as well as other conifers such as cedar and fir will have numerous healing effects.

Rhubarb

Cultivated around the world in moist fertile soil, **rhubarb** has been a favorite of pie makers for many generations. The herb resembles our ordinary garden variety, but attains a larger size. Avoid carefully the leaves, because of some poisonous properties. Small amounts of the powdered *rhizome* or root may be used for cleansing the intestines and colon. Rhubarb is one of the most mild laxatives, making it especially desirable in constipation associated with hemorrhoids.

Psyllium

Small **psyllium** seeds can be ground or soaked in water to form a mucilaginous substance. They are valued as a stool softener when taken with water. Commercial preparations, such as *Metamucil* or *Konsyl* are easily obtained, making it easy to try. One spoonful in a glass of water or fruit juice may be taken once or twice a day to improve the softness and ease of passage, especially for elderly, sedentary, or constipated individuals.

Smartweed

Another common wildflower growing in late summer is **smartweed**, of which there are several varieties. One type is quite mild, but the white flowered variety if crushed and rubbed on the skin will produce a definite *counter-irritant* effect. Poultices of charcoal mixed with smartweed and water have double value in reducing the inflammation of bruises and similar skin inflammations. These and other wildflowers can be easily identified from their descriptions and photographs, available in popular field guides.

Slippery Elm

A stately and beautiful tree, **slippery elm** has most interesting advantages, hidden beneath its bark. Carefully cut a section of slippery elm bark from the tree, then peel it back to disclose a mucilaginous substance. The gel may be scraped with a knife from the inner surface. Allowed it to dry and form a powder. Slippery elm can then be mixed with other herbs to prepare poultices, giving "body" and consistency to the medicinal herb mixture. With careful observation, you can find many slippery elm trees. Their growth should be protected by careful use of the valuable bark, allowing "healing" to occur after the material is harvested.

POISONOUS HERBS

A number of plants developed harmful properties, through amalgamation and genetic change. Some botanical substances are highly toxic and can quickly bring about death. Other agents have a slower action, yet are equally dangerous. I have chosen to list a number of these poisonous herbs, and recommend their identification in order to avoid accidental harm or poisoning that could easily come to the unwary.

Opium

From an oriental *poppy*, **opium** is refined into morphine or smoked as the "crude" substance. Having a profound addicting effect on the body, opium use is clearly harmful to society. It distorts mental perception. Although the use, possession, or transportation of opium or its derivatives in the United States carries penalties, opiates are nevertheless a big dilemma, both in medicine and in the influential underworld that permeates numerous large cities.

Marijuana

Common, but illegally grown in the United States and Mexico, the **marijuana** plant is a growing saboteur of youthful idealism. Frequently rolled into cigarettes called "joints" and smoked, marijuana has found its way onto college campuses, high schools, and even business circles. The active ingredient *tetrahydrocannabinol* (THC), produces a profound distortion of reality in both time and space.

In spite of the temporarily heightened imagination and false feeling of mental perceptions, regular use of marijuana is clearly associated with decreased mental acuity, a decrease of purpose and drive, and lack of interest and ambition. Marijuana use underlies many educational failures today, as well as leading into other serious addictions.

Tobacco

It is difficult to condense in a small reference book the insidious effects that have followed **tobacco** use. Tobacco is a major cash crop in the South, with a powerful industry and governmental lobby. Nevertheless, tobacco is without doubt a major health hazard. It is even more insidious because of its slow, malignant nature, the ability to create cancer. Many alkaloids that come from its combustion are capable of producing cancer in the lung, as well as the mouth, throat, larynx, stomach, and bladder.

Smoking not only contributes to cancer, it is a principle cause of heart disease, bronchitis, and emphysema. Tobacco use leads to depletion of the body's supply of a number of essential vitamins. **Carbon monoxide**, concentrated in the mainstream smoke of the cigarette's deadly "coffin nail," sabotages the circulatory system and leads to an oxygen deficiency. This impairs thinking, as well as opening the intracellular spaces in the lining of coronary vessels for cholesterol to deposit.

Nicotine is the primary addicting agent in the tobacco plant, which makes the smoker want to come back for more. Although smoking is the most common avenue of entry into the body, chewing or sniffing tobacco (*snuff*) is finding increasing entrance among the youthful generation and targeted minority groups. Smokers die eight years sooner than non-smokers and are sick 22 per cent more often. Non-smokers living with smokers suffer from more disease from the *passive smoke* to which they are exposed. All usage for the tobacco plant are harmful, unless it would possibly be employed as an insecticide.

Toadstools

A great many **mushrooms** are used for food. Some however, customarily designated **toadstools**, are highly poisonous. The *Amanita* species are among the most poisonous substances known to man. One small bite of this highly toxic mushroom may result in rapid death. It is easily recognized with its swollen base, the ring around the stem, and characteristic speckled cap. Learn to recognize the deadly *Amanita* and avoid them. A general rule in mushroom hunting should require positive

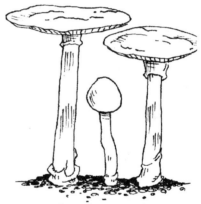

Amanita muscaria.
Watch out for this one!

identification of every species before using them as food. Some are delicious, many are healthful, but the presence of a few poisonous species among this interesting family of fungi makes caution quite prudent.

Poison Ivy, Oak, and Sumac

Notice the drawings which identify the characteristic features of these common skin irritant plants. A poisonous oil is present in each of these, called *urushiol*. It is the main ingredient implicated in the typical "contact dermatitis" produced by these poison plants. All parts of the **poison ivy, poison oak**, or poison sumac, including the roots, stem, leaf, and flower may inflame an allergic individual's sensitive skin. Although some people are seemingly resistant to urushiol's effect, one should never be too sure. Even burning clumps of the offending weeds has produced allergic eruptions. In spite of their beauty, one had better *look, but not touch* when these vines are encountered.

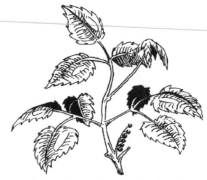

Poison ivy, *Rhus toxico dendron*.
Leaves of three, let them be!

Foxglove

The **foxglove** plants, of which there are many varieties, are a common source of *digitalis*. Of distinct medicinal value in patients with heart failure or rhythm disturbances, the foxglove plant, nevertheless, should be taken only under a physician's direction. Purified forms, with carefully regulated dosages, are available, when the use of digitalis is absolutely necessary. In general, however, the danger of rhythm disturbances and toxic effects with nausea, vomiting, or visual changes should confine the foxglove to its use as an ornamental flower, rather than a medicine.

Belladonna

Also called the **deadly nightshade**, this plant has a powerful inhibitory effect upon the autonomic nervous system. With dilation of pupils, drying of mucous membranes, and decrease of intestinal secretions, the *Belladonna's* properties are indeed powerful. Overdosage is likely with the use of this plant. Its common availability as a tincture should be avoided, because of the alcohol content.

Coffee

This popular beverage comes from a low bush-type plant, cultivated extensively in Central and South America. The beans are harvested when mature, and dried in the sun. Because of the habit forming nature of its principle alkaloid, **caffeine**, coffee is classed with the harmful herbs. Caffeine acts as a drug on the central nervous system. It irritates the stomach, adversely affects a number of organs, and contributes to heart disease, headaches, nervousness and high blood pressure. Caffeine is contained in tea, cocoa, sodas, and some medications, as well as coffee. Unfortunately, the decaffeination process used for most supermarket brands of decaffeinated coffees leaves behind traces of chemicals that may be more dangerous than caffeine. Herbal teas or grain beverages— like *Postum, Pero, Roma,* and *Caffix*— are healthier alternatives to coffee. You can buy them at most health food stores.

Jimson Weed

Classified in the same plant family as potatoes and tomatoes, the **jimson weed** is very toxic. Hallucinations and serious mental changes have been associated with its use, as well as sudden death from overdosage. Blooming in the summer season as a common roadside flower, jimson weed should be carefully avoided, and regarded as a most toxic plant.

EDIBLE PLANTS

Wonderful varieties of delicious and nutritious edible wild plants grow all around our world. Many species are more tasty than familiar foods. Some are as nutritious as similar garden vegetables. A few common ones are listed here for study, as well as to encourage you to try some.

Rose

After the **wild rose** has bloomed, fruit buttons form at the end of the stalk, an essence loaded with *Vitamin C*. **Rose hips** can be picked, made into jelly, or steeped for a tea or soup. In some parts of the world, rose hips are one of the most valuable winter sources of Vitamin C, well known for both keeping quality and delicious flavor.

Dandelion

The common **dandelion** grows in lawns everywhere. Its tender leaves may be made into a fresh tossed salad, as well as cooked for "greens." Some say that it has about four times the nutritional value as lettuce. Even the buds and blossoms are edible.

Plantain

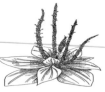

Common **plantain** should be cooked for best taste and palatability. The leaves can be blended with nettles for greater flavor. Gather the plantain in the spring, while the leaves are tender.

Common plantain.

Clover

The **red clover** is quite edible, including the blossom to the root. After drying you can steep the blossoms or leaves for a medicinal tea. Many edible species are known. They should be used in moderation. Even the cattle know that bloating occurs when they have overeaten of clover.

Lamb's Quarters

Goose foot or **lamb's quarters** makes delicious cooked greens. Often found between the rows in the garden, their leaf is shaped somewhat like a goose foot. The leaves are silvery underneath and have a crunchy feeling when you bite them. Like other greens, such as mustard, collards, chard, and spinach lamb's quarters are rich in calcium, as well as trace minerals and Vitamin C.

Chickweed

Chickweed grows in wayside places and around houses nearly everywhere. You will find it in a clump or extensive mat. It may be eaten raw, cooked as greens, or steeped for tea. This is a valuable plant.

Watercress

Watercress can be discovered in running streams, even during winter in the milder climate zones. Before using it in raw salads, soak the plant in chlorinated water for a few minutes to destroy disease producing germs. Some diced onions or leeks may be simmered with the watercress. With salt and lemon seasoning, this plant is delicious. Watercress may be boiled as greens or used in a delicious soup. Other cresses are also equally good.

Thistle

The **thistle** is not all prickles. It has several edible parts. The crisp young stems may be cut in early spring and eaten like celery. It tastes, however, more like grass. Under the faded flower is a white "meat" such as you find in artichokes. In fact, the artichoke plant is a thistle.

Milkweed

The ball-like flower cluster of the **milkweed** may be picked in the morning, while it is wet with dew. Steam them to obtain a sweet liquid, honey-like water. Avoid picking one with a reddish stem, as it is bitter and toxic. Some call it *wild broccoli.* The buds on top of the common milkweed may be cooked. It makes a good vegetable. Even the leaves may be boiled for greens.

Jerusalem Artichoke

Looking like an overgrown sunflower plant, the **Jerusalem artichoke** has smaller flower heads. Dig up the roots and look at the large nutritious tubers. They may be boiled, roasted, baked, or prepared in whatever way you would cook potatoes. The *inulin* content of these starchy tubers make them more healthful for diabetics.

Day Lily

The common **day lily** grows along roadsides, as well as in flower gardens. Orange, red or yellow blossoms may form. When the flower buds are closed and green, snap them off and boil them like string beans.

The blossoms may be baked in a batter for another tasty dish. Crisp white stems of the day lily may be snapped off and eaten raw or steamed. Diced and creamed they make a good dish. The roots are additionally edible.

Violets

The common **violet** is one of the most nutritious green plants that has been analyzed. It is rich in Vitamins A and C, and includes a number of trace minerals. There is more calcium than in your garden greens. The leaves and blossoms may be eaten raw, in a salad, or cooked like spinach.

Ferns

The young **fern** "fiddleheads" may be snapped off and cooked like asparagus. Bracken fern with its three curled prongs is the best, while several others are also good. Do not use the mature fern, as they may be toxic. Rub off the wool and hairs of the young fiddleheads and boil them in salted water. They may also be included in a tossed salad or dried for winter use.

Mints

Wild mint furnishes flavor in refreshing drinks. **Henbit** is an erect little plant with a beautiful flower. This may be eaten raw or boiled as a pot herb. All mints have square stems and clusters of snap dragon-like flowers. Some have medicinal properties, such as **peppermint** and **spearmint**. A cup of hot mint tea may provide a very refreshing beverage for the camper.

Nuts

Nuts are the most concentrated wild food. Many wild nuts grow all around the world, including walnuts, hickory nuts, chestnuts, pine nuts, pecans, hazel nuts, Brazil nuts, cashews, and butternut. They can be stored in the shell or outer hull for winter treats.

Acorns

The **acorn** of the white oak may be roasted and eaten, when picked in the early stages. *Tannic acid* can be removed by crushing the meats and soaking them in a cloth or boiling them in water containing wood ashes. Drained and rinsed, the acorn meat is then pressed thin and baked for crackers. It may be mixed with flour, or flavored with nuts and berries for a special fruit cake.

Elderberry

Black **elderberries** are edible either raw or cooked. Avoid the red ones, however. Growing in bushes along the roadside, the elderberry may be gathered and prepared like grape juice or canned and heated in the winter time with diced apples for a delicious elderberry soup.

Cattails

Growing in swamps, the **cattail** is one of the most edible plants known. The *pollen* found on the cattail spike in the spring may be used for flour, adding its delicious nutty flavor to pancakes or camp bread. Even earlier, look for the young spike hidden in the weeds. It appears like an ear of corn, and can be boiled like corn on the cob and served with salt and butter. It tastes more like the cob than the corn. The cattail *root* is more valuable and can be harvested in the winter, if you don't mind getting muddy. It is said to be 40% starch and 10% sugar. After being washed and peeled, it can be dried and ground to flour. A mixture of cattail flour and acorn meal with chopped wild nuts make delicious camping crackers.

Mushrooms

Most mushroom hunters start with one or two that are easily recognized. We suggest the pear-shaped **puffball**, as a good fungus for a starter. Break it open to be sure it is powder white like marshmallows. If it has lines in it, throw it away. Small egg-shaped puffballs are also good when white inside. No puffball is edible when it becomes old and the brown dust comes out.

A second type of fungus, which is unusual in appearance and easy to recognize, is the **morel**. Its wrinkled appearance makes it easy to identify. Look for the morel in deciduous woods or under apple trees. They are really good eating.

Most important, though, avoid the toxic species. **Do not eat any mushroom that cannot be positively identified**. Particularly, remember the *destroying angel*, or poisonous *Amanita*, with its characteristic cap, ring on the stem, and swollen base. Carry a field guide or take an expert with you in hunting for wild plants and mushrooms.

* * * * * * * * * * *

With a growing interest in plants, medical botany, and herbs, the most rewarding experiences come to the gardener. The cultivation of herbs can be a fascinating hobby, as well as a means of supplementing one's income. Many garden spots, backyard patios, and greenhouses have been devoted to herbs with a resulting beauty, as well as health. Contact with nature tends to enrich the soul, as well as the body. The simple life expressed, the object lessons learned, and the contemplative time spent in one's garden, cultivating herbs, or preparing the food, can bring a renewed awareness and appreciation for the harmony and infinite variety seen in the natural world.

CHAPTER NINETEEN

HEALTH

THROUGH

NATURAL

FOODS

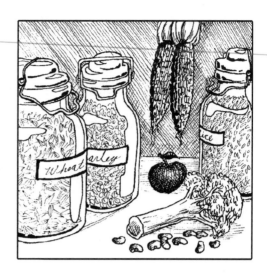

Everyone knows that health is more than diet. However, even physicians may overlook the fact that good food is essential for health. Some diseases are obviously related to nutrition. Obesity, vitamin deficiency syndromes, and malnutrition in underprivileged groups are examples of these. Other medical conditions are either caused or aggravated by poor nutritional practices, but seem less obvious to the nonprofessional. Arteriosclerosis and coronary heart disease, diabetes mellitus and hypoglycemia, and essential hypertension are examples of this latter class. Nevertheless, to have perfect health, our blood must be pure, and the circulation unobstructed. Obedience to the health laws that promote both mental tranquility and physical vigor is directly related to our habits practiced in the dining room.

As I have expressed earlier, our dietary practices established in infancy tend to perpetuate themselves long after teenage and adult years. Nutritional "seeds" planted in childhood bear fruit later, with resultant disease or a productive, happy life. In spite of numerous advances that medical science has made, more and more individuals living in our industrialized nation are "digging their graves with their teeth." This slow form of nutritional suicide is even more insidious than that of the tobacco smoker, but is nevertheless as sure.

Growing numbers of obscure and resistant infections, together with some common ones like colds and influenza, may be traced in part to dietary indiscretion. Many forms of cancer, especially those of the lower digestive tract are intimately associated with dietary habit patterns. I plan to examine in the paragraphs that follow several guidelines to aid you in choosing a more balanced diet. This introduction to the true science of nutrition can benefit you both through the supermarket and the "farmer's market." I wish to enable any homemaker in preparing a table set with the best of nutrients for each member of his or her family.

Choosing A Balanced Diet

Try to picture the body somewhat like a seesaw. When one side goes down the other side goes up. We experience a more pleasant ride when the two sides are balanced. Children then find enjoyment as they play. A balanced diet, likewise, does not come by accident. Careful planning is necessary to achieve the optimum results. We require a wide variety of foods in order to produce nutritional harmony in our bodies. Looking at nutrition from the viewpoint of a scientist, we observe foods divided into several groups. These supply various elements needed for the growth and maintenance of every cell.

Nutritional balance, then, involves a consideration of these elements and their proper interrelationship, aiding our quest for the best of health. Proteins, fats, carbohydrates, vitamins, minerals, fiber, and fluid, are the seven factors to be considered in obtaining this balance. A very simple way to obtain these involves choosing a wide variety of natural foods. These should be eaten at regular intervals, in amounts sufficient to maintain ideal weight. To elaborate further, I will consider these basic elements, including numerous perspectives for providing ourselves the most healthful nutrition.

Proteins

Proteins are the building blocks of the body. Like the brick wall of a house, they are built up of simple molecules called *amino acids*. There are over twenty of these, formed in the cells into long chains, and then coiled and intertwined to form the large structural *proteins*. Some proteins circulate in the blood, carrying valuable nutrients with them. Others transport such vital elements as oxygen to and from the cells. Proteins are used to form the structural wall of each cell, to bind cells together, to aid in the coagulation of blood, the formation of hormones and enzymes, and to contribute immensely to the identity of each species. Some most fascinating discoveries in biochemistry have been made in regard to the coding and regulating of this protein factory.

Most foods contain some protein. Some foods are high in protein and therefore are considered a major source. Vegetable foods that provide considerable protein for the body are legumes and whole grains. Nuts and dark green leafy vegetables also include a good quality of protein. In order to obtain the proper balance, we must get adequate amounts of the **essential amino acids**.

There are eight of them, and their relative proportions differ in various classes of food. For example, many whole grains are low in *lysine*, which is amply supplied in the legumes. The latter may be relatively low in sulfur-containing amino acids (*methionine* and *cystine*), which are supplied in a complementary relationship from the grains.

We look at many of the world's marginal diets with their corn and beans, or rice and beans, and see this essential combination supplying a proper balance. About the only **complete protein** in the vegetable kingdom is soy beans, an outstanding food, easily prepared in a variety of ways. Egg white *albumin* constitutes another excellent protein, one which forms the standard of comparison for all other types. Because of the toxic byproducts, cholesterol and saturated fat, present in meat, animal protein is definitely a second choice when it comes to building the most healthy bodies.

From an economic standpoint alone, a diet high in animal products is unwise. Land used to produce food crops for human consumption feeds nearly 14 times as many people compared to using it to grow food for animals, which are in turn used for nourishment. This is termed second hand food. Of the **protein** our common food animals eat, 1/4 is returned in milk, 1/8 in pork, and 1/10 in beef. Comparing **calories** returned to us by food animals, we find that milk returns 1/6 the calories the animal consumes, eggs return 1/14, and beef only 1/25. Perhaps in the United States we are not concerned, since our country is not yet overpopulated. But our birth rate is still relatively high—almost twice the death rate. If this situation continues, food will be in short supply some day, just as it now is in other countries.

A Swedish scientist, Dr. Per Olaf Åstrand, found that athletic endurance was much greater on a high carbohydrate diet than on a high protein or high fat diet. After three days on a high meat diet, the maximum work time on an exercise bicycle was about 60 minutes. Three times as much endurance (180 minutes) was seen in the same people after their three-day preparation using a high carbohydrate diet resembling more closely the vegetarian type.

Many people concern themselves with getting adequate protein. But even the U.S. government has revised its recommendations in a downward direction. The current daily **recommended allowance** of 56 grams per day for the average man reflects the trend toward a lower protein intake and is compatible with the best of health. Studies have shown that animals not only mature faster, but die younger, and have more cancers on a high protein diet as compared with a moderate one. Nevertheless, protein is important. We need some protein each day from foods such as beans, nuts, peanuts, whole grains, and the smaller but important contributions that fruit and vegetables make.

Fat

Fat, called *"lipid"* by the biochemist, is a complex of the three-carbon sugar, *glycerol*, attached to three long chains of *fatty acids*. Differences in the fatty acids, their length, and hydrogenation, contribute to the effect fatty foods have on your arteries. Just as protein is broken down in the stomach and small intestine to amino acids before absorption, fats are hydrolyzed by their fat-splitting enzymes. **Lipase** from the pancreas together with **bile**, an emulsifier, helps to break the oily forms of fat (called *triglyceride*) into more basic *diglycerides* and *monoglycerides*. A final breakdown to *free fatty acids* is followed by absorption. Fatty acids go first into the lymphatic channels, and finally into the bloodstream. Only the shortest fatty acid chains proceed directly into the blood.

The American-styled, high fat diet is associated with many health hazards. Fat, more than other dietary constituents, creates a milky appearance in the bloodstream, increasing the stickiness of tiny clotting factors called **platelets**. The contribution of fat to calorie intake is also enormous, with *nine* calories delivered for each gram, in comparison to about four calories for protein and carbohydrates. Fats, nevertheless, are useful to the body, forming layers of *adipose tissue*, which insulate, protect, and produce body contours. Some profiles, such as "spare tires," "love handles," and "double chins" are unwelcome, but the gentler curves are appreciated. Fat is furthermore used for storage of energy. Some fats convert into hormones.

Sterols are related to our common dietary fats. Some beneficial plant sterols (*egosterol, sitosterol*, and others) help block the formation of the harmful animal derived sterol, *cholesterol*. The latter is abundant in foods of animal origin, such as butterfat, egg yolk, organ meats, and so-called "red meats," and other animal foods. **Cholesterol** enters the bloodstream and forms deposits at critical points in the arterial walls. These *plaques* develop slowly over the years, and eventually produce the symptoms of *atherosclerosis*. This explains why Americans have such a high mortality from heart attacks and stroke. Most individuals today acknowledge that diet is crucial to the victory over hardening of our arteries. Millions of vegetarians, while eagerly awaiting additional research, enjoy the protective benefits of their natural vegetarian diet in lowering both cholesterol and triglycerides through these unrefined foods.

Profitable sources of dietary fat include both nuts and seeds. In warmer climatic zones, olives and avocados are valuable staples that contain beneficial oils. Almonds, filberts, and walnuts are superior to cashews, Brazil nuts, and peanuts when it comes to *polyunsaturated* fatty acids. All fats, however, should be used in moderation. Seeds such as caraway, pumpkin and sesame, and the whole grains bring not only with them excellent polyunsaturated fat, but also contain the antioxidant *tocopherols*, **Vitamin E**, that help to stabilize their oils, and benefit the body in additional ways.

It has been discovered recently that hormone-like substances called **prostaglandins** require several polyunsaturated fatty acids for their production. *Linoleic acid*, and its more polyunsaturated "cousin" *linolenic acid*, are needed to produce these important chemical transmitters. The availability of prostaglandin requires a modest, yet steady intake of polyunsaturated fats. Some doctors advocate a "no oil" diet. If sufficient olives, avocados, or nuts are consumed daily, this program is healthful. Current scientific evidence supports the "moderate" stand on fat intake with a substantial *reduction*, rather than the total elimination of these vegetable polyunsaturated oils. However, all animal fats, and *saturated* hardened (*hydrogenated*) vegetable fats and shortenings should be discarded, replaced of course with more natural alternatives.

Carbohydrates

Sugars and **starches** are called **carbohydrate** foods. Fiber, which is indigestible but most important for the smooth functioning of the digestion machinery, is also considered a type of carbohydrate. Carbohydrate is the fundamental food for most people in our world. Only in Western countries where cuisine is abundant, and this includes all affluent and wealthy nations, is fat such a mainstay of the dietary.

All natural foods contain some carbohydrate, as well as fat and protein. Nonetheless, it is from our grains, fruits, and vegetables that most food carbohydrate comes. Carbohydrate gets its name from its chemical composition, being formed of carbon, hydrogen, and oxygen. These are produced by the plant in the process called **photosynthesis**, where *carbon dioxide* is taken from the air, *water* from the soil, then combined by plant leaves in the presence of *ultraviolet light*, to form a carbohydrate.

The chemistry is fascinating. A basic building block for natural sugar is the simple *monosaccharide*, containing six carbon atoms. Blood sugar, **glucose**, is one of the principal varieties, coming from corn, fruit, honey and the breakdown of milk sugar. Two six carbon sugars appear in nature in pairs called *disaccharides*. There are three of these: **sucrose**, coming from sugar cane or sugar beets is a combination of glucose and fructose; **maltose**, composed of two glucose molecules linked together, is found in barley and other grains;

The inner part of the wheat kernel, called the ENDOSPERM, contains mostly starch and a small amount of protein.

These are the BRAN layers, in which are found large amounts of VITAMINS, MINERALS, and good quality PROTEINS.

The EMBRYO, or "wheat germ". This is the life-giving part of the wheat, one of the richest known sources of B and E vitamins.

In white flour about one-half of the fat is lost. This fat has a high food value, since it contains unsaturated fatty acids and vitamin B.

and **lactose**, present only in milk, in which glucose is joined to galactose. Long chains of sugar molecules are present in various fruits and vegetables. These are called *polysaccharides* and consist of the **dextrins**, **cellulose, pectins, glycogen** or animal starch, and **inulin** found in Jerusalem artichokes.

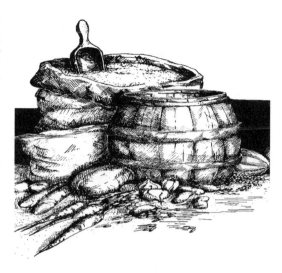

Every cell utilizes glucose as a principal form of energy. It is absorbed with the help of *insulin* circulating in the blood. The central nervous system, particularly the brain, functions on glucose and is in trouble when the level drops too low. Carbohydrates are used for **energy**, metabolized in the cell's *mitochondria*, which are miniature power houses. Four heat calories for every gram are produced from its complete digestion.

If sufficient carbohydrate is present in the diet, less protein needs to be consumed. Furthermore, the storage of fat is enhanced when our diet is adequate in carbohydrate. For this reason, in weight control, we must restrict both carbohydrate as well as fat.

Dietary **fiber** is necessary for normal function of the colon. *Cellulose, hemicellulose, gums, pectin*, and *lignin* are the various forms of these plant fiber carbohydrates. Although not digested, nor used for energy, this valuable "roughage" constitutes a significant part of our diet. Healthy peristaltic action of the small and large bowel is enhanced in the presence of adequate fiber, which produces a gentle laxative affect. Adequate bulk is thought to protect the colon against many diseases, including diverticulosis, appendicitis, and even cancer.

Vitamins

Trace amounts of certain essential chemicals are needed for the cell factories to operate efficiently. These "biologic catalysts" were discovered in the early 1900's, isolated and synthesized in the 1930's, and are now household words. Vitamin deficiency diseases and their characteristic features are discussed in Chapter Eight. Suggestions there are also given for the correction or treatment of these nutritional problems. Many enzyme systems of the body require vitamins for their operation. Some are synthesized by bacteria in the intestinal tract, but most are obtained from natural foods.

There are two basic classes of vitamins. **Fat-soluble** vitamins require **bile** for their absorption. They therefore are usually found in foods containing some fat, and are stored for longer periods in the body. Their excess is more likely to become toxic. Vitamins A, D, E and K belong to this fat–soluble vitamin group.

Vitamin A is important for proper vision, particularly at night. An adequate supply aids formation of our bones and teeth. Inflammation of the cornea (eye) is prevented by this vitamin. Blindness can result from its absence. Vitamin A is plentiful in most yellow and green vegetables, as well as yellow or orange-colored fruits. The deeper the color the more the Vitamin A is usually found. Vegetable sources particularly plentiful in this vitamin's precursor, called *carotene*, are apricots, carrots, cantaloupes, papaya, and yellow squash.

Vitamin D is called the "sunshine vitamin." When our bodies are exposed to sunlight, cholesterol converts to Vitamin D in the deeper layers of the skin. This is picked up and circulated in the blood, and thus aids in the absorption and conservation of **calcium**. The bones and teethe are all better mineralized in the presence of adequate Vitamin D. Fortified milk constitutes a supplied source of both A and D. Ordinarily, however, if adequate sunshine is permitted, such supplements are unnecessary.

Vitamin E is present in most seeds and oils. It serves as a *antioxidant*, preventing destruction or rancidity in the oil. A brain pigment (*lipofuchin*) which increases with aging, becomes more abundant in individuals who lack Vitamin E. Vitamin E is quite important in reproduction. Many claims have been made for its value in the treatment of heart disease. For vascular disorders, skin conditions, and cancer prevention, evidence is accumulating as to its therapeutic value. Ordinarily, a diet rich in whole grains, wheat germ, and healthful seeds—like sesame, pumpkin, or sunflower—will contain adequate amounts of this valuable vitamin. Although many Vitamin E–like substances, called *tocopherols*, exist in nature, the *alpha* form appears to be most active for humans.

Vitamin K is a coagulation factor. It is usually synthesized by bacteria. Present in many grains, tomatoes, and cabbage, adequate amounts of vitamin K are normally produced by our healthy intestinal flora. Breast feeding a newborn baby aids in establishing these healthful bacteria, making unnecessary the routine injection of Vitamin K to babies born in a natural setting. In fact this practice is rapidly being discarded, with most recent scientific findings. Finally, the babies get to feed on their own mother's milk as God originally intended.

Many other vitamins, just as important to the body, are **soluble** in water. These include the B complex group and Vitamin C. Most of these are important catalysts, promoting reactions in the cell and aiding in the production of energy. Adequate amounts of water-soluble vitamins help prevent many diseases, such as beriberi, pellagra, and scurvy.

The **B Complex** group includes many water soluble *coenzymes*. **Thiamine**, or **B₁**, is the most abundant. **Riboflavin**, also termed **Vitamin B₂**, occurs naturally in milk, but becomes rapidly inactivated in the presence of sunlight. **Niacin**, also named **Vitamin B₃**, is found in unrefined cereals, as are most of the other B complex vitamins. **Pyridoxine** and two "relatives," pyridoxal and pyridoxalamine, form the **Vitamin B$_6$** group that are essential to the nervous system, as well as our skin. **Biotin, folic acid, inositol**, and **pantothenic acid** are others of the B complex group. All of these are obtained in a well-balanced natural diet. Some are more abundant in green vegetables; however, all are adequately supplied when whole grains are eaten daily. The use of whole wheat bread, rolled oats, brown rice, millet, barley, and other cereals will give adequate amounts of the B complex group for any individual with normal absorptive capacity.

Vitamin B$_{12}$, although part of the B complex family, is quite different in character. Also known as *cyanocobalamin*, this factor is essential for the formation of the blood. Its absence produces anemia, where the blood cells become scarce, large, and poorly formed. Nerve conduction is also impaired when Vitamin B$_{12}$ is missing. This serious condition, called **pernicious anemia**, is discussed in Chapter Eight. A substance called **intrinsic factor** from the stomach and hydrochloric acid are necessary for the body to absorb this powerful vitamin. Although some B$_{12}$ is generated by friendly bacteria resident in the mouth and in the colon, it is not thought that the amounts are absorbed well enough to be adequate. Many people seem to live for years without supplemental B$_{12}$, and suffer no ill effects. Yet, the irreversible results of pernicious anemia are so serious that some form of B$_{12}$ should frequently comprise the daily diet. Milk and eggs constitute an substantial source for most people. Nevertheless, I recommend for complete vegetarians the use of fortified soy milk, nutritional yeast, or a supplemental form of B$_{12}$. This can prevent the only major nutritional threat to complete vegetarians, who commonly eat a variety of natural foods.

Vitamin C has one of the more controversial reputations among these interesting chemicals. Also called **ascorbic acid**, this valuable coenzyme is required to maintain the integrity of blood vessels and skin. It actually serves as the "glue" to bind cells, joints, and connective tissues together.

Raw fruits and vegetables are most important sources of Vitamin C, as are potatoes cooked "with their jacket on" or baked, cabbage—including Cole slaw— and tomatoes. Rose hips can supply Vitamin C during the winter, used especially by people living in northern climates. Some fresh vegetables, citrus fruit, or melon can be eaten daily to obtain adequate amounts of this vitamin. If one eats a natural diet including some of the above foods, it is not normally necessary to take large supplemental doses to prevent colds. Neither is the course of cancer appreciably altered by massive doses of this vitamin.

The conservation of Vitamin C, however, is very important. Prolonged cooking of vegetables will dissolve and oxidize many water-soluble vitamins. If this cooking water is discarded, the nutrients will then be lost. The use of cooking water should be kept to a minimum. However, it may be saved and used in preparation of gravies, sauces , or even used in baking bread.

Avoiding much food contact with oxygen to help conserve Vitamin C. Strawberries, preserved with their caps on, or eaten as soon as possible after picking, will have much more Vitamin C than those that are cut or stored for prolonged periods at room temperature. Shredded cabbage should be used fresh. When allowed to sit, particularly in an uncovered container, the Vitamin C losses are heavy. A little attention to vitamin conservation in fruits, as well as grains, will go a long way toward stretching the food dollar, helping it to yield the best nutrient dividends.

Minerals

Over sixteen different mineral compounds have been found to be essential for man's nutrition. Even more elements have been found in trace amounts in the "ash" of human flesh. Nonetheless their complete purpose and functions are as yet unknown. Four of these minerals are thought to be of major importance for our daily diet. These are calcium, phosphorus, magnesium, and iron. The others are called **trace minerals**, because of their much smaller requirement. However, they are by no means less essential. I will discuss a few of these in detail, because of their known importance to body health and the preservation of certain diseases.

Some minerals are called **electrolytes**, because of their importance in maintaining ionic composition of blood and plasma, the intracellular fluid, and the electrical voltage or "potential" in each living cell. The electrolyte elements are *sodium, potassium, chloride,* and the more complex ion, *bicarbonate.* The latter is in chemical equilibrium in the blood with *carbonic acid*, carbon dioxide, and water. Here is the chemical formula: $CO_2 + H_2O \leftrightarrow H_2CO_3 \leftrightarrow H^+ + HCO_3^-$

Calcium is one of the most abundant major minerals. It is essential in our blood-clotting mechanism, as well as several enzyme systems. Calcium is important for proper nerve transmission and for the contraction of muscles. Fundamental for proper hardness of the bones and teeth, calcium is absorbed in large amounts from many foods. Certain substances can interfere with the absorption of calcium. **Oxalates**, present in rhubarb and green leafy vegetables, bind calcium, forming salts to then be eliminated. Actually, the intestinal mucous lining has a safeguard mechanism to prevent flooding the body with calcium. Excessive IV administration of calcium could be lethal to the system, if no intestinal barrier was presented to absorption. Although only about 25% of the calcium is normally absorbed, in pregnancy this may go considerably higher. In infancy and early childhood, when the bones are forming, more may be absorbed.

Lactose and **gastric acid** enhance the absorption of calcium. Exercise aids in this reaction, keeping our bones harder when people are in the active years. Although an enzyme called *phytic acid* is present in the husks of many grains, the body quickly adapts to this substance, which would otherwise decrease the calcium absorption. **Phytase** is a valuable digestive enzyme elaborated to negate this otherwise deleterious effect. Stressful situations have been known to depress calcium absorption, even in the presence of mass supplementation! Peace of mind and body, at mealtime and around the clock, is therefore necessary for the proper utilization of calcium, a major mineral in the bones, the blood, the entire body.

Phosphorus is a mineral of considerable interest, usually absorbed with calcium. Present in our body as *phosphate*, it also forms a valuable part of many organic acids, including **DNA** (*deoxyribonucleic acid*) and the *phospholipids*, important in nerve transmission. Phosphates serve as valuable **buffers** of the body chemistry, keeping the acidity and alkalinity of our blood and body fluids in the most healthful range. Phosphate, moreover, acts as a storage form of energy, existing in the cells in the form of **ATP** (*adenosine triphosphate*). These high energy compounds help your body store the energy gained from the metabolism of carbohydrate and other foods.

Nearly everyone knows **iron** is essential for the healthy formation of good red blood. It is one of the more common mineral deficiencies, found particularly in women and children eating impoverished diets. When menstrual and pregnancy losses are combined with a borderline intake, anemia often develops. In spite of the "enrichment" of our grains with iron, it is all too common for people using refined foods to be deficient in this mineral. Foods high in **Vitamin C** aid in the absorption of iron. This mineral is particularly abundant in dark, green vegetables, legumes, prunes, raisins, nuts, and whole grains. Cooking in iron pots allows the release of some elemental iron to aid in securing our recommended daily allowance.

Magnesium is essential for the stability of muscles and nerves. It is involved in the conversion of glucose into energy compounds, and serves as a catalyst in many chemical reactions within the cell. Magnesium deficiency, like that of calcium, can produce *tetany*, a painful contraction of major muscles. Since most foods in their natural state contain some magnesium, deficiency is fortunately quite rare. High calcium supplementation, the chronic use of alcohol, drug use, and some less common disease states may induce a magnesium deficiency. In all but the most unusual cases, correction of an impoverished diet will result in stability of the important trace mineral elements.

The thyroid gland requires **iodine** to form its important hormones. Since some parts of the country produce vegetables in iodine deficient soil, it is recommended that iodized salt (or sea salt) be used to obtain adequate amounts of this essential element. Adequate testing of garden soil is required to determine if iodine is available. Most of the southern USA, the central plains, and the southwestern United States are outside the "goiter belt." Moreover, around the world, pockets of hypothyroidism exist from a dietary deficiency of this important element.

When most people think of **chromium**, they think of shiny bumpers. Nevertheless, the stability of the blood sugar and the prevention of diabetes pivot around the presence of this important trace mineral. I frequently recommend that people with either hypoglycemic tendencies or diabetes take a daily supplement of chromium for added assurance and sugar control. Whole grains are the major source of chromium, making your unrefined diet crucial in assuring this mineral's availability.

Selenium acts like Vitamin E in its service as an*antioxidant*. Grains and onions are the principal sources of selenium, which has been found to reduce the incidence of cancer. Excessive cooking or washing of foods, especially with the discarding of cooking water, will lead to selenium loss, and possibly that of other essential minerals, too.

Fluoride is the ionized form of the element fluorine. It is present naturally in some water supplies and supplemented in others. Fluoride helps to harden the bones and retards the development of osteoporosis. Whether the domestic water supplies in most communities need fluoride additives is a subject for considerable debate and concern. However, resistance to *dental caries*, or tooth decay, is a known fringe benefit of fluoride supplementation, when the amount is not excessive. Mottling of the enamel will occur when the water source of fluoride exceeds 3 parts per million. Usually only 1/3 of that amount is present in municipal supplies where fluoride is added. Present also in various toothpastes, and applied to teeth by dentists, fluoride may aid, together with other prudent dietary measures, in preventing dental decay, currently affecting at least 97% of our population.

A look at the other trace minerals, such as **zinc, cadmium, molybdenum, cobalt**, and **manganese** shows the great importance to emphasize eating unrefined foods. These trace minerals are found primarily in whole grains, fruits, nuts, and vegetables. When taken in their most unrefined form, without prolonged storage, excessive processing, or overcooking, these elements are available for your body's need and can help you resist many common degenerative diseases. Some minerals are toxic, even in small amounts. Warnings concerning these environmental hazards need to be considered, in the preventive nutritional care of our bodies.

TOXIC MINERALS

Lead

The amount of lead introduced into our environment since the beginning of the Industrial Revolution is enormous. More than 7 million tons of lead have been used as gasoline additives in the U.S. alone. Much of this lead is now widely distributed on the earth's surface. Urban soil and house dust can contain 33 to 500 times the normal concentration of earth lead. The bottom sediment of U.S. lakes now contains about 20 times more lead than they did just 100 years ago.

Lead is a slow, cumulative poison deposited eventually in the bones. The main sources of lead exposure include the production and burning of storage batteries, solder, paint, leaded gasoline, electric cable covering, pottery glaze, leaded glass, newsprint, ashes and fumes from burning old painted wood, black and colored inks, and drinking water that has passed through lead pipes. Fortunately, we have technology to avoid the use of lead in virtually all of the above industrial processes.

Lead exposure remains a major health problem for children today in the inner cities. Symptoms of lead exposure include colic and abdominal cramping, psychological and behavioral disorders, and decreased memory and learning ability. Greater levels of lead are associated with peripheral neuritis (inflammation of the nerves), paralysis, anemias, fatigue, and a serious type of encephalopathy (brain disorder) resulting in convulsive seizures, mania, delirium, stupor and coma. Elegant studies by Dr. Herb Needleman and others confirm that even lower doses of lead can result in long term learning impairment in children. This is frequent in children living in our inner cities.

Vitamin C and the trace element zinc both tend to displace significant amounts of lead in the body. Foods rich in zinc as well as ascorbic acid include the fresh vegetables, along with fruit and nuts.

Mercury

Thermometers, paints, felt, explosives, lamps, batteries, and dental fillings all may contain various amounts of **mercury**. Although environmental concerns about mercury in fish have surfaced in recent years, most fish seem to increase their selenium content to compensate and protect themselves from mercury poisoning. As with lead, we have probably underestimated the long term effects of mercury accumulation in the body. It does not have any known biological uses, and robs the body of sulfur-containing enzymes.

The most common human exposure to mercury is through silver amalgam dental fillings. Mercury accounts for about 50% of this compound by weight. The debate concerning safety of using silver amalgam in dentistry has raged for many years. The link between mercury exposure and symptoms is very complex. Nevertheless, many patients have appreciated a decided relief of joint pain, fatigue, stiffness and similar symptoms when the mercury-silver amalgams were replaced with acrylic fillings or gold.

Aluminum

The "shiny metal" that is seen so much in industry today is **aluminum**. With the widespread use of this metal in containers such as cans, a concern about possible toxicity to our human system constrains us to take another look at this trace mineral. Very abundant in the earth's crust, aluminum has found its way into a multitude of industries, from airplanes to automobiles from electronics to fine crafted jewelry.

Several years ago, researchers in Germany found a possible link between aluminum deposits in the brain and **Alzheimer's Disease**. Crossing readily the blood-brain barrier, aluminum deposits itself not only in brain tissue but also in bones. Its exact function isn't well understood. Careful evaluation of patients with mental deterioration and premature senility have found that aluminum concentrates itself in the *substantia nigra*, a specialized part of the brain that operates as a relay station. In cases of Alzheimer's Disease this substance becomes such a tangled mess of nerves (called *neuro-fibrillary tangles*) that memory circuits are progressively disrupted.

This finding naturally raises the question of how or where this misfortune occurs. Neurosurgeons in Germany discovered recently that antacids high in aluminum lead to enhanced absorption, with a definite increase of aluminum concentration in the brain! Twenty years ago these *best seller* antacids were considered non-absorbable, acting only on local organs such as the stomach, neutralizing gastric acid, thus relieving stomach pain.

A number of baking powders contain aluminum. Moreover, aluminum silicates are used to stabilize frozen deserts, cheese spreads, sauces, and confections. Most of the antiperspirants marketed today contain aluminum, which also very likely is absorbed through the pores of the skin.

In July 1992, Australian researchers reported their study of canned soft drinks and the aluminum content of the carbonated beverage inside. Fifty-two beverages from different parts of Australia, New Zealand, and Thailand were evaluated. The aluminum content of non-cola drinks was nearly **six times higher** in cans than in bottles. The content of aluminum in cola drinks was nearly **three times higher** in cans than in bottles.

Typically, the aluminum intake among Western Europeans, Americans, and Australians is less than 10 milligrams a day. Some researchers such as Dr. Gerald Spasmin, Ph.D. of Brandeis University in Waltham, MA hypothesize that aluminum may trigger a biochemical sequence that leads to the devastatingly progressive neurofibrillary tangles in the victim's brain. These concerns led them to recommend a maximum daily intake of less than 3 milligrams aluminum daily.

In the Australian study, soft drinks were find to contain up to **3.9** milligrams aluminum per can! The World Health Organization (WHO) and European Economic Community (EEC) recommend the maximum aluminum concentration of **7.4** mcM/l (micromoles/liter) in drinking water. The concentration of aluminum in bottled cola drinks (**8.9** mcM/l), cola drinks in cans (**24.4** mcM/l) and non-cola drinks (**33.4** mcM/l) all exceeded this recommendation.

Although Dr. John Dugan of Australia says there is "no cause for concern," I question this conclusion. Could it be that modern technology while attempting to benefit mankind is indeed contributing to destroy some of the very functions that it is meant to enhance? Aluminum in concentrated forms, baking powders, antacids, canned sodas is *clearly* a hazard to our health!

Arsenic

Despite its reputation, **arsenic** has a fairly low toxicity level, compared with other metals. Arsenic is used in insecticides, weed killer, paint, wallpaper, ceramics and glass. It is common knowledge that arsenic is extremely poisonous. It causes toxicity by combining with sulfur-containing enzymes (important in free radical control and detoxification) and interfering with cellular metabolism. Its toxic effects are cumulative. Chronic exposure to arsenic from ingestion or inhalation can lead to degeneration of the nerves in hands and feet (peripheral neuropathy) with numbness. Tingling and burning of the hands and feet, muscular weakness, hair loss, skin rash (dermatitis), headaches, fatigue, seizures, kidney or liver damage, or death are some of the other serious complications.

PLEASE REFER TO THE RECOMMENDED DAILY DIETARY ALLOWANCE CHART ON THE FOLLOWING PAGES, WHICH OUTLINES BASIC DIETARY REQUIREMENTS FOR FAT AND WATER–SOLUBLE VITAMINS AND MINERALS.

Appetite Control

We come now to factors that govern the intake and balance of various foods consumed. Modern advertising trends allure primarily our desire for gustatory satisfaction or taste. Technology adds a wide array of additives, condiments, and "non-foods" which appeal principally to the sight, smell, or taste buds. All this display advertises corporate attempts to "tickle" our appetite. Many unhealthful food additives are used in ignorance. Some produce real harm.

Certain spices, such as **black** and **red pepper** are actually corrosive to the delicate stomach lining. Most spices of tropical origin stimulate the appetite. Explorers have gone around the world in their search of these. In addition to pepper, some of the more harmful ones are **cinnamon, ginger, cloves, allspice, chili**, and **mustard**.

The proper use of many herbal seasonings may enhance the taste for natural foods. Thus, it is important for those who prepare food to understand their chemistry. Some trace minerals are found in various culinary herbs. Most herbs come from leafy plants growing in temperate or subtropical zones. Although some of these, such as **sage, turmeric, oregano**, and oil extracts, such as **almond** and **vanilla**, are considered relatively harmless, great moderation should be exercised in their use. As a general rule, a wise cook will *"season to taste, not to taste the seasoning."*

Food and Nutrition Board, National Academy

RECOMMENDED DAILY DIETARY

Designed for the maintenance of good nutrition

	Age (years)	Weight (kg)	Weight (lbs)	Height (cm)	Height (in)	Protein (g)	Vitamin A (µg R.E.) [b]	Vitamin D (µg) [c]	Vitamin E (mg α T.E.) [d]
Infants	0.0-0.5	6	13	60	24	kg x 2.2	420	10	3
	0.5-1.0	9	20	71	28	kg x 2.0	400	10	4
Children	1-3	13	29	90	35	23	400	10	5
	4-6	20	44	112	44	30	500	10	6
	7-10	28	62	132	52	34	700	10	7
Males	11-14	45	99	157	62	45	1000	10	8
	15-18	66	145	176	69	56	1000	10	10
	19-22	70	154	177	70	56	1000	7.5	10
	23-50	70	154	178	70	56	1000	5	10
	51 +	70	154	178	70	56	1000	5	10
Females	11-14	46	101	157	62	46	800	10	8
	15-18	55	120	163	64	46	800	10	8
	19-22	55	120	163	64	44	800	7.5	8
	23-50	55	120	163	64	44	800	5	8
	51 +	55	120	163	64	44	800	5	8
Pregnant						+ 30	+ 200	+ 5	+ 2
Lactating						+ 20	+ 400	+ 5	+ 3

Fat-Soluble Vitamins

a   The allowances are intended to provide for individual variations among most normal persons as they live in the United States under usual environmental stresses. Diets should be based on a variety of common foods in order to provide other nutrients for which human requirements have been less well defined. See text for detailed discussion of allowances and of nutrients not tabulated. See Table III (p. 4) for weights and heights by individual year of age. See Table III (p. 4) for suggested average energy intakes.

b   Retinol equivalents. 1 retinol equivalent = 1 μg retinol or 6 μg β-carotene. See text for calculation of vitamin A activity of diets as retinol equivalents.

c   As cholecalciferol. 10 μg cholecalciferol = 400 I.U. vitamin D.

d α tocopherol equivalents. 1 mg d-α-tocopherol = 1 α T.E. See text for variation in allowances and calculation of vitamin E activity of the diet as α tocopherol equivalents.

e   1 N.E. (niacin equivalent) is equal to 1 mg of niacin or 60 mg of dietary tryptophan.

of Sciences-National Research Council

ALLOWANCES, *a*Revised 1980

of practically all healthy people in the U.S.A.

	Water-Soluble Vitamins						Minerals					
Vitamin C (mg)	Thiamin (mg)	Riboflavin (mg)	Niacin (mg N.E.) e	Vitamin B6 (mg)	Folacin f (µg)	Vitamin B12 (µg)	Calcium (mg)	Phosphorus (mg)	Magnesium (mg)	Iron (mg)	Zinc (mg)	Iodine (µg)
35	0.3	0.4	6	0.3	30	0.5*g*	360	240	50	10	3	40
35	0.5	0.6	8	0.6	45	1.5	540	360	70	15	5	50
45	0.7	0.8	9	0.9	100	2.0	800	800	150	15	10	70
45	0.9	1.0	11	1.3	200	2.5	800	800	200	10	10	90
45	1.2	1.4	16	1.6	300	3.0	800	800	250	10	10	120
50	1.4	1.6	18	1.8	400	3.0	1200	1200	350	18	15	150
60	1.4	1.7	18	2.0	400	3.0	1200	1200	400	18	15	150
60	1.5	1.7	19	2.2	400	3.0	800	800	350	10	15	150
60	1.4	1.6	18	2.2	400	3.0	800	800	350	10	15	150
60	1.2	1.4	16	2.2	400	3.0	800	800	350	10	15	150
50	1.1	1.3	15	1.8	400	3.0	1200	1200	300	18	15	150
60	1.1	1.3	14	2.0	400	3.0	1200	1200	300	18	15	150
60	1.1	1.3	14	2.0	400	3.0	800	800	300	18	15	150
60	1.0	1.2	13	2.0	400	3.0	800	800	300	18	15	150
60	1.0	1.2	13	2.0	400	3.0	800	800	300	10	15	150
+20	+0.4	+0.3	+2	+0.6	+400	+1.0	+400	+400	+150	*h*	+5	+25
+40	+0.5	+0.5	+5	+0.5	+100	+1.0	+400	+400	+150	*h*	+10	+50

f   The folacin allowances refer to dietary sources as determined by *Lactobacillus casei* assay after treatment with enzymes ("conjugases") to make polyglutamyl forms of the vitamin available to the test organism.

g   The RDA for vitamin B12 in infants is based on average concentration of the vitamin in human milk. The allowances after weaning are based on energy intake (as recommended by the American Academy of Pediatrics) and consideration of other factors such as intestinal absorption; see text.

h   The increased requirement during pregnancy cannot be met by the iron content of habitual American diets nor by the existing iron stores of many women; therefore the use of 30 - 60 mg of supplemental iron is recommended. Iron needs during lactation are not substantially different from those of nonpregnant women, but continued supplementation of the mother for 2 - 3 months after parturition is advisable in order to replenish stores depleted by pregnancy.

Through hereditary and cultivated tastes for certain foods, an appetite may be created for substances which in reality are harmful. The appetite for salt and sugar, for example, as well as excess calories is often acquired from eating patterns established in childhood. Hunger and thirst are natural drives, stemming from the absence of food or water, respectively. But **appetite** is a much more complicated phenomenon, having to do with gratification of desire, the "need" to feel full, or merely a habit of overeating. The *hypothalamus*, a small bit of nerve tissue located at the base of the brain, has specific areas that regulate the thirst and hunger mechanisms. Controlled by reason, these function in their normal dominion. When, however, these lower centers are allowed to dominate the lifestyle, problems develop rapidly. **Obesity** represents one of the states where the "appestat" has been set too high, creating a most obvious health problem. Chapter Eight describes the best methods of control, victory, and restored health for the unfortunate victims of excess calorie consumption.

For good health, then, as well as gratification at the dinner table, these rules should be carefully observed. Cultivate a pleasant, contented disposition. Make mealtime a pleasant, social occasion, without stress, argument, worry or contention. Select a diet from as wide a variety of natural, unrefined, foods as possible. Include some of the "big four"— fruits, grains, nuts, and vegetables— in the diet every day. Emphasize thorough mastication, and a proper combination of these natural products. Choose a diet that will pay handsome dividends for many years, particularly during your golden ones. Balance the other health measures, such as exercise, rest, fresh air, and the use of sunlight. Finally, cultivate a trustful, unselfish disposition, relying above all on divine power as the **source** of true life. This brings to fulfillment the divine promise, *"I am come that they might have life, and have it more abundantly."*

CHAPTER TWENTY

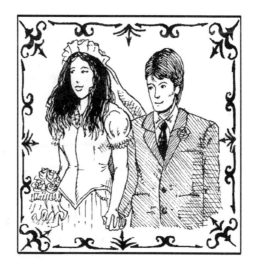

MARRIAGE

PROBLEMS

It is no secret today that our typical American home is in dire trouble. Statisticians eloquently advertise the rising divorce rate, with increasing rates of mental illness stemming from family strife. However, they offer no solutions. Teenage marriages increase in number, while more and more couples are just living together without legal sanction other than "common law." For many the marriage vows have become little more than a ring and a ceremony, while the "till death do us part" invisible ties are made only to dissolve and vanish in a vale of tears and broken hearts. In attempting to safeguard these most hallowed family ties, this chapter provides some guidance and common sense which could save, salvage, or heal your homes from the thousand perils that lurk around you.

First, let's turn toward the **setting** for marriage, as friendships are formed. A veneer of modern culture has supplanted ancient forms and customs leading toward the marriage altar. The most prevalent method of courtship is illustrated in the experience of the strong man, Samson. His words, "Get her for me, for she pleases me well," describe the modern trend in mate matching. Most young people today, following the trends of their parents and peers, look around to select life partners, as well as transient friends, on the basis of appearance, popularity, social standing, or wealth. Hence, today's campuses have developed the "dating game."

Special friendships are often encouraged in young children, as birthday parties find even parents matching boys with little girls, pairing them up as partners, and choosing fashions that are more alluring. This trend makes the child act "grown up" prematurely. Together with the bombardment of sexual stimuli from television, popular magazines, and storybooks, the youthful mind is bent toward early courtships and marriages. By the time high school banquets, proms, and sporting events take place, nearly all extracurricular entertainments revolve around a dating situation.

"Going steady" with an exchange of letters, trinkets, or even valuable jewelry has become increasingly common, followed usually by breakups with many tears, bitterness, and resentment. The trend toward "hands-on" contact from the simplest hand holding to the good night kiss, all tends to perpetuate early friendships, and deepen the emotional intertwining before reason has been allowed to speak its mind.

In a permissive society such as ours, the natural outgrowth of quasi-sexual activities becomes an intimate contact, reserved for and sanctified only in marriage. Restrictions of these liberties is deemed by many parents prudish, and by teenagers dictatorial. Nevertheless, there is a better way.

Another model for courtship finds expression in the Scriptures. The marriage of Isaac is one of these illustrations, an example of harmony and bliss which began in a heaven-directed fashion. An aging father entrusted to his most devoted servant the task of searching for a mate for his son. Isaac, the child of promise, was to be the father of many nations. His fulfillment of God's designs would have to be accompanied by obedience to the will of God.

Thus, in a providential manner the servant was guided to the very place where Rebecca, the "soon-to-be" wife, was working. In direct answer to his prayer and by "being at the right place at the right time," this trusted servant, Eliezer, found the woman and secured the consent of her parents. Today, it is appalling to think how many parents abandon their sacred responsibility to scrutinize a prospective suitor. They should take the lead in a kind, yet authoritative way to either accept or reject his proposal. Weakness on the part of parents, like the ancient priest Eli, produces untold tales of sorrow both in the home and in churches. Churches and communities are being devastated today with homes that have "gone on the rocks."

With this introduction, then, I offer an alternative plan for courtship that may seem very strange in the freedom-loving society we live in. It offers, however, an unusual amount of protection to the committed and submissive youth who will follow this way. First, please realize, **"it is the essence of all right faith to do the right thing at the right TIME."** There is an ideal time, as the wise man Solomon points out, for everything, including courtship. Being one of the three major decisions of life, it should follow two other milestones that mark a life pattern in preparation for marriage.

Primarily, and most essential, a young man or young woman should be completely committed to serve the lord. Only in a life of **service** is true marital happiness found. Only with a commitment to the nobler goals of life is a state of maturity reached that can endure the "winds of strife," the adversities, and the tests that try every married couple.

The second decision, equally vital, pertains to your life work. Too many young people are marrying with no thought of support, making themselves a burden to the burgeoning welfare system, or to their parents, who should be "cutting the apron strings" at that time. Young men should master a trade with which, if necessary, they could earn their livelihood. Women should be well versed in the practical arts of cooking, sewing, baking, housekeeping, including some fundamentals, background, or experience in the knowledge of physiology and rearing of children. A profession, such as nursing, secretarial work, or any similar skill is valuable, since at times sickness or death of the partner may result, requiring a young wife or mother to be her own support as well.

With these foundations laid and a mature personality developed, it **may** be time to consider a life partnership. How wise is the young person who consults the parents to secure, not their blessing, but their **counsel**; not the rubber stamp of approval, but words of wisdom that only years of experience can give. Counsel from pastors or teachers who understand the issues at stake and who themselves are examples of happy, secure homes is valuable at a time like this. Guard the affections and the emotions constitutes a valuable safeguard to "reason," which needs to prevail in the early decisions that could set the stage for success or failure in the choice of a life partner.

As these steps are taken, then, the young suitor is well advised to **consult the parents** of the young woman to whom he has been attracted. For in reality, the young lady belongs to them. Fathers have a God-given responsibility to guard the interest of their daughters and to insure, if possible, their future happiness. Parents should consider carefully, via correspondence or interview, the young man *before* allowing steps to be taken, either in dating, intimate correspondence, or outright courtship that may rapidly intertwine a couples emotions and lead to the marriage altar. At every step from this point forward a courtship should be carried on in a spirit of reverence, prayer, and calm deliberation, with the highest respect shown for the counsel and wishes of parents, ministers and other trusted counselors.

These measures, when followed, are **guaranteed** to slow the rising divorce rate, the heartbreak, and the smoldering tensions that threaten to pull apart many marriages today. And, may I say, these principles are not just for teenagers, but for one who at any age is contemplating marriage. Questions like these should be asked: Will this honor God? Can it advance His cause? Will our proposed marriage help us to be of greater service to others? Otherwise, why not remain single? Unmarried life, by the way, isn't as frustrating, undesirable, or disastrous as many would make it seem to be. Remember the apostle Paul, who writing from the viewpoint of a missionary, advocated, *"I wish that ye may be as I am."* (I Cor. 7:20-29)

Some people would say that this "restrictive" method of courtship would simply prevent marriages altogether. Nonetheless, I personally know many couples who have gone this "route," admittedly infrequently, with resulting happy homes and secure lasting relationships. These friends, in contrast with others, show not the slightest remorse for romances which, although for the moment sincere, did not turn out "for real."

Marriage Customs

It has become quite fashionable for marriages to be consummated with a great expense and display. Borrowed from the popular operetta a century ago, our **wedding march** has been embellished with many modern customs, and instrumental and vocal music. Florists, photographers, and fashion designers all have their share in the profits, as parents, not infrequently, sponsor the "show," backed by credit cards, mortgages or bank loans. On the other side of the economic spectrum is the justice of the peace, with his simple "service" and the marriage license costing only a few dollars.

Somewhere between these two extremes lies the balance for a Christian wedding — enough simplicity to make it genuine, and a touch of originality for interest. It is most unfortunate when the focal point of a wedding service becomes a kiss, an exchange of rings, or a grand march. Rather, let us hear a simple message from a God-fearing pastor, followed by sincere vows which can be memorized. Let the attire be made more practical, clothes designed to be worn more than once. Thus, means are saved for establishing a home. Furthermore, by using fewer flowers, candles, or photos, the bridal couple will have means to share unselfishly with others who, unfortunately, have no home at all. What a benefit society would reap from the change! Then it could truly be said, *"A prudent wife is from the Lord."* Proverbs 10:14.

We look now at the home itself — its location, furnishings, and schedule. The modern trend is toward country living. A rural location has many advantages. There is less noise, smog and other pollution in secluded country-sides, hills, and valleys. Water supply is usually pure, and a well can be prepared if desired. Fertile land for cultivation is invaluable. The planting of an orchard and yearly cultivation of a garden brings dividends, not only in healthful exercise, but the pleasure of eating fresh produce. Many young couples find even greater joy in "do-it-yourself" projects, such as building a log cabin, remodeling an old home, or their own start-to-finish home building. This adds construction experience to their individuality expressed in a uniquely personal design.

Secrets Of A Happy Marriage

For certain couples, sad to say, marriage is the end of happiness. It need not be so. Follow a few simple rules, and you will let the sunshine of God's love lighten your family circle. You can make a heaven out of any humble cottage, if love dwells there. Without that simple ingredient, even a palace may become a prison, and tears continually flow.

First, to every married couple, **continue the early attentions**. Remember the thoughtful remembrances for his or her birthday, and always your anniversary. The magic words "thank you" are like nectar to a honeybee.

Special words of kindness and appreciation— after a delightful meal, when the house is squeaky clean, when the neatness of shrubs and lawn bear witness to hours of diligent labor— these should never be neglected. Acts of kindness can do much to lighten the load that every housewife or mother carries, and make the home a preferred place for husband to spend his leisure hours. These little expressions will benefit health, as well as home and heart, often bringing smiles to relieve tears or trials.

Second, as far as possible, a couple should **do things together**. Pray together, work together, worship together, study together, and very important — walk and talk together. Communication barriers often arise in a marriage. They must be broken down by determined effort, "oiled" with shared love. Never allow anything to come between the two partners. Secrets, for example, should not be withheld from husband or wife to be shared with others. The management of your household should be, from start to finish, a team effort. Mutual discussions in regard to major purchases — a new car, a house, vacation plans, or the raising of children— are extremely important to marital harmony. Where frankness in communication exists, suspicion cannot develop. Mutual trust grows daily with exercise.

Set reasonable goals for the family. Aspirations to be rich or famous often lead to a false display of affluence. In the purchase of new cars or homes, stay within your budget. **SHUN DEBT LIKE THE PLAGUE!** Sometimes the galling yoke of debt drives many a breadwinner to despair, while big monthly bills testify to poor planning. The bondage of financial stresses often lead to unkind accusations behind closed doors. Try to cultivate the same trustful, confiding atmosphere within the inner circle of the home that casual visitors see when they drop in for a few moments. **Be genuine**, not only with your friends, but with each other.

Next, **enlarge the circle** of your influence and benevolence beyond your special "twosome." Selfishness in society can breed like algae in stagnant swamps. Cultivate true benevolence, with mutual giving of time, money, counsel, and service to benefit many others. It will make the home a happier place to live. The exercise of true sharing brings out the best in people, nurturing that which is noble, enduring, and worthy of admiration. Simple entertainment for guests, inviting your neighbors for a meal, or lodging a stranger, all will bring rich dividends for a little time spent in this unselfish hospitality. The patriarch Abraham one time even entertained *angels* unawares (Heb. 13:2), because of his spirit of kindness habitually expressed to strangers.

Many of today's youth need secure **homes**, a place where harmony and devotion prevail. Lacking this privilege in childhood, some teenagers become rebellious, disenchanted both with religion, and the people that profess it. These do not need a lecture, but a demonstration. Sincere unselfish love manifested in this way may turn their lives around. Enlarging your family circle to take in these youth might even strengthen family ties. However, the special "inner circle" of confidence, love, and sharing should always be preserved and carefully guarded.

Family Worship

Many drive past colorful freeway billboards, and see the slogan *"The family that stays together, prays together."* Yet, too many households give no more than lip service to the sacred worship service that was fundamental in the home of the Israelites, the Waldenses, the reformers, and the founding fathers of America. Numerous individuals frequently forget God at mealtime, except to utter a memorized phrase before beginning to eat. The wise couple who wants a spiritual influence to prevail in their new home will safeguard carefully the time set aside for family devotions. A devotional service before breakfast is a fine way to start the day. It need not be long, but ideally complete, to include reading the Scriptures, singing a hymn, followed by some comments on the day's Scripture theme, then a fervent prayer offered by one of the family members. A father's prayer for his children and wife helps to place a hedge about them, to guard them in the path of right doing.

Worship should not just be prepackaged, like opening a box of ready-made cereal. A little time spent in preparation, prayerful thought, and study will reward the "priest" of the family with an enthusiastic response to this special time. Worship need not be boring, routine, or a drudgery. A hymn or two sung as a family, a few special testimonies, with the texts chosen by the children on occasion, helps to bring variety into the service. You may make it one of the happiest memories that the offspring carry with them through life. Evening services may be different, choosing a Bible lesson, a bedtime story of a character-building nature, or a personal time with husband and wife studying their Bibles and praying together. Couples that habitually pray together before going to bed each night need never allow misunderstanding, grudges, or barriers to arise in their home. Happy is the family that is united in religion, and makes theirs last seven days a week!

Family Finances

Many unhappy household experiences arise over disagreement in the spending of money. The budget for family spending needs mutual discussion. Usually, one member of the family is more skilled at money management or bookkeeping than the other. Nevertheless, a team relationship should always be encouraged. Even if the husband is the "breadwinner" and provides through his work the family livelihood, every wife should have some money that she can call her own, that she is able to spend as she sees best. Budgeting helps to keep the income and outgo balanced, with appropriate amounts allotted for utilities, housing, food, clothing, tithe and offerings, gifts, recreation, education, medical expenses, taxes, etc. This should be carefully analyzed on a periodic basis. Remember the adage, *"If your outgo exceeds your income, then your upkeep may be your downfall."* Most important, keep the channels of communication open. Never let suspicion smolder to mar the happiness of your marriage partnership.

Vacations and Recreation

Vacation plans and periodic recreation should be considered in the needs of the family. Let these decisions be mutual ones also. A drive in the park, a picnic, a hike in the hills, or an excursion to the ocean may provide those "golden moments" that bind husband and wife together, and bring happy memories to reflect upon in later years. Especially after children arrive, your plan for family outings should be sure to take in all their needs, bringing the blessing of the Lord upon the money spent, as well as the time expended. Camping trips, or excursions of a missionary nature to foreign countries, are particularly unifying. New skills can be acquired, such as swimming, wilderness survival, or the intensive study of nature. Family attitudes fostered on such occasions will be reflected in self-reliant youth and more stable homes for the next generation.

Birthdays and Christmas

Birthdays and Christmas pose interesting challenges. Never forget them, but remember the true Giver of "every perfect gift" on these occasions. Thank the Lord who has spared the life of wife or husband for another year. Rather than falling for the commercial veneer society has thrown over the Christmas season, make it as its name implies, a special season of rejoicing for the birth of Christ and His gift to the world. Give Him your highest and best society during the holiday seasons. All–night parties, social drinking, and foolish games should be avoided. They often leave an aftertaste of bitterness and remorse, to say nothing of the drain on checkbooks, pocketbooks, and the sad tales of woe that are recorded concerning those unfortunate victims of intemperance and vice.

Birth Control

A topic frequently introduced after marriage, but which preferably is discussed in advance of the altar, is the subject of childbearing. It is advisable for a couple to become acquainted with each other for a year or more, before taking on the responsibility of pregnancy and childbirth. From a financial standpoint, as well as for social reasons, a couple's preparation for childbearing is best achieved when marital adjustment has been completed and the home well established. For this reason I discuss some of the concepts of birth control and their best implementation in marriage relations.

Remember that sexual experiences are given of God, being illustrated in the Bible as a symbol of the union of Christ and his church (Eph. 5:25). For too many, the popular press, sentimental songs, and sordid accounts of movie star licentiousness have distorted the beautiful conception of marital relations and the sacredness in which they are to be regarded. Tenderness and compassion on the part of the husband, as well as the wife will bring forth happy dividends to such couples.

Birth Control provides for appropriate spacing of pregnancies, and to enable a couple to have those children for whom they can afford, feed, educate, and care. Therefore, the following family planning considerations should be kept in mind. The most basic method to appropriately space the arrival of children requires self-control in the frequency of marital privileges. Too many couples, in ignorance of the sacred beauty surrounding their sexual relationship, give rise to indulgence of lustful passion, making the marriage vows cover even vile practices, which God's Word condemns. Notwithstanding, there is an appropriate use of this privilege. And, under the blessing of God, heavenly angels may hallow the sacred chamber.

From a medical standpoint, there are some basic features of a woman's menstrual cycle which makes conception more likely at certain times. The interval between menstrual periods usually occupies three or four weeks. It is commonly spoken of as a "monthly" cycle. This interval can be best calculated from the onset of one period to the beginning of another. The time when fertilization is most likely is in the middle of this cycle, during a time period called **ovulation**, when the egg is released from the ovary. This egg (*ovum*) is then picked up by the nearby *Fallopian tube* in the pelvis, and conducted toward the womb. If marital relations occur during this interval, millions of vigorous *spermatozoa* may traverse the cervix, enter the womb, and migrate to the Fallopian tube. Then, fertilization takes place. Although it takes millions of sperm to generate the enzyme (*hyaluronidase*) required to penetrate the ovum, only one actually fertilizes the egg! With millions of possibilities for a unique child, how wise are the parents who make this conception a matter of prayer.

The rhythm method of birth control, then, consists simply of abstaining from intercourse during the "danger period." This extends from about one week after the menstrual period ends for another ten days or so, corresponding to at least five days past ovulation. An interval of abstinence between the 10th and 18th of a 28 day cycle usually suffices for birth control.

A woman may take her oral temperature early in the morning before rising or drinking fluids. Through a monthly cycle, she will usually notice a pattern. At the time of ovulation the morning temperature (called *basal temperature*) increases about 0.5° to 1° F. This change marks the day of ovulation. Examination of mucus from the cervix may help to further pinpoint the unsafe time. The basal temperature measurement, moreover, helps couples wishing to conceive to evaluate an apparent infertility problem. They can thereby time intercourse, so as to increase the chances of conception.

Numerous mechanical barriers proliferate to prevent pregnancy. The **condom** is a sheath-like latex device designed to fit over the male organ and entrap the sperm during *ejaculation*, preventing their deposition within the birth canal. Provided the condom is intact, and does not slip off after intercourse, the method works quite well. Notwithstanding its widely advertised usage in the prevention of venereal disease, the condom is an effective means of birth control if used faithfully each time. For controlling **AIDS** and to contain the spread of the HIV virus, I do not recommend reliance on condoms. It is **fidelity** to one marital partner, and the avoidance of all illicit and high-risk sexual contacts that protects people. **Chastity** is the means God has ordained to avoid these life-threatening exposures.

A similar mechanical barrier may be temporarily placed in the birth canal just before intercourse. This is called a **diaphragm**. They must be fitted by a physician, for several sizes are available. The diaphragm must conform to the structure of the vagina, serving as a obstructive barrier to the mouth of the womb. Coating the diaphragm with a jelly (*spermicidal gel*) to inactivate and destroy the sperm will increase its effectiveness. With regular use according to manufacturer's directions, the diaphragm may function successfully for many years. More recent development of the *female condom* still awaits testing.

Foam, spermicidal gels, and other vaginal inserts such as the newer **cervical cap** are available for birth control. These utilize the same principle as the diaphragm, namely the chemical destruction of the sperm, united with a barrier to sperm penetration, rendering them inactive. Some recent reports have indicated that these substances, if absorbed, may have some detrimental effects. However, with convincing evidence still lacking as to their danger, it is your author's current opinion that these methods may be employed with safety if used appropriately. Some ladies may be sensitive to the chemicals involved. Others decline their use because of inconvenience. Nevertheless, if faithfully used, these methods are effective for most couples in preventing unwanted pregnancy. All of the mechanical and chemical methods of birth control have some "failures," sometimes associated with a failure to use them properly. Nonetheless, occasions of fertility may happen, making none of these methods completely "fool proof."

Two other more controversial forms of birth control are the "**pill**" (oral contraceptive) and the **IUD** (intrauterine device). These methods have some harm associated with their use. The **oral contraceptives** or birth control pills utilize a combination of synthetic *estrogen* and *progesterone*. Synthetic female hormone substitutes produce a "pregnancy-like" effect over the hypothalamus and pituitary gland, inhibiting several hormone cycles that produce ovulation. Breast tenderness, headache, high blood pressure, visual changes, depression, nausea, menstrual spotting, lack of menstruation, an increased risk of *thrombosis* or clotting of the veins, even stroke and heart attack— these are some of the hazards associated with the available birth control pills. All these symptoms and risks are detailed in the drug package inserts. The potential side effects should be carefully scrutinized by potential users. **Smokers**, particularly, have a very high risk, at least five times greater than the nonsmoker for thrombotic complications associated with the pill. Increasing controversy over hormone therapies should make consumers more uncertain of its use, even for short periods.

The **IUD** (called an *intrauterine device*) is becoming more popular in underdeveloped countries. A carefully performed pelvic examination is required for its insertion. Barring complications, it may stay in the uterus for a long time. However, the IUD operates differently from any other form of contraception. It does not **prevent** fertilization of the egg, but rather makes a fertilized egg that arrives in the womb unwelcome. Preventing implantation of this multicelled "child," the IUD actually performs a *"microabortion"* when it acts to prevent pregnancy. From ethical and religious standpoints, more and more concerned Christian ladies avoid this means of family planning. Medical complications frequently result, with increased vaginal bleeding, infection of the womb lining (endometritis), migration of the IUD through the womb into the pelvic cavity, and the increased risk of *tubal pregnancy*. In spite of their widespread use by public health officials, my clinic has always discouraged IUD use for contraception.

Many couples desire a more permanent method of birth control, especially after completing their family. After multiple pregnancies, with several children, they investigate the possibility of sterilization. The simplest form of sterilization involves an operation performed on the husband. Called a **bilateral partial vasectomy**, this operation involves the removal of two small segments of the *vas deferens* from the scrotum. These small tubes conduct the sperm, produced by the testes, to pelvic storage sacs called *seminal vesicles*. In conjunction with the secretions of the prostate and accessory glands, a sticky substance called *semen* is discharged during intercourse. The interruption of the vas deferens by this operation makes the passage of sperm impossible. Very difficult to reverse, this operation should be regarded as essentially permanent. Precaution to preserve a man's health requires that the surgery be performed by a competent surgeon. The removed specimens should be analyzed by a pathologist. Follow-up *semen analysis* after six weeks can assure the success of any vasectomy designed to produce sterility.

The counterpart for a woman's sterilization is the so-called *tubal ligation*. This operation may follow immediately after a normal delivery, at Caesarean section, or at other selected times. More and more frequently the **laparoscope** is employed to perform this procedure. The instrument consists of a lighted fiber-optic tube, inserted through a small incision just below the umbilicus. After carbon dioxide inflation of the abdominal cavity, the Fallopian tubes are visually identified, then cauterized, and divided. Although no specimen is removed, the success rates with this procedure equal that of the more traditional tubal ligation. Even though reversal has been attempted in these procedures, sterilization operations on both men and women should be regarded as permanent, for all practical purposes.

A final type of surgery that produces permanent sterility is a **hysterectomy**. This operation should never be performed solely for the purpose of preventing pregnancy, however. When other medical indications exist, such as excessive bleeding, presence of *fibroid* tumors, or severe pelvic pain from the disease called *endometriosis*, a hysterectomy may be an imperative last resort for regaining the woman's health. Many pelvic operations, however, are not necessary at all. If any question persists, we recommend a second opinion before considering this major surgery. If during childbearing years a hysterectomy becomes necessary, the ovaries should be retained, if possible. Thus, a cycling female hormone effect may prevent premature symptoms of the menopause.

The After Years

Finally, we look briefly at the medical aspects of the *climacteric* or the "**change of life**." Both men and women go through emotional as well as physical changes in their middle years. Women usually stop menstruation between the ages of 46 to 52. Some go longer; and others quit sooner. The cessation of menses is called **menopause**. Associated with this are a number of symptoms, most of them related to estrogen deficiency. Excessive dryness of the birth canal, hot flashes, emotional changes of a psychosomatic or depressive nature, and lack of energy or increased fatigue often occurs during these years. An active exercise program, a careful diet, with the cultivation of a positive attitude, especially trusting in the Lord, will help many women through these difficult years.

Fundamental to this adjustment, however, is the understanding spirit of her loving, committed husband. Consideration for his wife's special needs for rest, relief from stress and worry, and the presence of her mate with his continued affection will go a long way towards minimizing adverse health consequences during the change of life. Men themselves, at times, go through periods of adjustment as with declining strength, increasing weight, and growing waistlines, their previous athletic prowess or intellectual abilities appear to wane. A most powerful remedy for these ills is a continued active, unselfish interest in the lives of others.

When children leave to form homes of their own, parents may consider the needs of other youths who need a home. Volunteer service in hospitals, churches, and other civic organizations brings great personal satisfaction and fulfillment. Special vacation times spent together— in camping, gardening, or travel— or personal study around the fireside helps keep the home happy, even when healthful vigor does not seem to be as perfect as in former years. Outdoor exercise is vital for a healthy body. It aids in the pursuit of peaceful reflection for one's soul as well. Do not give up the quest. Seek counsel, and pray, whenever you are perplexed.

CHAPTER TWENTY–ONE

MENTAL

HEALTH

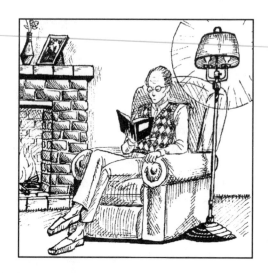

A great epidemic of mental illness is spreading across the country today. Medical statisticians report that at least half of our available hospital beds in the United States are occupied by sufferers from various mental diseases. Great variations exist in both the cause and manifestation of mental disorders. Some mental patients, for example, have disrupted their peace and thought processes. Others victims express their anger in deeds of violence, or the most bizarre behavior. Some appear totally devoid of normal contact with reality.

Physician psychiatrists, such as Dr. Szatz of Syracuse University, regard **mental illness** as largely a myth! Others interpret these disturbed thought and behavior patterns as a disease, classifying them in detail, much like the infectious and malignant conditions are categorized. In an attempt to better understand the working of the mind in both health and sickness, this chapter presents the more common mental problems and a number of simple home remedies which have been tested and found helpful in my own medical institutions.

ANXIETY

One of the more common disrupters of a tranquil mind is the process we term **anxiety**. This has been defined as an "irrational fear" that comes on suddenly, with the associated thought of impending doom or harm, either to one's self or others. This fear will persist and grow unless prompt measures are taken to combat the disturbed thought patterns. In its full-blown manifestation, anxiety causes total loss of volitional control of body actions. This, then, is usually called a *"panic attack."*

There are many potential causes for anxiety. One of these is the very *real* threat of danger, though dwelt upon at length and magnified by the imagination. A common type of mild anxiety is **worry**, associated with fear of what *might* happen. For example, your husband arrives home late from work, your child is playing in the street, unusual variations appear in the Dow-Jones stock averages, gasoline becomes scarce, or food availability is threatened— all of these fears may engender such preoccupation with excessive worry that they disturb your peace or mind. It is for such reasons that nervous Americans turn to tranquilizers.

Sedative drugs, sleeping pills, and nerve calmers have become a way of life to many. Others turn to alcohol as an escape from the tensions and stresses of everyday living. It is obvious that these so-called "remedies" are never *solutions* for they do not address the underlying cause. Our problems of life that evoke anxiety cannot be solved by a capsule or a bottle. In reality, these chemical "crutches" tend to cover up the situation, producing only a illusory *feeling* of tranquility. Meanwhile, the deep inner strife persists unabated. Fortunately, there is a better way.

Exercise is a most valuable remedy for people distressed with anxiety. A quiet walk on a wooded trail, meandering down a country lane, or even strolling with "man's best friend" around the block, or in the city park—these activities offer time for calm reflection and invite the return of peace. "Mini– vacations" in a state park or other remote rural setting also afford time for repose. Fishing on a quiet lake, bird watching with binoculars, or cultivating flowers and vegetables in the garden—all these tend to put life back into perspective.

Soothing instrumental **music**, with a slow, regular rhythm, can help to bring tranquility in the place of tension. The young boy David, playing on his harp, soothed the mind of troubled King Saul. He in deep depression, was lacking a solid spiritual foundation for his kingdom, thus was burdened over the affairs of his nation. David was able, temporarily, to bring peace of mind to the king through the harp and sacred song.

However, there is a modern type of music which brings no peace at all, but rather engenders more anxiety. Rock rhythms, the music of the discotheque, and even much "country western" religious rhythms are far from beneficial to the nerves. Psychologic research discovered that a fast beat and a syncopated rhythm tend to raise the pulse and jangle the nerves. This contrasts with smooth flowing beauty emanating from an orchestral symphony, a pipe organ, or even hymns played on the family piano. With music and melody, the words should also be considered. Listeners should replace frivolous and sentimental songs with messages that are true, noble, and enduring. Fortunate are the children who grow up in a home where mother sings them to sleep, hums a tune in the kitchen, and makes simple sacred music a way of life. It really brings the family close together.

Reading also may bring peace, when the articles or books are true, helpful, and character building. Much of today's literature that fills people's minds is fictitious, trivial, or downright vulgar. Try studies with meditation from the Scriptures, or biographies of great religious leaders, essays by reflective naturalists, and sublime poetry that has stood the test of time. This will serve to promote that quality reasoning and a philosophy of life that helps better to weather the storms of stress.

Yet, with all of these natural approaches to the relief of anxiety, we must *never* forget the supernatural. Above time and space, above the problems and perplexities of man's existence lies an unseen, all–powerful Creator God. The One who hung the worlds in space, continually sustains them by His power. He has the ability to uphold His children, who by celestial design were created in the image of God. Remember daily that *"all things work together for good, for them that love God, to them that are called according to his purpose,"* (Romans 8:28). This realization will help the space–age Christian to endure surprises, disappointments, and the concerns which come to every soul.

The ancient Jewish prophet Isaiah summarized this meditative plane of living succinctly when he said, *"Thou will keep him in perfect peace whose mind is stayed on Thee, because he trusteth in Thee."* (Isaiah 26:3). Yes, without question your **trust in Divine power** lies central to a tranquility of mind which not only can cover but cure the anxious brow, the troubled heart. This serenity brings smiles instead of tears, joy in place of sorrow, and peace to every worried, doubting soul.

DEPRESSION

Despondency and **depression**, although common, and seen at all ages, has diverse specific causes and various practical remedies. Any depression seen in childhood is usually transient. Most children appear to have unusual buoyancy enabling them to rise above feelings and grief, unless surrounded by an atmosphere of gloom. In teen years, depression is more common. It occasionally lingers for months to years. This may be associated with tragedy, or continued elusive expectations, when romantic imaginations are shattered. Marital strife in the home disrupts the routine. Sudden illness likewise requires unforeseen adaptation.

The **postpartum "blues"** constitutes a type of depression seen after childbirth and delivery. It often follows the arrival of a baby, but does not seem to be related to the incidence of Caesarean section, any deformed offspring, or other obvious cause. The "baby blues" may last for days or develop into a deep-seated depression, requiring superhuman effort to pull out of the gloom.

In the middle years of life, however, depression finds its most common expression. Although menopause need not necessarily be associated with this emotional disaster, nevertheless it is not uncommon. Occasionally depression persists in a subliminal state—where life does not seem to have the same meaning, time slips away without the usual things being accomplished, and thoughts tend to be morbid, centered mostly on self. Occasionally, this depressive syndrome becomes so chronic that hospitalization is necessary.

One most serious complication of longstanding depression is attempted **suicide**. This takes an increasing toll among both adults and teenage youth. Ranking within the top ten causes of death, suicide is an obvious, but most self-centered, escape from the psychic pain of deep depression. Some suicides occur without warning. However, most patients leave telltale signs of their mental distress. Letters, notes, or words that express hopelessness, such as wishing to die, are usually a "cry for help." Such signals should be heeded with prompt response. For this reason, studiously avoid depending on sleeping pills, tranquilizers, and other sedatives or mood affecting drugs so that can easily be used to overdose, or prove fatal to the user. Newspapers are replete with accounts of movie stars, politicians, and wealthy, apparently well-adjusted neighbors who just came to "the end of their hope," and were found at the end of a rope. Being unable to cope any longer, they tragically took their lives. Crisis intervention at a time of deep despondency, when death wishes are expressed, may save a life for time and eternity.

In spite of prevailing philosophies among psychiatrists and counselors, it does not seem reasonable to cast, in Freudian fashion, the entire blame on traumatic childhood, punitive mothers, absentee fathers, or marital conflict when deep depression ensues. With due medical regard for the exigencies of life that bring about grief, remorse, and distress, we know that within the human heart there is a desire for goodness and a hope for better things. If cultivated, this innate quest can make even the worst of circumstances turn out to be a blessing. Illustrations in the Scriptures abound, when pressing circumstances brought out deeper faith and trust in God. Examples such as, Daniel in the den of lions, and Paul and Silas in prison, as well as Jesus in His trials and crucifixion—all were calculated to inspire faith and hope in the face of apparent disaster.

Some very real **chemical causes** may lie at the root of depression. An overuse of **caffeine** or other stimulant drugs, either in liquid or tablet form can provoke a depression. For caffeine's unnatural stimulation of the central nervous system is, as it were, a borrowing of energy reserves which must be repaid to keep the nerves in balance. Following each stimulation, whether caused by reading sordid, exciting stories, seeing the latest movies, or drinking caffeinated beverages, the aftermath of depression is inevitable. Sometimes this is transient and primarily of a physical nature. But on other occasions the nerves are affected for many days.

Drugs, particularly the tranquilizer and sleeping pill type, can produce depression, especially when the dosage is increased and the usage prolonged. The use of mind-altering drubs must be stopped to overcome this type of despondency. Chronic illness, particularly if painful, may lead to depression. Patients with chronic back disorders, amputees, and others convalescing from mutilating surgical procedures are often victims of depression. Alcoholics are also not uncommonly depressed and drink to "drown their sorrows," only to wake up with *hangovers* and to find their troubles once again looming on the horizon. In fact, alcohol tends to compound most difficulties, since coping mechanisms are impaired and the tolerance for stress is handicapped under the chronic influence of this socially destructive beverage.

Some people eat to satiate their depressed feelings. In such cases, food becomes a tranquilizer. One authority on weight control stated, "It doesn't matter much what you eat, but it matters more what eats you." Most specialists in the treatment of obesity recognize that it is next to impossible to control weight without attending to emotional needs, particularly to the relief of depression.

Let us look at several simple remedies that can be applied to the depression problem encountered in an ordinary home. Our first approach in treating depression consists in a thorough evaluation of the cause. If possible, any identifiable precipitating factors should be removed. Such things as chronic illness, divorce, or grief over a death in the family may not go away for many months, or even years. Such eventualities require a firm determination to cope with the immediate crisis. Finally, with the help of God, we must rise above the inclination to become despondent. Research studies have shown that **going to bed early** is helpful in resisting depression. Most commonly the despondency appears associated with morning hours. Usually, depression improves during the course of a day. Rising early and becoming busy with household or shop projects—cooking, sewing, reading, auto maintenance, or handicrafts—will help to "put your mind in gear" early, diverting it from the self–destructive habit of centering thoughts on self. The exercise of will power goes with the labor of the hand. Thus, the more occupied any person can be in useful employment, the easier depression is to cope with.

Active physical **exercise** is a great reliever of depression. Vigorous walking, jogging, calisthenics, aerobics, bicycle riding, swimming, and other similar recreational outlets help in the cure of depression. It is important, however, to avoid the unnatural overexcitement associated with contact sports, competitive games, or the "carnival atmosphere" that stimulates, only to leave a hollow, empty aftermath when the stimulus is no longer there. Try cultivating flowers, small fruits, or vegetables. Horticulture helps divert the mind, and relieves depression by occupying the body in a satisfying, rewarding type of activity. Gardening is full of learning possibilities and object lessons that illustrate the Creator's love.

The real cure for depression, however, lies in a confiding **trust** in our great Creator, God. This firm confidence can keep a person steady, even cheerful, under the most forbidding circumstances. It can smooth life's troubled waters, banish grief and psychic pain, and lift the spirits when all around is apparent disaster. In fact, to brave the future when our pressures, disappoint-ments, and trials will be greater than we have ever seen, we people in America, as well as other nations, need the "faith of our fathers living still, in spite of dungeon, fire, and sword." Our steadfast confidence should be based upon the Word of the living God. Daily meditations in Scriptural precepts will be like a life preserver, holding us poised in the whirlpool of doubts, grief, or temporary depression.

One final remedy that also is needed for many depressed souls, is **confession of known sin**. It is not unusual to find what the Bible calls the "transgression of the law," lying deep within as a fundamental cause for long-standing depressive reactions. Marital infidelity, theft, extortion, a failure to care for the needs of aging parents, or the deep inner conflict of "respectable sins," such as inordinate pride and covetousness, produce their natural results in many disturbed minds. The early apostle and Christian leader, James, put it succinctly when he wrote: *Confess your faults one to another, and pray for one another, that ye may be healed. The effectual fervent prayer of a righteous man availeth much."* (James 5:16). The experience of peace that comes to an individual who has experienced this assured forgiveness can be measured in eternity when the joy of Jesus is seen, who saw "the travail of His soul" and will be satisfied. Yes, friend, there is a cure for depression.

FEARS AND PHOBIAS

Nearly everyone is subject to certain fears. Unforeseeable events, such as accidents and natural disasters, commonly produce a sudden overwhelming concern called **fear**. Sometimes it becomes excessive and imaginary, akin to anxiety. On rarer occasions, the chronic nature of fear develops a pattern of bizarre behavior, which may lead to a disabling *obsession*. Such irrational responses are called **phobias**. Several types are described.

Acrophobia is the fear of heights. **Claustrophobia** is a fear of closed, tight spaces. **Hydrophobia** involves a fear of water. Phobic responses often occur on the edge of a cliff, the end of a diving board, or with the sight of blood. **Obsessive reactions** may be associated with fear of germs, occasionally leading to symbolic and excessive hand washing, compulsive wiping of doorknobs, or bizarre eating habits.

Many phobias have their roots in childhood trauma, where fear was "planted" by well-intentioned, but misguided parents, siblings, or relatives. School teachers might further exaggerate the fear response. The imagery of television, comic books, and fictitious stories do their damage, too. Since the root of the disease lies in the diseased imagination, stern self-discipline, as well as keen parental insight, are required to overcome any phobic reaction.

Some psychiatrists resort to "shock treatment" (called *electro-convulsive therapy* or ECT) in order to stifle phobic responses. Rarely does this therapy cure on a long–term basis. Moreover, it may produce hostility or even intensify the symptoms. Throwing a child who is afraid and unable to swim into deep water, or threatening to push an individual off a cliff, only lowers the child's confidence in those close to him or her. Such abuse can nullify the spirit of trust so important to a well-balanced life. **Counseling** has a role in developing improved understanding of these fearful circumstances. Too often, however, insight comes slow. The counselor, if he or she becomes frustrated and impatient, can never achieve any therapeutic goal.

In order to overcome a particular phobia, one should focus on developing a trusting relationship with our all-wise heavenly Father. God's Word declares, *"The Lord has not given us the spirit of fear, but of power, and of love, and of a sound mind."* (II Tim.1:7). Also from I John 4:18 is the declaration, *"There is no fear in love, but perfect love casteth out fear."* These and other Bible promises should be memorized, repeated, and claimed to help overcome any deep-seated phobia. Just as a child begins to tiptoe first to the lake's edge, then wades into the water, and goes deeper until he or she finally swims, so a person can be gingerly coaxed into activities that formerly were terrifying. This must always be done in the context of a warm, trusting human relationship. Often when some friend provides this security, the individual, in their mind at least, instinctively minimizes the risks and becomes more daring. Most phobias can be controlled and channeled into useful productive activities, if not be completely cured.

SCHIZOPHRENIA

How unfortunate it is when a person becomes so disturbed that all contact with reality is disrupted. Many of these disorders are called **schizophrenia**, a term which means "splitting of mind." Although there are many psychotic variations, medical science has yet to find a cure for this disruption of thought processes. Some professionals, with psychoanalytic insight look to childhood experience for causes. Others look for spiritual explanations, regarding some cases as "demon possession." Whatever the cause, the results are not pleasant. Numerous children and adolescents are affected. Some who have used drugs such as LSD have suffered long-term consequences, even permanent mental derangement, from their youthful drug experimentation.

Several types of mental illness are described. In some cases, **paranoia** is the most prominent manifestation. This is a type of thought disorder where deep suspicion exists. Sometimes the symptoms of **delusions** fit so perfectly together that almost anyone would be convinced as though persecution were directed to the affected individual. It may be the Mafia, the communists, or more tragically the delusions may be directed against a husband or wife, who is at a loss to know how to make amends. Except for the paranoid delusions, the remainder of a patient's life may function normally, making his or her disease all the more difficult to diagnose.

In one common type of schizophrenia, the affected individual becomes completely irrational. Sudden onset of destructive behavior may ensue, while on other occasions screaming, insane babbling, or bizarre physical manifestations may give evidence of strange voices he or she is hearing *(auditory hallucinations)* or the totally disrupted state of the person's mind. Disgraceful disrobing is not uncommon, with eccentric exhibitions that cannot be tolerated in a respectable society.

A not so common, but very perplexing, type of mental disruption is the **catatonic** state. In this mental condition a sick individual will assume a posture and often hold the position in a waxy state of inflexibility, while remaining entirely mute and unresponsive. It is difficult to distinguish this from drug reactions or brain tumors. Careful neurologic investigation is indicated.

Some have thought that the habit of **masturbation** lies at the root of diverse forms of schizophrenia. Scientific investigation does correlate the resulting zinc deficiency with mental aberrations. Usually, however, progressive disorder of thought processes, bizarre behavioral mannerisms, and the unpredictability of a patient's verbal response makes mental illness the more likely diagnosis. The real problem is: *"What do we DO about it?"* Generally, the earlier any diagnosis can be made and the treatment instituted, the more likely a successful outcome. Always avoid excusing the behavior as "just a stage" he or she will grow out of. Take such happenings seriously.

One basic therapy for improvement in mental disorders is good nutrition. Adequate quantities of all B–complex vitamins should be obtained with a strong emphasis on foods which are high in trace minerals. Fresh fruit and vegetables, whole grain cereals, and nuts, with a strict avoidance of spicy foods, sugar, and stimulating caffeinated drinks should help the affected person's diet. **Regularity** in mealtime should be habitual and as far as possible tensions should be minimized.

* * * * * * * * *

Many mental breaks are the result of sleep deprivation. As far as possible a person suffering from mental disease should be encouraged to **retire early**. Often a long period of uninterrupted sleep will be rewarded by renewed balance to the mind. *"Early to bed and early to rise"* with an active program of physical labor during the day can bring relief. Long walks in the woods, particularly when accompanied by a sane, understanding, sympathetic person can help to direct the thoughts and conversation back to real life.

Several hours each day should be devoted to some type of physical activity. Table games, television watching, and idle daydreaming should be curtailed, with the mind kept busy on useful, pleasant diversions. Sometimes weeks to months are required for the nervous system to regain its balance. Nevertheless persisted in, these natural remedies will produce results.

As far as possible, recourse to mind–affecting drugs, shock therapy, or hospitalization in a mental facility should be avoided. The stigma attached, as well as the sights and sounds experienced in contact with the insane, may only serve to reinforce the abnormal behavior. Psychotherapy can even prolong mental illness, rather than effecting a cure. In my experience, those afflicted with schizophrenia who have been institutionalized for years and have undergone numerous shock treatments as well as heavy sedation with tranquilizers are *almost* impossible to bring back to a normal state of thinking and mental function. Here are cases for the healing power of our Creator to cure.

All the above simple measures are best instituted in a rural setting. The tranquility and quiet of country life, the contact with domestic animals or agricultural products, as well as the necessity for the stern discipline of useful outdoor labor will help those whose minds are breaking under stress of life. Furthermore, with all of these things, good as they may be, patients with mental illness should be approached with much prayer.

The Maker of our mind knows best its needs. Reading the Word of God will bring stability to all health workers, with a balanced treatment of the physical, mental, and spiritual ills that cannot be perfected in any other way. Sing simple gospel songs, pray fervent prayers, read Scriptural promises, and the narrative of Christ's healing others who also were oppressed in mind. Thus, a parent, friend, or relative can work with confidence, persistently applying the measures that, blessed by the Lord, bring mental health. A clear intelligent eye, and words of deepest gratitude will evenutally come as your reward from the recovering victims of emotional or mental illness.

CHAPTER TWENTY–TWO

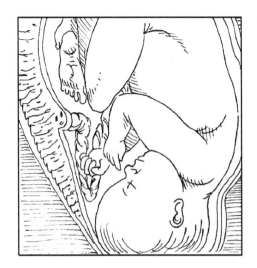

PREGNANCY

AND

CHILDBIRTH

The arrival of a newborn baby is an exciting moment for the entire family. After months of waiting, not a little expense, and the experience of labor and childbirth, the newborn baby is a welcome sight indeed. Many items must be considered in planning for the baby's arrival. First, the mother's health together with the presence or absence of genetic diseases in the family should be scrutinized carefully. Financial questions should be asked, since the current costs for obstetrical care and delivery in local community hospitals is formidable. Next remember, with the arrival of your baby, expenses have just begun. The costs of feeding, clothing, and educating children are all subject to inflation. This should, ideally, be considered before conception occurs. For many reasons today, financial and philosophic, numerous couples contract with midwives and plan for home deliveries.

In this context, the following description of pregnancy and childbirth applies especially for **home birthing** experiences. However, I do not want to be understood as recommending that *every* baby be born at home. Nonetheless, a long experience involving most western European nations attests that a home delivery, if performed by a competent midwife or medical practitioner, can be safe and beneficial to all concerned. Barring unforeseen complications, home birthing proves extraordinarily satisfying to both the newborn's parents.

Evidence of this modern trend toward natural home-like deliveries is evident in an increasing number of "birthing rooms" placed inside modern progressive hospitals. A definite trend toward breast feeding, "rooming–in," and maternal–infant bonding also advertises the modern mother's interest in personalized, home–like approaches to those sacred moments when her off-spring takes his or her first breath. I will depict first some problems of early pregnancy, with many simple remedies that can be applied in the home. Then, with a description of prenatal care I will offer several suggestions on the delivery of a child in the home, its aftercare, and the successful initiation of breast feeding.

PROBLEMS IN EARLY PREGNANCY

One of the earliest predicaments to confront a woman who has missed one or two periods, involves this all absorbing question, "Am I pregnant?" There are several simple techniques to determine pregnancy with reasonable certainty, right within one's own home. A suspicion arises when there is a miss of the normal menstrual period. If menses have been regular for several months, then the intuition heightens. Many women have months when they skip the cycle normally. Others have periods too scant to notice. Then the diagnosis of pregnancy becomes more difficult.

Symptoms of pregnancy may be present. You may experience a feeling of *nausea*, typically in the morning. This is occasionally associated with prolonged vomiting lasting throughout the day. The breasts may swell and become more tender than is usually associated with the premenstrual state. A slight change may occur in the vaginal discharge. Occasionally, a woman who has had previous children just "feels pregnant." In pregnancy after three to four months, a "lump" may actually be felt above the pubic bone, located in the lower abdomen. This is probably the enlarging womb. By five months gestation it will usually reach to the navel, with an obvious rounded prominence in the lower abdomen. Fetal movements may be sensed at four to four and a half months, though they are sometimes detected earlier by experienced mothers carrying their second or third child.

In most pharmacies today, you can purchase a urine pregnancy test kit. This analysis very simply measures the amount of HCG *(Human Chorionic Gonadotropin)*, a hormone secreted by the developing placenta. A positive test for pregnancy develops within three to six weeks after conception. Use a concentrated morning urine sample for best reliability. If performed according to directions, these tests are quite dependable in confirming the suspicion of pregnancy.

Vague abdominal pains are sometimes felt in early pregnancy. Pelvic pain may occur from pressure on an enlarged ovary, or from a "tilted" uterus. As it enlarges, the organs become tighter in the pelvis, while the womb has not yet risen into the abdominal cavity. Pain could be related to constipation, or to **cystitis**. Usually, a bladder infection is characterized by burning combined with a frequent urge to urinate. Stretching of the ligaments that support the uterus may produce pain. In later months, the pressure of a fetal part on a pelvic nerve or a sudden shifting of the baby within the womb may give rise to such symptoms. Usually reassurance is all the patient needs. Severe pain or sudden changes in health status should be called to the attention of a physician immediately, however, since it could be an **ectopic** (*tubal*) **pregnancy**. If this goes unrecognized it could rupture, with internal hemorrhage and potential disaster. Appendicitis may occasionally be superimposed upon pregnancy, requiring early diagnosis and prompt surgical treatment as usual.

Vaginal bleeding sometimes occurs, even after pregnancy begins. Usually this appears scant and transient, but at times it may be profuse. When an actual hemorrhage develops after pregnancy has established, this constitutes an obvious threat of **miscarriage**. The presence of regular contractions and pelvic pain, combined with vaginal bleeding, should alert to this possibility. At times a miscarriage may occur with the complete passage of the placenta and the subsequent stoppage of bleeding. If incomplete expulsion of the placenta or fetal tissue occurs, a simple operation, called a **D and C** (*dilation and curettage*), should be performed, so the bleeding will stop and the uterus can return to its normal size. Fever in the presence of a miscarriage is a more ominous sign, as it probably indicates the presence of pelvic infection.

For treatment of threatened miscarriage, bed rest is always advisable. The absence of straining, standing, or moving about lessens the flow and usually decreases the likelihood of a miscarriage. Sexual intercourse should be avoided in early pregnancy, particularly near the times when a menstrual period would otherwise occur. Uterine cramping and the likelihood of miscarriage is greater at these cycles, for reasons yet unknown. Hormones are no longer given routinely to mothers threatened with miscarriage. They are powerless to stop the inevitable. Furthermore, progesterone concentrates may cause damage to the fetus, if it is carried to term. Scientists believe that many spontaneous miscarriages are the result of some chromosomal defect, which otherwise would have led to congenital deformity. They are eliminated by nature before the pregnancy goes too far. This is of considerable consolation to parents, suddenly disappointed by the premature loss of a long-looked-for baby. Most couples can wait a few months, then try again.

One of the more troublesome conditions of early pregnancy, sometimes lasting for months, is an upset stomach. Called "morning sickness," for obvious reasons, nausea and vomiting tends to herald the onset of pregnancy. Although only a few ladies find it incapacitating, these symptoms tend to hinder proper nourishment, so important in the early months of pregnancy. This nausea may last throughout the day. On the other hand, it may be relieved by eating some crackers or other form of dry food. Frequently, the appetite completely changes, and the "lady-in-waiting" craves foods that were formerly disliked. In extreme cases this so-called **pica** (abnormal craving) is manifested by the "clay eating" habit of southerners, or the strange love for "pickles and ice cream" that ordinarily seems like a repulsive combination. Mothers need to be careful that their appetites are controlled by reason when such cravings become abnormal.

Where vomiting in pregnancy becomes persistent, hospitalization may prove necessary. One or two days of intravenous feedings is normally sufficient to bring back a normal digestion once again. Emotional contributions to this gastric problem are frequent. These can be related to ambivalence about being pregnant, or an underlying temperament of nervousness manifested in an unusually sensitive stomach. Nevertheless, the physiologic and hormonal changes that occur are profound. Such endocrine considerations may well explain these early digestive symptoms. A tolerance for food usually emerges by the fourth month, enabling a normal digestive tone to continue for the remainder of pregnancy.

Adequate fluid intake is vitally important from the start. It is suspected that the common, insufficient intake of water is one principal cause of persistent nausea and vomiting. Drink at least six to eight glasses of water per day, at whatever temperature is best tolerated by the sensitive stomach. If the mother avoids soups and creamed mixtures, and chews thoroughly a rather dry meal of whole grain crackers, breakfast cereals, or raw vegetables, her food will stay down better and permit the best nutrition at this critical stage.

Vaginal discharge is often troublesome during the latter months of pregnancy. This may be due to the parasite *Trichomonas*, but is more commonly caused by a buildup of yeast or **Monilia** *(Candida albicans)*. Hormone changes combined with increased perineal moisture and warmth, create an environment favorable to the growth of these organisms. Diabetes mellitus, particularly aggravates the tendency to develop yeast infections.

Administration of hormones such as the birth control pill may produce a diabetes-like state in non-pregnant women. However, pregnancy increases this trend. Nylon underwear, panty hose, and tight slacks tend to increase the propensity for vaginitis. This is because greater warmth and moisture are produced in the perineum when one wears those synthetic fabric materials. Air circulation around the body and "breathing" of the skin is impeded. Then it leads to the rapid multiplication of yeast germs with such unpleasant symptoms as discharge, burning, itching, and skin rash. Gentle vaginal *douches*, with a dilute vinegar solution (one tablespoon of white vinegar to one quart of warm water) can help decrease the discharge and restore normal acidity to the birth canal. Specific agents are available to help in acute stages (such as *Massingill* products). However, the intestinal tract always harbors these germs, so it is impossible to completely escape from them. Therefore, you will find it preferable to build up resistance and let improved health of the body create its own defense.

Marital relations should be avoided, not only when discharge or infection is present, but during any time of spotting or uterine cramping. Moreover, for at least four to six weeks prior to the birth of the baby, intimate relations should likewise be curtailed, since a significantly increased risk of infection in the amniotic fluid surrounding the baby has been linked to intercourse at this stage. Sexual continence at this critical time will be rewarded with better health, as well as peace of mind.

PRENATAL CARE

Before your baby arrives, a great deal of care needs to be maintained to preserve the your best health. Although pregnancy is a normal physiologic event, many physicians treat it as a disease, and attempt to control too closely the behavior of the mother. Most women, however, can be taught the basics of hygiene during pregnancy. That means taking take responsibility for your own health.

During the monthly visits a pregnant lady makes to her midwife or physician, she will have a urine test for protein and sugar. Sugar in the urine raises a suspicion of diabetes. The diabetic mother is at increased risk during pregnancy, and has a greater likelihood of difficult labor, due to the predictably excessive size of her baby. Blood incompatibilities and hemorrhagic problems are more severe in a baby born to a diabetic mother. In addition, the stability of a mother's diabetes is greatly influenced by her pregnancy. It could even trigger the death of a baby *in utero*, or a miscarriage, if care is not taken to control the diabetes with appropriate levels of insulin. Still, one can perform the simple test for urine sugar right in the home with commonly available strips of *Tes Tape* or *Clinitest* tablets, available at any pharmacy.

Toxemia in pregnancy has several facets. With the mother's excessive accumulation of body tissue, fluid overload becomes generalized edema. Her weight may go up several pounds within a few days, creating puffiness not only in the ankles, but the hands, eyes, and occasionally her entire body. Along with this dilemma, the kidneys show signs of damage, losing large amounts of protein. A simple dip–stick urine test for protein may show 2+, 3+, or 4+ protein, implying heavy losses of this important substance. Third, the blood pressure rises, frequently producing symptoms of headache, painful pressure behind the eyes, or outright nosebleed. When these three manifestations of toxemia (*hypertension, proteinuria, edema*) occur late in pregnancy, it is crucial to evaluate the reflexes. Tap gently, for example, with the doctor's little hammer on the tendon just below your knee. Then, for preventive treatment, secure a calm, quiet environment, strictly limit your salt intake, and eat adequate protein to replace the heavy losses. Prolonged bed rest in a darkened room is occasionally prudent to prevent external stimuli that could trigger seizures. **Convulsions** are the most frequent cause of death (for mother *and* child) when toxemia develops. This grave complication should be prevented, whenever possible. Modern management with I.V. administration of magnesium sulfate (Epsom salts) prevents most serious and life-threatening convulsions that could occur without warning.

For many timely reasons, during every pregnancy I recommend the routine measurement of weight and blood pressure on a monthly basis. Mothers, be sure to limit weight gain during pregnancy to approximately twenty five to thirty pounds. Extreme austerity in diet is not necessary, but neither is overindulgence and its resulting obesity a boon. Mothers who later breast feed their infants, find their weight returning to normal much sooner. Nursing helps because it utilizes significant numbers of stored calories to manufacture milk. As a general rule, very little weight gain is advisable during the first three months of pregnancy, about two pounds per month in the second trimester, and one pound or more per week during the final three months. This adequacy of weight gain provides for a mother's and child's needs with plenty of nutrients that will build bone and blood, muscle and connective tissue. Even more importantly, good nutrition promotes health to the nervous system and brain of each developing *fetus*.

Proper diet for every pregnant mother is vital. You should strictly avoid **all** use of alcoholic beverages, because of their toxic effect on your baby. Moreover, beverage alcohol sabotages your brain and will power. Tobacco should also be eliminated, for numerous reasons mentioned above. Coffee and tea are unnecessary, as every pregnant mother needs a calm environment without stimulants or any chemical that would weaken the nervous system. Recent research shows caffeine definitely harmful to the unborn child, capable of transmitting a legacy of irritability to the high–risk offspring.

The mother's diet should ideally be unrefined, with a unequivocal emphasis on whole grains, fresh fruits and vegetables, along with adequate amounts of water. Calcium intake can be secured through a liberal use of whole grain cereals, green leafy vegetables, and skim milk. The iron needed to maintain healthy red blood comes from such foods as: cereal grains; fruits— such as raisins, prunes, and strawberries; and dark green and yellow vegetables. At times, supplements are needed for those with deficient absorption of these important trace minerals. All other needed vitamins and minerals can be obtained easily from a diet of unrefined natural foods.

The mother should eat a substantial breakfast. Energy needs for the day are best obtained at its beginning. One or two pieces of fresh fruit, a slice of whole wheat toast with peanut butter, a bowl of cereal such as shredded wheat, oatmeal, or granola, topped with fruit and soy milk make an excellent breakfast. For variety a healthful waffle, apple crisp, fruit sauces or muffins may be substituted. The mother who starts the day sharp with a good breakfast will keep going longer and maintain far better health than those who sleep in, nibble a little, then make up for it with evening snacks. Lunch should be carefully planned, so that the noon meal is as generous as breakfast. A vegetable or two, a baked potato, a bowl of soup, or a sandwich on whole wheat bread, with tossed salad, or a vegetable entree are some of the variations that bring the best of natural nutrients for better health to mothers. Vegetarian recipe books abound with suggestions for cooking these natural foods. Suppers should be light—fruit, fruit soup, *zwieback*, or homemade crackers are ideal. The evening meal should be completely digested several hours before going to bed.

Exercise should be carefully planned, to keep the muscles strong and the joints limber. "Tailor sitting" helps the perineal muscles to relax and loosens the ligaments of the thighs. Arch the back from the hands and knees position to strengthen the postural muscles. This so-called "pelvic rocking" exercise is excellent for late pregnancy to minimize low back pain. Moreover, it helps promote an erect standing and walking posture. "Sitbacks,"— in which a person sits on the floor with the legs outstretched and leans back, then forward, then back, repeating several times—is an exercise designed to improve tone in the abdominal muscles. It benefits the tummy, while avoiding any danger of back strain so common in more traditional sit-ups. Practice a general routine of warm-up calisthenics each day to prevent muscle cramps and joint tightness, which could otherwise create problems later during labor.

The very best exercise, however, for any pregnant mother is **walking**. Walk briskly one, two, or even three miles per day with your shoulders back, the arms swinging comfortably from the sides, and your head erect. This will pay dividends in fitness, health, and a feeling of vigorous well-being. The mother who walks during pregnancy may well breeze through labor. On the average, labor and delivery requires less time in a physically fit mother, when you can relax and cooperate with these forces of nature. Swimming, bicycling, gardening, and other mild activities are likewise beneficial during pregnancy to keep the muscles firm and the disposition gentle.

With the physical culture of your body, remember to cultivate the mind. Pregnancy is an ideal time to read books on child training and natural childbirth. You can secure the best mental preparation for motherhood in a context of Christian commitment that makes motherhood a partnership between you and your Maker. Such encouraging books as *Child Guidance* by Ellen G. White and *Natural Childbirth and the Christian Family* by Helen Wessel constitute valuable resources to every parent who is serious about successful child**rearing**, as well as child bearing.

HOME DELIVERIES

In European countries most babies are delivered at home. Until recent years in the United States, the same custom was true. Among idealistic college youth, natural living enthusiasts, and those with no insurance, home delivery still holds an attraction. Midwives and occasionally physicians usually attend these patients. Husbands, wives, nurses, and family physicians should all become acquainted with the techniques of a home delivery. Either through planning or in an emergency, this knowledge may prove most useful.

First in importance is the **recognition of labor**. For several weeks prior to delivery there may be painless, irregularly spaced contractions. These so-called *Braxton–Hicks contractions* serve to firm up the uterus and, as it were, "prime" it for the main event. The baby typically "drops" several weeks before labor is to begin, as the head descends into the pelvis, creating a "lightening" sensation. Slight cervical dilation then follows, with increased secretion of mucus–like discharge.

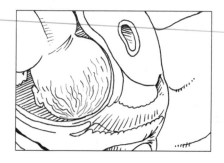

When labor actually ensues, however, one of three changes heralds its onset. The loss of the mucus plug, at times coated with blood (*bloody show*), may coincide with the onset of labor. Second, the cervix begins to thin (called *effacement*) and dilate. Regular contractions then commence, usually coming every eight to ten minutes, lasting at least sixty seconds. They then increase in frequency, becoming quite intense. Labor contractions located in the low back may be extremely painful. They are commonly associated with an "occiput posterior" delivery. In this more challenging type of labor, the back of the head orients toward the mother's back, making passage through the birth canal during labor more difficult. The "bag of waters" (*amniotic sac*) may burst, causing a sudden flood of warm clear fluid. Occasionally, the escape of urine or a vaginal discharge may mimic the breaking of the water. This must be tested with **pH** paper (litmus or nitrazine). The amniotic fluid is always alkaline, turning nitrazine paper blue. When labor initiates itself by the breaking "bag of water," it normally proceeds faster. In fact, it is important for the delivery to be accomplished within twenty four hours after the water breaks, to lessen any risk of infection in the mother's womb.

Labor usually progresses steadily through three distinct stages. The first stage consists of progressive cervical dilation and thinning (*effacement*). When the cervix is completely dilated, the opening is 10 cm. in diameter, the average diameter of a baby's head. The second stage of labor begins when the head passes through the completely dilated cervix, and descends into the birth canal (*vagina*). The first appearance of the baby's head between the *labia* is called **crowning**. Progressive dilation of the vulva then occurs, requiring special self-control on the part of the mother. Periodic panting with each contraction, helps to avoid pushing the baby out too fast, thus preventing laceration of either vagina or cervix. If all goes smoothly at this point, the baby enters the world into the waiting hands of an attendant midwife or physician.

Your first maneuver, after the baby's head emerges, should be to clear its mouth and nose of mucus. A rubber suction bulb works excellently for this

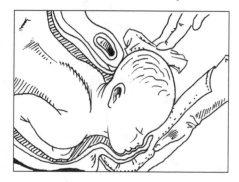

purpose. Clearing the airway of mucus should be performed thoroughly, with the baby's head in a downward position (for a normal "face down" delivery). Quickly check the baby's neck for the umbilical cord. If a loop of the cord is discovered, slip it gently over the head to make the delivery of the shoulders and trunk easier. This helps prevent its strangling the baby, or accidentally tearing the cord. A hemorrhage would then result, depleting the baby of its precious blood. The upper shoulder of the infant is usually delivered first, followed by the lower. Finally, the rest of the body slips out easily.

Continue holding the baby in a head down position, and suction the mouth and nose again. Wait "patiently" for the first cry and a few deep breaths that ventilate the lungs and bring a healthy pink color to the newborn body. The pulsing umbilical cord should be left alone for a minute or two, to allow further blood flow from the placenta into the baby. This acts as a mild "transfusion" to give the baby some of its own blood, which would otherwise be lost. "Stripping" the cord of its blood in this fashion retards the later development of anemia, commonly seen in babies a few months old. When the cord quits pulsating, it can be tied or clamped. In a normal home-like setting it is convenient to boil a clean white shoelace, and use this to tie the cord. About ¼ to ½ inch from the skin of the navel, tie the cord securely, with care taken to avoid pulling or traumatizing the umbilicus. Place two ties about an inch apart, the second one being further from the baby than the first tie. Then use a pair of **sterilized** scissors to cut between the cord ties.

The third stage of labor involves the **delivery of the placenta**. The "afterbirth" follows within five to forty five minutes, and usually separates on its own accord with no manipulation required. If necessary, use your hand to gently massage the uterus. Another "push" on the mother's part, and the placenta comes easily.

The uterus should again be massaged carefully. The baby can be positioned to nurse at mother's breast. This enables both hormonal and neural mechanisms to contract the uterus and lessen the likelihood of hemorrhage. Periodically, for the next hour massage the uterus to keep it firm and minimize bleeding.

If there has been a laceration of the perineum during the delivery, it should be carefully inspected. If the tear is extremely small and not bleeding, it may be allowed to seal by merely lying still with the mother's legs together for a few hours. All deeper lacerations, particularly those involving the muscle of the rectal sphincter should be sutured. Even if this means a trip to the emergency room or doctor's office, it should be repaired, so complete healing will occur. Then the rectum and birth canal will not lose their normal anatomic relationships, leading to incontinence or discharge.

One most important qualification for a successful nurse-midwife is the ability to remain calm under pressure. The delivery of a baby is an exciting time. All the attendants should continually remain alert, interested, and composed. Encouragement to the mother during the strenuous pushing stage can make all the difference between a successful home delivery and one that needs obstetrical assistance in a hospital. The use of forceps can often be avoided if mothers receive the proper coaching and encouragement during this labor stage. Patience in waiting for the placenta will likewise be rewarded. Although excited viewers may request to take pictures, it is much more important to attend to the physical needs of the newborn than obtain a few precious snapshots.

The newborn baby needs immediate care once the cord has been divided. He or she should be wrapped in warm dry blankets, and the head gently covered. A small cap made of stockinette helps to prevent heat loss from the scalp as well as the baby's body. Prompt breathing and rapid delivery of oxygen to the tissues are enhanced when the newborn is kept warm. If the home is unusually cold, the child should be placed "skin-to-skin" upon the mother. Then, both should be wrapped in a blanket. The use of insulating "aluminum foil" may be helpful, but in such cases monitor the child's temperature frequently with a thermometer to prevent overheating. Some newborns enjoy the experience of suckling, and will lay at their mother's side to nurse for several minutes. A newborn baby who has been delivered with minimal trauma will have its eyes open, looking around. He or she may recognize the mother and "imprint" her image in their mind within hours after birth. This "bonding" is very important for the mother-and-child interaction, often conditioned by the immediate experience of the postpartum period.

Several emergency situations should be kept in mind. Their possibility, although rare, may require immediate intervention. The **prolapse of the umbilical cord** is one urgent complication. If the umbilical cord appears before the baby has been delivered, emergency rescue measures may help to save the infant's life. The head should be firmly pushed back into the birth canal, to prevent its pressing tightly against the cord, and thus obstructing the flow of blood to the baby. Usually a *Caesarean section* is indicated in such cases. If performed soon enough, surgery may save the life of the child.

Breech delivery sometimes presents unexpectedly. Either a foot, both

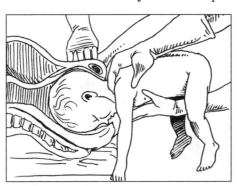

feet, or the rump of the baby will appear at the opening of the birth canal. If this was the first pregnancy, the baby is particularly in danger. Ignorance concerning the size of the "aftercoming" head leads most physicians in a hospital setting to do a *Caesarean section* on the mother whose firstborn baby is a breech presentation. However, if the mother has delivered previous children, this baby could be delivered with the feet grasped and held by an assistant, elevated above the mother's abdomen. Then, the baby is rotated so that the head can be delivered face down. Exert a *gentle* pulling with a finger in the baby's mouth. When its chin appears at the entrance of the birth canal, help to deliver the head with minimal trauma.

At times, **premature** babies come unanticipated in the home. They are particularly sensitive to heat loss, and should be kept very warm and close to the mother. Usually the tiniest ones are unable to suck well and must be tube fed. With practiced skill, this small feeding tube can be placed in the baby's stomach with each feeding. Give a small amount of breast milk for nourishment every two or three hours. Most premature infants should be cared for in a hospital with facilities for newborn intensive care.

Hemorrhage involving the mother is a serious emergency. Usually, this will occur immediately after the birth of the baby or within the first few hours. When the blood flow is bright red, there exists the possibility of an overlooked laceration. Look for it carefully. Pressure may help stop the bleeding until the patient can be transported to an emergency room. If there is no laceration, then the bleeding usually originates from the uterus. Firmly massage the softened dome of the uterus immediately, while applying an ice pack to the lower abdomen. This may help the uterus to contract. Place the infant at her breast to nurse and stimulate the release of *oxytocin*. This hormone aids in uterine contraction and shrinkage (*involution*). However, if bleeding is not immediately controlled, the mother should quickly be taken for emergency care. Blood transfusions and medications designed to contract the womb may be lifesaving.

Fever occurring immediately before or after childbirth may be ominous. It may indicate infection in the bladder, particularly if a catheter has been used. Occasionally, fever may be due to unrelated conditions, such as influenza or respiratory illness. However, it could emanate from infection of the womb itself. Urgent treatment may help to prevent blood poisoning and serious complications. Cooling measures, such as the hot blanket pack, will open the pores. On the other hand, a dripping wet sheet for evaporative cooling may be beneficial, as described in Chapter 17.

Maintain careful **records** of the delivery, including the weight of the newborn, and the time and date of birth. Birth certificates may in most states be filed and signed by the individual who attended at the delivery, whether they are husband, friend, nurse-midwife, or physician. A drop of antibiotic ointment or *1% silver nitrate* solution should be put in each eye of the newborn baby, required by state law to prevent gonorrhea infection.

After a brief rest the mother should walk, go to the bathroom, and take a shower if she feels able. Early physical activity after the delivery of a baby will enable her to gain strength as soon as possible. Exercise also helps to prevent complication such as venous clots (*thrombosis*), that formerly were common with prolonged bed rest. Textbooks of maternity nursing and midwifery describe in more detail the equipment needed for a home delivery and the most efficient setup of the bedroom.

BREAST FEEDING

Many benefits transpire from choosing nature's method for infant feeding. Popularized by the **La Leche League** in a book called *The Womanly Art of Breast Feeding*, this routine is finding increasing acceptance among

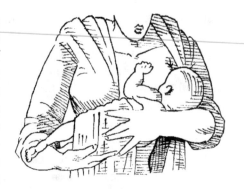

educated mothers and the thinking classes of society. Many scientific facts have amplified our understanding of the superiority for breast feeding over formula. In spite of infant formula propaganda, motivated by economic considerations, human milk and cow's milk are *very* dissimilar. Only the water and lactose (milk sugar) contents resemble each other. The protein is different, with amino acid ratios that are quite distinct. Much less *phenylalanine* (a factor in the PKU syndrome, called **phenylketonuria**) is present in breast milk. The principal protein of cow's milk is *beta-Lactoglobulin*, while those of human milk are *lysozyme* and *lactoferrin*. The *casein* in the two milks are quite different. Fat content, cholesterol levels, and vitamins are likewise dissimilar.

Although technological tinkering has modified cow's milk to make it less inappropriate for the human baby, hindsight proves the story of formula production to be a procession of errors. Additions and subtractions of Vitamin B_6, Vitamin E, protein, sodium, and other substances have occurred. Various additives are employed in baby formulas, such as emulsifiers, thickening agents, and antioxidants. Although these are known not to be essential for nutrition, they seem for the most part to be lacking in normal breast milk.

Breast feeding affords considerable protection against infection, particularly the diarrheal diseases. Lack of cleanliness and contamination of bottles and formulas has produced a high mortality in developing nations where bottle feeding was introduced. Human milk is, moreover, rich in a wide range of "host resistance factors." It contains **Immunoglobulin A**, which protects against a number of infections. **Lysozyme**, an enzyme particularly effective against viruses and bacteria, is rich in milk from the baby's own mother. Factors that regulate the micro-organisms in the intestinal tract, as well as white blood cells (called *macrophages*), are there to combat disease-producing germs in the intestinal tract. A breast-fed baby develops a flora primarily of *Lactobacilli*, much different and more harmless than the normal germs resident in the intestine of a bottle-fed baby.

Cow's milk protein is the most common food allergen in infancy. About 1% of bottle-fed babies are affected by **allergies** to cow's milk. These foreign cow (bovine) proteins enter the body through the relatively "open" young intestinal wall. In later childhood and adult life, these foreign proteins are normally broken down. However, in early infancy they are absorbed intact. Breast feeding and the avoidance of semisolid foods—particularly eggs, meat, and wheat—until four to six months of age is considered the best protection against food allergies in infancy.

Child spacing is relatively successful when the baby is breast fed full time. When the baby is totally nourished from his or her mother's breast the menstrual period ordinarily does not return until at least six months after birth. A hormone called **prolactin** is secreted by the pituitary gland. This inhibits the onset of mother's menstrual cycle. World estimates indicate that *"lactation amenorrhea"* has a larger statistical effect on large scale birth control than any other available contraceptive program! Breast feeding in Western cultures consists of a limited number of feedings, usually only in the daytime. Often the early use of solid foods will negate further this protective effect, explaining why many breast-feeding mothers become pregnant within the first year.

Breast feeding has great economic implications. In all communities this form of nourishment conserves resources. Not only concerning the ingredients used in cow's milk formulas, but in canning tins and bottles, energy is consumed in production. Formula manufacturers have turned largely to the third world to promote their wares today. Sales personnel, dressed in white uniforms (*milk nurses*), enter the hospitals to give free packages of their artificial nutrition to mothers as they are about to leave. When mothers finally realize that they can neither afford the formula, or that it is unavailable, their breasts have already dried up. Then, thousands of babies lose their lives.

One most important benefit of breast feeding, however, prevails in the emotional realm. An intense attachment between the mother and her infant was shown to be related to early contact. Called "bonding," this occurrence is most significant during the first twenty four hours of life. Maladjustment developing later in the child, may be traced to the absence of this "mother–baby interaction" within the first few days after birth. Closer contact is more likely to occur when the mother breast feeds. She holds the baby more, cuddles it more, and is less likely, according to a number of surveys, to abuse the child physically subsequently.

In summary, then, we realize that there are many rewards to a natural birth and a natural feeding program. Whether the baby is born in a hospital or at home, reared on a farm or in the city, fed at the mother's breast or cradled at her side, both parents and babies will find happiness, health, and security in these simple, natural, satisfying approaches to parenthood. This, Biblically speaking, is a fitting prelude to raising their children *"in the nurture and admonition of the Lord."* *Ephesians 6:4.*

CHAPTER TWENTY–THREE

OUTLINE

OF

BODY

STRUCTURES

AND

FUNCTIONS

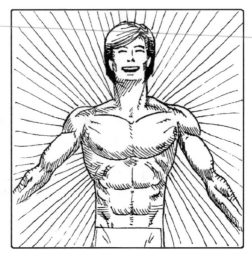

"Fearfully and wonderfully made" was the testimony of David the psalmist, after reverently studying the human structure. Here are some of the various medical terms that describe the science and study of the human organism: **anatomy**, the study of structure; **physiology**, the study of function; **pathology**, the study of disease process; and **genetics**, the study of heredity and inherited influences. An introduction to this knowledge is essential for any parent or health worker who desires to understand and treat various diseases.

It immediately becomes apparent, when we scrutinize the intricacies of the human form, that our bodies are highly organized. When God said, *"Let us make man in our image, after our likeness,"* the orderly principles of the universe were concentrated in designing the human structure. As the task reached completion, man was *inspired* with the breath of life. The genesis of our human race is embodied in this simple Biblical declaration, *"Man became a living soul,"* (Genesis 2:7). From the viewpoint of creation, then, we will ponder the organization, design, and purpose for our various body parts, which together make up a whole man.

The "hierarchy" of the body is usually illustrated by four general classifications: cells, tissues, organs, and systems. **Cells** are the "building blocks" of which our body is made. There are trillions of them, some functioning for a lifetime, while others are shed and replaced every few days. The concept of the *simple cell*, that satisfied foremost biologists a generation ago, is no longer adequate today. Cells are miniature factories with complicated enzyme systems and little organs (called *organelles*) that manufacture, store, package, defend, design, and even reproduce cells after their kind.

Central to the design of each cell is its **nucleus**. This specialized inner portion contains the hereditary material we call **DNA**. Containing the code for structural proteins, as well as its master plan for reproduction, this DNA (*deoxyribonucleic acid*) is wound in the shape of an alpha-helix, containing four basic groups of nitrogenous rings (*guanine, cytosine, adenine, thymidine*) linked through phosphate bonds to the five-carbon sugar, *deoxyribose*. This combination of genetic codes makes possible practically an infinite variety of human beings. Simple features of hair color, body shape, and native intelligence, as well as the more complex human features which give us our individuality, are determined by the DNA molecule.

Reproduction involves the genetic combining of one-half the DNA structure from the sperm and the other half from the ovum. In reproductive cell division, called **meiosis**, the number of chromosomes (usually, human cells contain 46) is reduced by half, allowing two germ cells to combine and make up a full chromosome complement for the fertilized egg (called the *zygote*). Cell division then occurs to create the beginnings of an embryo. This follows the usual plan of **mitosis**, where identical "daughter cells" are produced with each division. It has been estimated that the possibility for variations and differences in the hemoglobin molecule alone is of the order 1×10^{146} (this means the number one followed by 146 zeros). Thus, the probability of this marvelous event occurring by chance or evolving over long eons of time is virtually nil!

Other parts of the cell are equally marvelous. The **mitochondrion** is a tiny "organ" within the cytoplasm of the cell. It is in this structure that food processing takes place for the production of energy. For that reason, it is sometimes called a "power house." Oxygen is required to utilize various vitamins and minerals as cofactors in the conversion of food to energy. The **Golgi apparatus** is a packaging plant where enzymes, mucus, and other products of the cell's metabolism are stored in parcels, ready to be released. Closely related to protein synthesis in each cell is the **endoplasmic reticulum**, which provides a operational base for the **ribosomes**. These small packages of RNA (*ribonucleic acid*) constitute the location for our structural genes, that direct the manufacture of protein molecules. They, seemingly, are "turned" on or off like a thermostat in a type of *servo–control* mechanism. **Repressor genes** act in this manner to regulate the process of protein synthesis. It is estimated that there are approximately 175,000 genes derived from the DNA of each living human cell! This is represented along the more that eight million base pairs, comprising the numerous DNA molecules present in each cell's nucleus.

The second level of organization is our **tissues**. These are groups of similar cells, organized together for a common purpose. Examples of tissues are found in the following areas: **adipose tissue** is the storage form of fat, comprised largely of foamy appearing lipid–laden cells. **Epithelial** or covering tissues are the linings of the body. The skin is an example of **stratified squamous epithelium**, in which the cells are layered and flattened, with an external layer of horny (*cornified*) cells providing a waterproof covering for our body's surface. The skin contains sweat glands, hair follicles, and oil-secreting **sebaceous glands**, as well as the following: nerve fibers for perception of temperature, pressure, pain, and touch; blood vessels for proper nutrition; and an under layer of elastic supportive tissue, fatty insulation, and lymphatic vessels that give the skin its contour, warmth, color, and texture. The respiratory membrane is lined with a **pseudo–stratified columnar ciliated epithelium**. This long term refers to the tall column-shaped cells lining the respiratory tract, each of which contains tiny hair-like **cilia**. These move in a wave-like fashion, transporting a layer of mucus toward the throat, carrying dust particles and other debris that must be eliminated daily. The lungs, for example, completely cleanse themselves by this *mucociliary escalator* approximately every twenty minutes, bringing any inhaled particles up to the cough area, where they can be expectorated or swallowed. Muscular tissue, nervous tissue, and blood–forming (*hemopoietic*) tissue are other examples of this hierarchy of organization within the body.

The various tissues of the body become more highly organized to form **organs**. These may be extensive, as represented by the skin, or solid organs, such as our liver or brain. The stomach and intestines are examples of hollow organs.

Various organs, functioning together to accomplish a common purpose, constitute the **systems** of the body. There are nine of these systems, some of which will be illustrated in the sections that follow. The **nervous system** has to do with the electrical connections and general oversight or control of all body functions. The **circulatory system**, comprised of the heart and blood vessels, enables nutrients to reach the cells, oxygen to be delivered, then removes waste products, and maintains hormonal connections with all parts of the body. The **skeletal system** provides support, structure, a framework for contour, and protection to nearly all our body parts. In vertebrate animals, such as humans, the skeletal system comprises bones and muscles that move across the joints, keeping the spine erect, and creating the possibility of numerous facial expressions, as well as innumerable other actions. These muscles, of course, are controlled by nerve connections, to enable the body to move. Locomotion with functions as diverse as walking, running, sitting, eating, typing, or playing a musical instrument are coordinated with skills programmed for us by our muscular system.

The **respiratory system** includes our lungs, the voice box (*larynx*) and amazing air passages. This network governs the exchange of vital gases— oxygen and carbon dioxide. The **digestive system** includes our entire digestive tube and its related glands. However, we think of digestion especially involving the stomach, our liver, the intestines, gallbladder, and pancreas. Beginning in the mouth, digestive physiology embraces all our nutritive processes. The

urinary system provides for the excretion of liquid and soluble wastes, the conservation of sodium and various vital nutrients, and numerous diverse functions of our two kidneys. The paired ureters, a urinary bladder, and urethra act as final excretory organs. The **reproductive system** preserves our human race, with hormone functions controlled by the hypothalamus and other command centers in our brain. These are mediated through the **gonads**—the ovaries and the testes—giving rise after puberty to the distinguishing sexual characteristics of women and men. Finally, there is the **endocrine system**, that most fascinating collection of *ductless* glands, which send hormones through our bloodstream to influence organs at considerable distance from the parent gland. The growth and development in our body, feminine menstrual cycles, and our rate of metabolism are examples of marvelous functions controlled through this somewhat mysterious hierarchy of physiologic functions.

BONES AND JOINTS

Just as a tall building is supported by a foundation, and its framework of girders and steel supports, so the body uses its framework, called the skeleton. Our bones give structure and shape to the human form, as well as providing a protective case around certain vital organs, such as the brain and heart. Bones provide for the larger share of our calcium storage, and constantly sustain a blood-forming mission. Most outstanding, is our locomotion provided through the skeletal system, enabling us to stand erect and move.

There are two general divisions to the skeletal system. The **axial skeleton** consists of the *cranium* or skull bones, the spinal column, and our twelve sets of paired ribs. Several smaller accessory bones, such as the **hyoid** in the neck, and the tiny bones of the middle ear, the *malleus, incus,* and *stapes* (hammer, anvil, stirrup) are also associated with our axial skeleton. We have twenty eight distinct bones in our cranium. Four of these contain air–filled **sinuses**—two frontals, two maxillary, the ethmoid air spaces, and the sphenoid sinus. In the temporal bones on the side of the head are **mastoid** air cells arranged to allow equilibration in ambient air pressure with that in the middle ear. Abnormal blockage of the channels to any of these air-filled cavities can produce severe pain, or result in an infection—sinusitis or mastoiditis. The most vital parts of the body are encased in the skull. In addition, functions such as speaking, chewing, thinking, and breathing are intimately associated with this system.

The **vertebral column** provides for the erect posture of our human race. There are curvatures in the lumbar, thoracic (chest), and cervical (neck) portions. These form naturally during the normal developmental stresses as a baby sits, stands, and walks. There are seven cervical vertebrae. Interestingly enough, this number is equal in all mammals, the giraffe included! His neck bones are just longer. Twelve vertebrae delineate the chest or thoracic portion. To each of these is attached a pair of ribs, one on each side. So we have twelve pairs of ribs. Most of them connect to each other in the midline anteriorly through the *costal* *cartilage* and our breast bone, or **sternum**. There are two paired ribs on each side that are unattached in front; hence they are called *floating* ribs. Five **lumbar** vertebrae support the low back. They are the largest and heaviest, since they must bear the most weight. The **sacrum** is a set of five vertebrae fused together. The **coccyx**, our tailbone, connects its two or three bones at the lower end. Our sacrum forms the posterior wall of the pelvic girdle.

We look now at the second portion of the skeleton, the **appendicular** bones. These comprise the upper and lower extremities. The **shoulder girdle** includes the collar bone (*clavicle*), the shoulder blade (*scapula*), to which is attached the long bone of the upper arm (*humerus*). There are two bones in the forearm, the *radius* and the *ulna*. The latter hinges at the elbow, while the radius, the larger, pivots at the wrist. It is located on the thumb side. The wrist bones (*carpals*) are attached to five hand bones (*metacarpals*) in the palm of the hand. To these attach the bones of the fingers (*phalanges*).

The pelvic girdle is composed of a basin-like set of bones—the *ilium*, the *ischium*, and the *pubis*. These fuse to form the pelvic (or *innominate*) bone. United with the sacrum, they constitute the pelvic girdle. The *femur*, the longest bone in our body, is attached to the hip via a ball-and-socket joint. This bone articulates at the knee with the *tibia*, the largest bone of the lower leg. The kneecap (*patella*) increases the mechanical force of our leg straightening muscles. The *fibula*, a small accessory leg bone, aids ankle stability and provides the attachment of muscles traversing the lateral side of our lower leg. Ankle bones are called *tarsals*. The bones of the feet are the *metatarsals*, and our toes are called *phalanges*. There are an equal number of phalanges, fourteen, in both the hands and the feet.

The **articulations** or joints of our body enable these bones to move against each other. Some of the joints, such as our hip and shoulder, are *ball-and-socket* type. Others, like the elbow, are *hinged* joints. In the fingers we have *saddle* joints, in the wrist *gliding* joints, while in the axial skeleton the bones are relatively fused. The skull bones join together by fibrous tissues and are comparatively rigid; whereas in the spine the cartilaginous joints allow considerable motion. In fact, our vital intervertebral discs are thick plates of fibrous cartilage. They function as shock absorbers to enable considerable running, jumping, and other forms of gymnastic "horse-play" without the danger of trauma.

The structure of any joint is closely related to its function. Most of these movable joints are bound together by fibrous connective tissue. This allows considerable elasticity, while providing for conservation of space and energy. Each joint surface is lined by cartilage, which acts as a cushion to absorb pressure. The movable joints are lubricated through a lining of **synovial membrane** and its enclosed fluid (*synovial fluid*). This fluid contains a large amount of protein, to keep the joint moving smoothly without friction. Disturbances in this synovial fluid, the joint lining, or the cartilage can give rise to various forms of arthritis.

There are several interesting differences between men and women in the structure of their skeleton. A male skeleton is usually larger, with heavier bones to accommodate his increased strength. Primary differences are found in the pelvic girdle. The female **pelvis** (a word meaning *basin*) is shaped to allow the cradling of a developing child and its passage through the birth journey. The male pelvis is more funnel-shaped with a narrowed opening. These contrasts develop during puberty.

The ratio of our head circumference to body height differs considerably with aging and maturity, being 1:4 in a baby and 1:8 in an adult. A cross–section of a child's thorax (chest) is round, while in an adult it is oblong. Comparisons among other vertebrates can make the study of anatomy fascinating, where function is always reflected in the design.

The Scripture records, *"God made man upright,"* and God's design is best obtained when our posture is erect. The positions chosen for lifting, sitting, and standing should be selected with regard to the necessities of our system. A body in motion is less likely to become stiff and arthritic. The benefits of exercise to bone structure and joint flexibility are incalculable.

THE MUSCLES

Lending graceful form to the body contours, muscles are primarily for movement. When you are active, your muscles use more oxygen than any other part of the body. They store the carbohydrate **glycogen**, a type of starch for energy. The contraction of muscles is initiated by the nervous system. Coming from the brain, long nerve fibers unite (at the *synapse*) in the spinal cord with nerve cells connected to the muscles. Some muscles, such as in the eye, have such precise control that one nerve fiber innervates each muscle fiber. Other large muscles in the back have hundreds of muscle fibers controlled through one nerve. There are actually three basic types of muscle tissue.

Cardiac muscle, as you might expect, is found in the heart. These specialized muscles have microscopic filaments of contractile proteins (called *actin* and *myosin*), somewhat similar to those found in our skeletal muscles. Consequently, they appear *striated* viewed under a microscope. However, the muscle cells of the heart are much more interconnected than the skeletal muscles. The fibers connect with one another through a branching network, enabling the heart to contract as a whole. Moreover, the cardiac muscle is under a non-voluntary **autonomic** control. Fortunate for us, it does not require a decision of the will to initiate each heartbeat.

Smooth muscle fibers are found in our gastrointestinal and genitourinary tracts, the walls of each blood vessel, and the air tubes (*bronchi*) leading to the lungs. These muscles are likewise controlled through the autonomic nervous system. Contraction is either speeded up or slowed down by a modifying action of these nerves. Stress influences the autonomic nerves in profound ways.

However, they are separated from the conscious (volitional) control of our central nervous system.

Third, we come to the **skeletal muscles**, long fibers of *striated* muscle tissue, all under voluntary control. These are the muscles that bulge when we exercise, and with which we move our limbs. All skeletal muscles, nevertheless, work in cooperation. When a muscle, such as the *biceps* in our upper arm contracts, other opposing muscles must relax, to permit a smooth coordinated movement. Along with this action, other muscles join in and assist, giving us the terms "prime mover," "antagonist," and "synergist"—names for the synchronized muscle groups described above.

Looking closer at muscle contractions, we see that each fiber contracts according to an **"all or none" law**. This means that either the fiber is contracted or it is relaxed. Additional strength is obtained by the phenomenon of "recruitment." Additional available muscle fibers unite to give the desired action added force. If contraction occurs repeatedly and the glucose supply is exhausted, *fatigue* sets in. Overstimulation of the muscle produces a sustained tonic contraction, called **tetany**. It is usually quite painful. A muscle *cramp* illustrates simply this phenomenon.

Motions of the major skeletal muscles are described under six general headings: **Abduction** involves a motion away from the body, as when your arm is raised from the side. **Flexion** is a forward motion of the arm, or a drawing upward at the elbow or knee. **Extension** is the opposite of flexion, where the angles of the extremity open completely. **Adduction** is the opposite of abduction; the limb is moved *toward* the body. Bringing the arm down to the side, is one example. The forearm **pronates** when the hand is turned inward, palm down. The opposite of this motion is called **supination**. Finally, we have **circumduction**, in which the ball-and-socket joints of the shoulder and hip rotate in a circular motion. These joints, of course, can circle either clockwise or counterclockwise. These six actions constitute the major directions of motion that our skeletal muscles make. The accompanying table lists the major muscles of our extremities and the basic functions of each.

Muscles that are not often used lose their strength. Then, progressive **atrophy** results. Complete absence of muscle function, either from nerve damage or disuse, is called **paralysis**. This may occur from injury to the central nervous system, as in a stroke, or from traumatic injury.

Muscle strength may be acquired through two types of exercise. **Isometric** exercise involves an increase of tension in the muscle without actual change in length. An example of this would be the mutual clasping of your hands, then pulling back on each arm, without any actual movement taking place. **Isotonic** exercise, on the other hand, is motion with constant tension. This occurs when a weight is lifted. Isotonic movements tend more to promote endurance than simply to develop muscle bulk. Most exercises, regardless, combine the two forms. Swimming, running, walking, and cycling, for example, produce our greatest build-up of strength, flexibility, and endurance.

Large muscles in our back and neck serve primarily the function of **posture**. These are designed to possess a resting *tone* that maintains our body position without the necessity of continual thought. Proper standing posture is attained when your shoulders are back, the head erect, your belly, buttocks, and chin tucked in, and your knees very slightly flexed. A straight rod should line up with the tip of the ear, mid-point of your shoulder, the hip bone, the back of your knee, and the ankle bone. Walk with your arms swinging side to side; keep the shoulders and spine erect, and hold your head up. Proper posture contributes greatly to a free respiration, a healthy disposition, and an inner self-confidence, and poise. Correct sitting and standing posture will help promote all these attitudes. This attribute of nobility is something that corsets, girdles, braces, or body casts could never provide.

THE NERVOUS SYSTEM

Just as every army needs a general and every country a president, so the body has built-in methods of leadership and control. The "headquarters" for all body functions reside in the **central nervous system**. A brief overview of the nervous system shows it to consist of the brain, the spinal cord, and the peripheral nerves. The **autonomic** nervous system is involved in the regulation of blood flow, hormone production, responses to stress, and other functions not under voluntary control. Recently, a hormone-producing (*endocrine*) branch of the nervous system has been discovered. This, likewise, has profound regulatory effects on the body as a whole.

Transmitting nerve fibers, called **axons**, carry messages from the brain to every part of the body. Sometimes a sequential connection of *neurons* (nerve cells), with their transmitting axons, is required to reach a distant organ. The junction or connection between neurons is called a **synapse**. Chemical trans-mitters, such as *acetylcholine*, are used to transmit the electrical impulse, conducted first through the nerve fiber, then across the synapse to stimulate the second arm of the "final nerve pathway." Nerves bringing impulses to the brain are called **afferent nerves**. Those carrying impulses away from the brain to distant parts of the body are called **efferent nerves**. A simple illustration of how this works is seen in the *reflex arc*.

The **reflexes** of the body involve both the reception and the reaction of the spinal cord to sensory signals. This may be a pin prick, a tap on a muscle tendon, a burning sensation, or a loud noise. In the spinal cord and brain stem these impulses are integrated and connected with outgoing nerves that react to preserve the body from harm. An example of this occurs when you step on a tack. Immediately there is a *withdrawal response* in the affected foot and leg, while the other one extends to support the body and prevent a fall. The withdrawal of your hand from a hot stove, eyes blinking in response to loud noise, and the general startle response are examples of these protective reflexes.

331

The second type of reflex occurs when a tendon is stretched. Perhaps you remember your doctor taping on the patellar tendon, just below the kneecap. Your knee jerks in response to the sudden stretching of the tendon. These reflexes can either be accentuated or diminished, depending on the modifying nerve impulses that affect the spinal cord. For an example, a stoical individual may be able to endure much more pain without flinching than one who is sensitive or scared. Under certain conditions an athlete can perform feats of near super-human strength which in other circumstances would be virtually impossible.

The Spinal Cord

The **spinal cord** extends from the brain stem down to the lower level of the lumbar spine. Nerve filaments, appearing like a horse's tail (*cauda equina*), extend downward to exit through their individual openings. Discrete tracts of nerve bundles connect the brain to our extremities, supplying motor control and coordination. In turn, there are numerous ascending fibers bringing sensory impulses for the perception of touch, pain, temperature, and location. Position sensitivity allows for the integration of smooth motion, in conjunction with the cerebellum. Accidentally disrupting the spinal cord will produce paralysis and anesthesia below the level of the severed nerve roots. A pinched nerve occasionally develops when there is protrusion of the central portion (*nucleus pulposus*) of an intervertebral disc.

Gradual degeneration of the spinal cord occurs in such diseases as **multiple sclerosis** and **amyotrophic lateral sclerosis** (sometimes called Lou Gehrig's disease). In both of these conditions the nerve fibers lose their insulation. With demyelinization, a short circuiting of the electrical current results, producing patchy loss of muscular (motor) function, sensation, or both. In multiple sclerosis the condition is more progressive, diffuse, widespread, and subject to periodic remissions. The cranial nerves and sensory organs may similarly be affected.

The Brain

Headquarters for our body control system resides in an organ called the **brain**. Protectively housed within the skull bone, this three pounds of gelatin-like, gray substance operates as a powerful miniaturized computer. It is here that the **mind** dwells, our **personality** is integrated, **memory** storage takes place, and smooth control of all muscular activity begins. Humming a tune, playing the violin or piano, ice skating, reading *Braille* with the finger tips, learning a foreign language, the meticulous skill of a surgeon, and a warm handclasp by a loving friend— all these experiences, emotions, and sensations find their origin here. Let us examine the brain's various parts that make up the whole.

Cerebrum

The highest level of organization of the human brain is found in the **cerebrum**. The **cortex** (from a word meaning *bark*, as of a tree) consists of at least 15 million individual nerve cells! Many interconnections between these nerves (*synaptic junctions*) allow for the storage of an unlimited amount of information. Most of our increase of brain size occurs here, during the first year of life, making that period critical for the development of intelligence, personality, and a happy, productive existence. The **frontal** cortex is thought to be the "seat of the soul." It is here that the willpower, reasoning processes, and judgment find their home. Damage to the frontal lobes may occur with a severe head injury, surgically as in a *lobotomy*, or through the influence of mind-affecting drugs, such as alcohol and tranquilizers. Our sense of right and wrong, the desire to please others, and our ability to love—all reside within the frontal lobes. Just behind this area is the "motor strip," so called because the fibers that control all the muscles in the body are arranged here. An *association area* just adjacent to this set of "pyramidal neurons" provides for the integration of smooth muscular function, the ability to memorize a musical composition, and the proficiency to reproduce accurately one's signature for a lifetime.

The **parietal lobes**, just behind the frontal cortex and above the ears on each side, are areas primarily devoted to sensation. An *association area* nearby allows one to remember and accurately distinguish the feel of a nickel and a dime, the positions of the keyboard notes on the piano, and remember (hopefully) what it was like to touch the hot stove. In the **occipital cortex** of the brain is located our visual area. The imprint of visual images may be stored for a lifetime, although fortunately for us, some memories are soon forgotten. Our sense of awe when looking at a beautiful sunset, the happiness expressed as children play, and the pictures of childhood that bring back memories— all are integrated as the visual impulses traverse first our eyes, then lodge in the memory bank of the occiput. A blow to this area causes one to "see stars." Developing a cancerous tumor that destroys this part of the brain causes a characteristic type of blindness.

The **temporal lobes** contain the auditory receptors. One of the earliest experiments in brain function involved the electrical stimulation of this part of the brain. The patient, awake at the time, reported hearing a symphony which could be started or stopped as though one would remove the needle from a phonograph disc. This occurred as the electrical connections were initiated and withdrawn. Our ability to memorize a composition, sing a song, give a speech, and communicate in several languages is a tribute to the amazing engineering design of the temporal lobes.

333

Deep inside the cortex of the cerebrum, lies a pair of **basal ganglia**. These areas integrate the smooth flowing gait and enable fine finger motions. One type of *Parkinson's disease* stems from the degeneration of these areas. It is characterized by a shuffling gait and pill-rolling tremor, along with rigidity of the muscles.

The **thalami** are located more central to the midbrain. They function as relay stations. Sensory impulses are distributed to the brain from receptors in the skin, through ascending nerves of the spinal cord. Stimulation of the thalami, however, produces a *generalized* sense of discomfort. The localization of pain is accomplished within the parietal area of the brain.

Just below the thalamus on each side is a specialized part of nerve tissue called the **hypothalamus**. It is this area that secretes the *releasing factors* for many pituitary hormones. The headquarters for appetite and its control through the *satiety center* are located here. Some of its hormonal interactions will be presented as we study the pituitary glands and endocrine system.

The **reticular formation** in the brain stem regulates our level of arousal and alertness. Nicotine and caffeine affect this influential center, as well as impacting the hypothalamus.

The **cranial nerves** govern many functions of the face, including its sense organs, the muscles of expression, and the sensation of taste. These twelve paired nerves are as follows:

I.   Olfactory nerve — Sensation of smell.
II.   Optic nerve — Vision.
III.   Oculomotor nerve — Eye muscles.
IV.   Trochlear nerve — Eye muscles.
V.   Trigeminal nerve — Sensation to the face and taste of the
            anterior two thirds of the tongue.
VI.   Abducens nerve — Eye muscle.
VII.   Facial nerve — Muscles of facial expression and mastication.
VIII.   Auditory nerve — Sense of hearing and balance.
IX.   Glossopharyngeal nerve — Swallowing mechanism, taste of
            the posterior one third of the tongue.
X.   Vagus nerve — Swallowing reflex and parasympathetic fibers
            to the lungs, heart, stomach, intestines,
            gallbladder, and pancreas.
XI.   Spinal accessory nerve — Muscles to shrug the shoulders and
            move the neck.
XII.   Hypoglossal nerve — Movement of tongue.

These nerves may be affected by infections such as bulbar *polio* or degenerative conditions such as *multiple sclerosis*.

Cerebellum

Located at the base of the cerebrum in the back of the head is a specialized portion of nerve tissue called the **cerebellum**. Functioning like a miniaturized analog computer, it monitors the state of muscle contraction and the positions of all our muscles simultaneously. These bits of information are integrated into a pattern that smoothly controls the movement of muscles. The ability to feed oneself, play an accordion, type a letter, or walk a tight rope are all due to the special services provided by the cerebellum. Disease in this area often manifests itself in a staggering gait, an inability to point and accurately touch an object, with total loss of coordination when the eyes are closed.

The Autonomic Nervous System

The "automatic" (in the sense of being unavailable to *volitional* control) or **autonomic nerves** function as modifiers of organ function. There are two divisions to this system, the **sympathetic** and the **parasympathetic**. Sympathetic nerves exit from spinal roots in the thoracic and lumbar portions of the spinal cord to be distributed into all parts of the body. The adrenal medulla is affected, its stimulation producing the secretion of *adrenaline*. Blood pressure rises with the contraction of smooth muscle fibers in the blood vessels, all attributed to a "second cousin" of adrenaline, *noradrenaline*. Stimulation of the sympathetic nerves inhibits peristalsis in the intestinal tract, decreases blood flow to the stomach and its acid production, and inhibits the secretion of digestive enzymes. Dilation of the bronchial tubes leading to the lungs occurs when the sympathetic nerves are stimulated. The pupils dilate, the heart rate increases, and sweating occurs. All of these responses are typical of the "fight or flight" mechanism that we see manifested during periods of stress. A frightening "growl" heard while walking in the woods, the first tense ride in a jet plane, stage fright, or pressure in the operating room when one is performing unfamiliar surgery— all involve the secretion of this fascinating stress hormone, adrenaline.

The **parasympathetic** nerves exit through the sacral plexus, as well as via the cranial nerves. The voiding reflex of the urinary bladder, healthful digestion after a good meal, and clear vision through constricted pupils are all mediated by the parasympathetic nerves. The heart rate is slowed, salivation enhanced, and blood flow to the major internal organs increased through the media of parasympathetic nerves. In contrast to the chemistry of the sympathetic nerves whose transmitter is primarily noradrenaline, the parasympathetic nerves use the transmitter *acetyl choline*. This balance between the "gas pedal" and the "brake" in our body infrastructure is profoundly influenced by *nicotine*, which adversely stimulates both systems simultaneously. Imagine driving a car that way. No wonder the body is affected and life span shortened by this "wear and tear" phenomenon of tobacco addiction.

NEUROENDOCRINE CONNECTIONS

Within the last decade a fascinating new family of body chemicals has been discovered in the brain. The **endorphins**, located in certain portions of the midbrain have been related to many powers, including our threshold for pain and the stability of the emotions. Every year another brain peptide gets discovered, stimulating fascinating research in stress control, mental illness, and the relief of pain. Corresponding hormones have been found in the stomach and other abdominal organs, revealing to scientists the Creator's wisdom and the complexity of body design. Surely, we are *"fearfully and wonderfully made."*

Moreover, all of these integrated functions help produce a unique person with characteristics that no other human being possesses. This is partly what makes us so precious, not only to our friends and closest companions, but in the sight of God, our Creator.

The ability of a human mind to restore and retrieve information is just amazing. Some philosophers maintain that, because of this, the memory should be carefully guarded, putting nothing into it that we would not choose to retain. To carry out this aim, we really should **"guard the avenues of the soul,"** and avoid reading, seeing, or hearing things that would suggest impure thoughts. You might have to turn away from a thousand topics which invite attention in order to keep your God–given *computer* from being filled with "garbage" which only confuses, never edifies. To develop in children and youth the type of mind that can give our world what it needs—Josephs, Esthers, Daniels, Carvers, Whites, and Lincolns—will require forethought and stern self–discipline. The television set may have to be discarded, so that study becomes more relevant. Furthermore, the labor of your hands should be such that it will help build character. Believe me, it is possible. Growing numbers of Christian youth are here to testify.

Our character does not come by accident. It develops by careful attention to the laws of the mind—laws which our Creator has written on every nerve fiber and brain cell, and which He sustains and upholds continually. *"In Him we live, and move, and have our being,"* (Acts 17:28).

THE ENDOCRINE SYSTEM

Most people at some time in their lives have observed midgets, giants, and excessively obese people. Although we know that some instances are genetic, other cases are certainly acquired. Significant numbers of people are affected by disease of their endocrine organs. The word **endocrine** refers to *ductless glands*, which discharge their secretions directly into the blood. This distinguishes them from other glands (called *exocrine*), which have channels (ducts) to discharge their secretions at a body surface location. For example, consider the sweat glands and the breasts.

The purpose for our endocrine glands is similar to that of the nervous system, namely communication and control. Through the **hormones** secreted by these glands our body maintains contact with many distant organs. Several of these hormones will be described as we consider the individual glands and their functions.

Pituitary

The **pituitary gland** is located at the base of the brain, just beneath the hypothalamus. It is encased in a bony cradle called the Turkish saddle (*sella turcica*). The two parts of the pituitary gland exhibit different functions: the anterior pituitary (*adenohypophysis*) secretes several hormones via a feedback mechanism which functions like your household thermostat. **ACTH** (*adreno-corticotropic hormone*) controls the secretion of cortisone from the adrenal gland. This increases in certain conditions such as accidents, surgery, burns, and major stress. Over secretion of ACTH will cause adrenal gland enlargement and a clinical picture called**Cushing's syndrome**. In this case, there is a moon-faced appearance, with obesity of the trunk and relatively thin extremities, violet-hued striae on the abdomen, and general loss of mineral from the bones. Glucose intolerance resembles that of diabetes. Hypertension often develops. Along with the characteristic appearance come personality changes.

Deficiency of ACTH will lead to atrophy of the adrenal cortex and the onset of **Addison's disease**. In this syndrome there is low blood pressure, increased pigmentation of the body, weakness, and profound loss of salt. Eventually, the patient will collapse if the condition is not recognized and treated.

Several pituitary hormones stimulate the sex organs. **FSH** (*follicle stimulating hormone*) helps in the monthly development of an *ovum* by the ovary. It also plays a role in men in stimulating sperm production.   **LH** (*luteinizing hormone*) aids in the ripening of the ovum prior to ovulation. It also promotes the production of *progesterone* by the ovary, just as FSH stimulates estrogen secretion. These two female hormones are potent in producing the impressive feminine changes of puberty. Another hormone, **prolactin**, helps to stimulate milk production and aids during pregnancy in the development of the breast for this purpose. In fact, all of these three hormones influence the breast, with resulting growth in size and proliferation of milk glands and ducts to prepare a pregnant mother to nurse her baby.

In the posterior portion of the pituitary (*neurohypophysis*) two hormones are secreted. **Oxytocin** is actually produced in the hypothalamus. It travels down tiny tubules to the pituitary where it is stored. Oxytocin is the hormone that stimulates the onset of labor and regular uterine contractions associated with the delivery of a baby. It also causes the "let down" reflex in a nursing mother, to permit the expression of milk that has been formed. The other hormone, **ADH** (*antidiuretic hormone*), is also produced in the hypothalamus. Its action, however, is primarily on the kidneys, where it helps our body retain water to aid in the conservation of body fluids. This hormone (ADH) is closely related to our thirst mechanism. It definitely tends, as do other endocrine functions, to help preserve our lives.

Pineal Gland

The **pineal gland** is located deep within the brain substance. Until recently, its function was a mystery. A hormone called **melatonin** has been found to influence the *estrus* cycle in animals and the human menstrual cycle, as well as other body rhythms. It also plays a role in the pigmentary changes that occur in our bodies. A prime stimulus to melatonin production is the presence of light transmitted through the eyes. Many mysteries have yet to be uncovered in regard to body rhythms. However, one thing is clear—regularity of eating, sleeping, and working are important for normal utilization of these hormones.

Exciting research into the **Seasonal Affective Disorder** (SAD) reveals the vital role that sunlight plays in our hormones, our biologic rhythms, and our emotional stability. In climates where the long winters and northern latitudes create shorter days, some without much sun at all, eating disorders and depression are much more common. During the darkest months this syndrome may affect up to 10% of the population! Exposure to bright light, even for only a few minutes a day, helps to shut down the melatonin hormone production, relieving depression and the so-called "winter blues."

Thyroid

The **thyroid gland** is located just below the "Adam's apple," in the front of the neck. It regulates the *metabolic rates* of the body—that is, the speed at which food substances are burned to produce energy. Over-activity of the thyroid gland produces a rapid heart rate, weight loss, a fine perspiration, tremor, and nervousness. In one type, called **Grave's disease**, serious problems with the eyes may develop. The opposite side of the hormone "coin" is **hypothyroidism**, a disease where the production of *thyroxine* (called T_4) is deficient. In this condition characteristic lassitude, fatigue, dullness, and apathy are seen. The body becomes colder, the digestive tract slows down, and constipation develops. Edema accumulates in the skin (*myxedema*). Along with personality change, an almost "bovine placidity," and heart failure may occur from thyroid hormone deficiency.

Actually, the production of thyroid hormone is regulated by the anterior pituitary gland (*adenohypophysis*). **TSH**, the **thyroid stimulating hormone**, is produced there. Like the ACTH mentioned above, TSH serves a regulatory purpose to maintain the body in metabolic balance (called *homeostasis*). Supplemental forms of these hormones are available. Accurate laboratory blood tests can determine their body serum levels. The examinations are needed to make the proper diagnosis.

Parathyroid

Four small glands are found in the neck behind the thyroid, two on each side. These **parathyroid glands** help to regulate the calcium levels in our blood. Their hormone, called *parathormone* (short for parathyroid hormone), is able to draw calcium from the bones, as well as increase its absorption in the gastrointestinal tract. When the calcium level of our blood drops too low, **tetany** develops. This occasionally occurs as a serious complication following thyroid surgery.

Adrenal Glands

Two small organs, each perched like a three-cornered hat on top of a kidney, are called the **adrenal glands**. These have two main divisions: the outer part is called the **cortex**, the inner substance the **medulla**. The medulla is supplied with sympathetic nerves, stimulation of which evokes the *"fight or flight"* response discussed above. The production of either **epinephrine** (*adrenaline*) or **norepinephrine** speeds up the pulse, raises the blood pressure, dilates the pupils, and produces sweating. This is the hormone, that in an emergency, enables a ninety pound mother to lift an automobile off the ground, when it rolls over on her three year old. It also helps hikers to run away from bears, whether real or imaginary.

The adrenal cortex is much more complex, producing three distinct types of hormones. The stimulation of **ACTH** from the pituitary gland enhances the adrenal's production of **cortisone**. This hormone, widely known for its relief of arthritic pains, is considered a normal stress hormone. It stabilizes the blood pressure, increases our resistance to infection, and aids in growth and maturation. Excessive function of the adrenal cortex results in the *Cushing's syndrome*, mentioned above.

Second, the adrenal cortex secretes a hormone called **aldosterone**. In contrast to cortisone (a *glucocorticoid*), this hormone functions to safeguard minerals (thus termed a *mineralocorticoid*). It primarily conserves sodium, which is retained as urine flows through the kidney. With retention of sodium comes fluid retention (*edema*). Occasionally an adrenal-cortical tumor will develop, that secretes excessive amounts of this hormone. Aldosterone produces not only fluid retention, but high blood pressure as well.

For its size, the adrenal receives the richest supply of blood of all the organs. It is essential for having vigorous health. In fact, our survival is unlikely without at least one functioning adrenal gland.

Pancreatic Islets

Microscopic sized islands of specialized tissue in the pancreas were discovered by Langerhans, while a medical student in Vienna over a century ago. These specialized glands, called **Islets of Langerhans**, contain unique cells which secrete two hormones. The *alpha cells* produce a secretion called **glucagon**, which raises the blood sugar, by mobilizing it from liver **glycogen** (animal starch). The *beta cells* are producers of **insulin**. This fascinating hormone was isolated by Doctors Banting and Best in Montreal during the early 1920's. The fortunate discovery of insulin has lengthened the lives and productivity of millions of diabetics, who otherwise would have died early, or at best been unable to have families.

Insulin is a protein-like hormone (actually a chain of *amino acids*) whose primary function is the constant regulation of blood sugar. When a person eats a meal containing carbohydrates the elevation of blood sugar (or *glucose*) is modified by the influence of insulin. This helps all sugars to pass from the blood into our tissues. It "knocks" on the cell membrane for entrance, expecting its welcome admission into our cells. There it is processed, and converted to energy or stored as fat. Insulin, furthermore, aids in producing glycogen for the liver, and it affects the metabolic reconversion of fats and proteins into available energy.

Excessive amounts of circulating insulin produce **hypoglycemia**. This is periodically seen in the body's reaction to prolonged stress, especially when combined with a diet high in sugar and/or caffeine. Occasionally, through hereditary or viral causes the pancreas loses its ability to produce insulin. This gives rise to elevated blood sugar levels and the clinical syndrome called **diabetes mellitus**. Recent evidence points to the early use of cows milk in babies for this pancreatic failure, at least in the juvenile forms of diabetes. Excessive amounts of glucose spill over into the urine, and feelings of lassitude, excessive hunger, increased thirst, frequent urination, and cloudiness of vision ensue. The administration of insulin corrects these problems, bringing normality to the body's metabolism again.

The Gonads

The reproductive organs likewise serve an endocrine function. These glands, both male and female types, secrete hormones that profoundly influence sexual maturation during puberty. The **testes** (male) secrete a hormone called *testosterone*. This is the amazing steroid chemical which leads to voice change, muscular development, and sexual maturation in earliteen boys. It is additionally necessary for the formation of **spermatozoa**, permitting reproduction.

Three female sex hormones are known. **Estriol, estrone**, and **estradiol** are *estrogens*, feminizing substances produced at puberty, again during pregnancy, and throughout the childbearing years. These hormones contribute to adolescent female maturation, to normal breast development, and a woman's cyclic menstrual periods. The ovaries also secrete *progesterone*, a hormone which also contributes to a normal monthly cycle during the years of menstruation. These biologic rhythms will be further explained as we consider the reproductive cycle (page 353).

DIGESTIVE SYSTEM

Proper assimilation and processing of our food is essential to life. Since all of us "are what we eat," the proper understanding of nutrition and the physiology of digestion is basic to the maintenance of excellent health. This process begins in the mouth.

The **teeth** are most important organs of digestion. Thorough mastication of our food mingles it with enzyme-rich saliva, aiding the initial digestion of starches. The skillful care of our teeth and simple approaches to prevent dental decay are discussed in Chapter 16.

The **salivary glands** are additionally located in the head. Two, called the *parotid glands*, lie just in front of our ears at the approximate angle of the jaw. These are the glands that enlarge frequently when a person has mumps. Their secretions, thin and watery, contain a rich enzyme **ptyalin** (*salivary amylase*), which begins to digest complex carbohydrates. The mucoid secretions of the submandibular and sublingual salivary glands are similarly important in the proper lubrication of well-chewed food. In addition to grinding our breakfast and mingling it with saliva, **mastication** initiates, through vagus nerve pathways, secretion of the gastric enzyme *pepsin*, with its teammate, *hydrochloric acid*.

The **esophagus** is a ten-inch long tube that conducts the food from our swallowing area down to the stomach. It lies behind the windpipe (trachea) in the upper portion of the chest and behind the heart, piercing the diaphragm to enter the stomach. There is an area of increased pressure, called the *lower esophageal sphincter*, which normally prevents the regurgitation of food into the esophagus. A **hiatus hernia** sometimes develops in the diaphragm, permitting a portion of the stomach to crowd into the chest. This leads to regurgitation and the inflammatory symptoms of heartburn.

The **stomach** is an expandable pouch, capable of accommodating about 2-3 quarts of liquid or solid food, when it is stretched to maximum capacity. Of course, with adaptation, the capacity of the stomach may be increased. For example, the stomach, given a steady diet of heavy foods, changes form into a "J" shape. This phenomenon is taken advantage of by sword swallowers. In the membrane lining the inner surface of our stomach there are about 62,500 gastric glands per square inch! These mostly secrete **mucus**, providing a protective, coating effect. There are also specialized cells that produce **pepsinogen** (called *chief cells)* and **hydrochloric acid** (secreted by the *parietal cells*). The precursor enzyme *pepsinogen* is the forerunner of our best protein-splitting enzyme, **pepsin**, to which it is activated in the presence of acid. Thus, pepsin plays a significant role in the breakdown of protein into simple *peptides*. A small amount of the fat-splitting enzyme, *lipase* is also present. In the stomach our food is thoroughly mixed by a **peristaltic** churning action, while considerable absorption of water takes place.

The **small intestine** consists of three parts: the **duodenum**, about twelve inches long; the **jejunum**, five to eight feet long; and the **ileum**, sixteen to twenty feet long. The inner lining of our small intestine is much folded, giving it an enormous surface area (called *valvulae conniventes*). The tip of each cell ends in many *microvilli*, which constitute a so-called "brush border." These keep busy producing enzymes to enable our efficient enzymatic digestion to take place just before absorption. These enzymes digest the *peptides* into *amino acids*, and break up many of the fat molecules into *monoglycerides* and *diglycerides* as well as *fatty acids*, so they all can be quickly absorbed. Long-chain complex fatty acids usually enter our lymph system through channels called *lacteals*. Lymph appears as a milky fluid, migrating slowly up into the chest (*thorax*), where it is enters the circulation to mingle with our blood. This lymphatic vascular system enables the breakdown products of absorbed fat to bypass our liver for several minutes, and thereby be distributed to other tissues, notably the *adipose* (fat) cells. End products of carbohydrate and protein digestion are absorbed directly into the bloodstream, transported by the portal veins to our liver. Minerals and vitamins, such as **iron** and $\mathbf{B}_{12}$ are absorbed in the small intestine, together with most of the water we consume.

The **large intestine**, or **colon**, consists of the following six segments: *cecum, ascending, transverse, descending, sigmoid,* and *rectum.* The **appendix** attaches to the cecum. It contains a specialized type of lymphoid tissue, as does the small intestinal lining (*Peyer's patches*). In our colon the final absorption of water, and formation of the stool (waste products) takes place. **Constipation** occurs when the intake of dietary fiber, your physical exercise, inadequate fluid intake, or other habit patterns are out of balance, preventing regular perstalsis and evacuation. **Hemorrhoids**, dilated veins in the rectal area, then may develop, with irritation, pain, or bleeding.

The **pancreas** is an accessory organ to digestion, cradled in a curve of the duodenum, and lying behind the stomach. It secretes into the second portion of the duodenum juices rich in fat-splitting enzymes (*lipase*), protein-digesting enzymes (*trypsin* and *chymotrypsin*), and a starch splitter (pancreatic *amylase*). Further digestion of carbohydrate occurs in the intestine with the disaccharide-splitting enzymes (*sucrose, lactose,* and *maltose*), as described in Chapter 16.

Bile is produced by the liver and stored in the **gall bladder**. Under the influence of a stimulating hormone (*cholecystokinin-pancreozymin*), the same substance which stimulates pancreatic secretions, the bile releases. By a strong gallbladder contraction bile squirts through the common bile duct into the duodenum. Bile aids in fat emulsification, making the fat droplet particles small enough to permit entrance into our lymphatic system. Occasional stones can form in the gallbladder, producing chronic irritation (*cholecystitis*). When gall stones block the bile duct, jaundice develops, with the very severe pain of a gallbladder attack.

The largest "gland" of our body is the **liver**, filling the upper right section of the abdominal cavity and extending across to the left. One of its important functions is to secrete bile. This juice drains out of the liver through the hepatic duct and is stored in the gallbladder, as mentioned above. After a big dinner, glucose, amino acids, and some of the breakdown products of fat are absorbed into the blood, passing through the portal veins to our liver. The hepatic cells of the liver help maintain the quantity of sugar in our blood at a normal level, and also make various blood proteins. This organ produces, for example, the blood clotting factors, so important in coagulation. Detoxification of various drugs and other harmful substances is carried on in the liver. Disease of the liver can produce serious consequences. **Hepatitis** is a relatively common infection caused by one of several viruses. Cancer may develop in the liver, either secondary to malignancies elsewhere in the body (called *metastasis*), or as a primary tumor, related to chemical toxins. Contamination of water with carbon tetrachloride and other poisons, as well as molds which produce *aflatoxin* have been associated with liver cancer.

In summary, the science of digestion holds fascination. Nevertheless, much more important is the **eating** of good food. This kind of study should always be carried on in the context of nutrition and the intriguing science of healthful cookery. For, remember, **we are what we eat**.

RESPIRATION

No one needs to be told how important his or her **respiratory system** is, for you cannot live without breathing for more than a few minutes. After only four or five minutes without oxygen, brain damage occurs. *"Air is a precious boon of heaven,"* having an invigorating influence over the entire body, as well as helping to soothe our nerves. Laden with fresh inspired oxygen, our blood circulates energetically through the system, refreshing our organs and keeping the body strong and healthy.

Recent evidence has shown the vital importance of *outdoor* air, particularly abundant under evergreen trees. Beneficial influences of negative air ions (called *aerions*) have been demonstrated in many scientific studies. They enhance a quickened sense of well-being, including a lessened risk of disease. Air ions, moreover, enhance several cellular enzyme functions, enabling them to help kill germs floating in the atmosphere. The influence of negative air ions is lost in an artificially air-conditioned, indoor environment. Closed windows in schools and offices are one frequent cause of the boredom and frustration that exists in so many sedentary jobs. Modern science, therefore, highlights the original plan of our Creator, who situated His first children in a garden.

The respiratory organs are the nose, pharynx, larynx, trachea, bronchi, and lungs. Their basic structural plan is that of a wind tunnel or tube, with many branches ending in tiny thin-walled sacs called **alveoli**. Capillary networks, appearing like hair nets, surround each microscopic *alveolus*. The purpose of such an arrangement is to bring inspired air within reach for the blood cells to extract enough oxygen and release carbon dioxide. This delicate membrane barrier is less than 5/1000 of an inch thick! With millions of alveoli per lung, an enormous surface area is presented, in the neighborhood of 1,100 square feet.

The **nose** is the first organ of respiration we encounter. Air enters through our nostrils (or *nares*) into the nasal cavity, which is divided by a membrane (*septum*). The paired nasal chambers are lined by mucous membrane, which traps duct particles. Mucus secreting cells produce a powerful enzyme, **lysozyme**, that efficiently kills most harmful germs. The **pharynx** is what most people call the throat. It serves the same purpose as your hallway does in the house. Two pairs of **tonsils** and **adenoids** are located in the pharynx. It connects with the middle ear by way of the paired *Eustachian tubes*.

The **larynx**, or "voice box," is located just below the throat. It is composed of several pieces of cartilage. The one we feel (the so-called "Adam's apple") is surrounded by other laryngeal cartilages, with the *epiglottis* acting as a lid to close our larynx when we swallow. If this does not function properly, we may cough and choke, because food or liquid enters where only air should go. *Vocal cords*, tensed by attached muscles, stretch across the interior of the larynx. When our vocal cords are short and tense, the voice sounds high pitched. On the other hand, longer relaxed cords vibrate with a lower tone.

Feeling your neck just below the larynx, you will encounter the **trachea**. Its framework is made of almost noncollapsible material, namely 15 to 20 C-shaped rings of cartilage. Air has no other way of getting into the lungs. Therefore, any complete tracheal obstruction causes death in a matter of minutes.

The **bronchi** appear like a miniaturized upside down tree. These smaller air tubes branch and divide approximately twenty-three times! They finally terminate in the **bronchioles**, then into tiny microscopic *alveolar sacs* resembling a cluster of grapes. These vital alveoli further the final exchange of oxygen.

Our two **lungs** are large organs, filling almost the entire chest cavity on each side. They are covered with thin, moist, slippery membranes that enable each lung to slide smoothly against the chest wall as they expand and deflate with each breath. When fluid accumulates in this pleural space, one feels the effects of an inflammation of the pleura, called *pleurisy*. It is best treated with hot packs.

Respiration involves a rapid molecular exchange of the gases *oxygen* and *carbon dioxide*. As blood flows through the delicate and alveolar walls, carbon dioxide (CO_2) leaves the blood to diffuse into the alveolar air sacs. Oxygen molecules, simultaneously, enter our blood. This two-way gas exchange is carried on continually. Oxygen is transported speedily to our tissues by millions of microscopic red blood cells.

The **hemoglobin** molecule (part of the red blood cell) is responsible for carrying most of the oxygen. Carbon dioxide, a waste product of cell metabolism, dissolves principally in the plasma. **Hyperventilation** occurs when one breathes too fast. This lowers the carbon dioxide level of the blood, producing several uncomfortable symptoms. Tingling, drawing of the hands, and dizziness can occur. These may be relieved after a short period of shallow breathing into a paper bag, quickly reversing the abnormal gas exchange in the tissues.

Breathing, furthermore, involves the brain, skeletal muscles, and even some bones. Ordinarily we take about a pint of air into our lungs with each breath. This is referred to as the **tidal volume**. The largest amount of air that we can breathe in and out in one full inspiration is known as the **vital capacity**. In most adults this amounts to approximately 4.5 to five quarts (or *liters*). A special diagnostic device, called the *spirometer*, is used to measure the amount of air exchanged in breathing.

THE CIRCULATION

Scriptures declare that *"the life of the flesh is in the blood,"* (Leviticus 17:11). However, without the circulation of blood, life as we know it, would be impossible. As we consider the **circulatory system**, let's look first at the blood and its constituent elements. Our survey of clotting factors and blood types will be followed by a close look at the heart, the blood vessels and their vital functions.

Approximately four to five quarts of blood constantly circulate in an average man or woman. The time required for our blood to traverse throughout the entire system can be measured. When a bitter substance, such as bile, is injected into a vein of the arm, it can make its circuit through the heart, the lungs, back to the heart, then be tasted by the tongue, all within 10 to 15 seconds! So, it is no wonder that each hormone produced by the body, every morsel we eat, and all the oxygen inhaled are all rapidly distributed throughout the body.

When blood is centrifuged or allowed to stand for several hours, it normally separates into two distinct layers. There is a layer of blood cells that settles first, being heavier than the *plasma*, which is primarily fluid. If we first allow the blood to clot, then separate the liquid portion, we have *serum*, which is basically blood plasma minus the clotting factors. This ratio of blood cells to plasma is measured in the laboratory with the **hematocrit** test. A small capillary tube of blood is centrifuged. Allowing for slight variations between men and women, the blood cellular elements will usually constitute 38 to 46% of the total volume. Lesser figures indicate the presence of *anemia*.

Two major types of cells distinguish themselves under the microscope. The **red blood cell** is our oxygen carrier, deriving its name from the crimson pigment *hemoglobin* which gives blood its characteristic red color. These red cells are produced in the bone marrow. After several stages of maturation, mature red blood cells (*erythrocytes*) are sent on to the circulation. Normally there are 4 1/2 to 5 1/2 million red blood cells in every cubic millimeter of blood. Seen under the microscope, these appear as biconcave discs, a peculiar shape which provides maximum surface area for any given volume. Their flattened shape enables them to pass through the tiny capillaries, where they optimize their surface area by folding in two, like an apple turnover. Their life span is approximately 120 days.

The **white blood cells** are produced in the bone marrow also, all except for our *lymphocytes*. By producing powerful *antibodies*, lymphocytes defend against many kinds of infection. These cells develop in our lymph nodes and spleen, as well as the thymus gland in children. Other lymphoid tissues—located in the ileum, appendix, and tonsils—aid in this important secondary "line of defense" against many abnormal cells, numerous germs, foreign proteins and other extraneous material.

The most numerous white cell in our blood is called the *neutrophil*. It gets its name from its microscope staining characteristic, and appears as a multi-lobed, nucleated, granular cell. Several members of the white blood cell series contain granules, little packages of potent enzymes that help them in their job of body protection. These granule containing defender cells include the neutrophil, the *basophil*, and the *eosinophil*. Lymphocytes and *monocytes* (another scavenger cell) do not contain granules.

The neutrophil is really quite interesting. Living only around eight days, it frequently gives its life to defend our body. More than any other circulating cell, neutrophils (sometimes called "polys") are able to surround a germ, take it within the cell, eat it (termed *phagocytosis*), then discharge its potent "suicide bags" (*lysosomes*) of powerful enzymes to kill the invader, then finally digest it. Large numbers of these cells migrate into a wound, and ultimately give their lives to defend the body. The outcome of this defense reaction produces a substance known as *pus*. Nearly five to ten thousand white blood cells per cubic millimeter circulate in the blood at any given time.

During most bacterial infections, the white blood count increases. Viral infections, on the other hand, depress the white blood count, or leave it normal. In the laboratory one will see a "shift" toward more lymphocytes, the body's prime defenders against virus. During a normal, healthy state, many white blood cell lie "marginated." That is, they spread themselves along the blood vessel walls, moving slowly, or even resting while the main stream of the circulation moves on. Vigorous exercise, the *sauna* bath, a very cold shower, or a *cold mitten friction* increase the white blood count, mobilizing all our available blood "soldiers" to the "battleground."

Less is known about the other white blood cell's activities. Eosinophils appear to play a strategic role in allergic states and parasitic diseases, since their numbers are often increased in those conditions. Unusual forms of white blood cells are additionally seen. In **leukemia**, a type of blood cancer, many bizarre white blood cell characteristics appear, as well as a proliferation of immature forms. **Mononucleosis**, an infectious disease of viral origin, is likewise characterized by the appearance of unusual white cells.

In studying blood transfusion science we encounter several distinct **types** of human blood. **Antigens** on the surface of each red blood cell give rise to these characteristics, categorized as follows: *type A* blood contains the antigen classified "A," with antibodies to type B circulating in the plasma. Blood *type B* contains just the reverse, the "B" antigen and the anti-A antibodies. *Type AB* contains both antigens, "A" and "B," attached to the cells, but has no anti-B or anti-A antibodies. For this reason *type AB* blood is called the **universal recipient**. *Type O* blood contains neither "A" or "B" antigens, but has circulating anti-B and anti-A antibodies. This type is called the **universal donor**. The accompanying table summarizes these characteristics.

TYPES	ANTIGENS	ANTIBODIES
A	A	Anti-B
B	B	Anti-A
AB	A and B	O
O	O	Anti-A and Anti-B

Another blood factor was discovered in research on *Rhesus* monkeys. Called the **Rh factor**, it is present in 85% of the adult population. The other 15% have no Rh factor. Precisely as the *ABO type* classifications must be compatible for a blood transfusion to be given successfully, so also must the *Rh factor* match. This is determined by a laboratory process called "crossmatching" in which a few donor cells are placed in some serum from the potential recipient's blood. If antibodies in the patient's serum coagulate the donor cells, that blood cannot be used to transfuse that particular patient.

During pregnancy, the Rh factor becomes extremely important. A mother who is *Rh negative* may be married to a man who is *Rh positive*. If the baby born to them is also Rh positive, sensitization of the mother's placental blood cells can occur. Subsequent pregnancies may result in newborn *jaundice* and *hemolysis*, a serious condition in which the baby's blood cells are destroyed by circulating maternal antibodies. In recent years, not only has the cause of this **hemolytic disease of the newborn** (*erythroblastosis fetalis*) been determined, but its prevention likewise assured. A small injection of *gamma globulin* high in the anti–Rh antibody (marketed as *RhoGAM*) will prevent the mother's sensitization which otherwise would occur in subsequent pregnancies. This has been a tremendous breakthrough for safer obstetrical care of babies born to Rh negative mothers. **Exchange transfusions** for the newborn are necessary at times to prevent severe jaundice with its danger of brain damage (*kernicterus*).

Blood Coagulation

The speedy **clotting** of blood is a marvelous study in cooperation. When injury occurs to a blood vessel, the damaged tissues elaborate a chemical called *thromboplastin*. This triggers the activation of a whole "cascade" of enzyme reactions, with the final production of *thrombin* to activate the clot. Thrombin forms in the liver, under the influence of *Vitamin K. Fibrinogen*, another circulating coagulation factor, is ultimately converted into *fibrin*, which is stabilized into a network of fibers, securing the clot. Another extremely minute, strategic element circulating in the blood is the **platelet** (*thrombocyte*). This smallest blood cell presents in large numbers, 250,000 to 400,000 per cubic millimeter. They are essential for normal coagulation to occur. Platelet stickiness, which contributes to abnormal clot formation, is enhanced by eating animal foods. Eating cholesterol-rich meats increases the production of a potent chemical, *thromboxane A_2*, which spurs on the coagulation sequence. Normally, it is optimum to have our platelets negatively charged, so that they repel each other. They should not be inclined to stick together. This would endanger our heart or brain by clot (*thrombus*) formation. Research in animals has shown that one meal of meat can alter the electric charge on the platelets, making them dangerously sticky.

The Heart

"Keep they heart with all diligence; for out of it are the issues of life," (Proverbs 4:23). These were the words of the wise King Solomon, as he meditated on the sublime wisdom evidenced in the human body. The **heart** is a pump designed to circulate blood throughout the entire system. Carrying nourishment to the tissues, warmth to our limbs, and oxygen to billions of cells, our "pump" performs a marvelous function. It beats over 100 thousand times a day, pumps six to thirty quarts of blood per minute through more than 60,000 miles of blood vessels! The human heart does this by beating sixty to eighty times per minute, never stopping for one's entire lifetime! Actually, the pumping phase takes about one-third of the time (*systole*), with a resting phase of two-thirds that allows time for re-filling

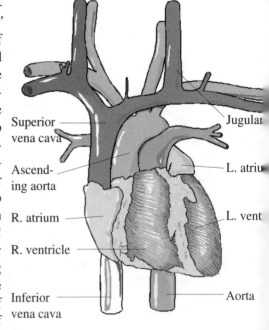

Superior vena cava

Ascend-ing aorta

R. atrium

R. ventricle

Inferior vena cava

Jugular

L. atriu

L. vent

Aorta

the cardiac chambers (called *diastole*). A healthy heart is capable of increasing its output five or six times normal during strenuous exercise.

Four chambers compose the heart, much like four rooms in an apartment. Blood enters the heart through the superior and inferior *vena cavae*, two large veins that collect blood from the upper and lower parts of the body respectively. These enter the right *atrium*, a mixing chamber through which the blood passes on its way to the *ventricles*. As blood passes through the door (*tricuspid valves*) between these two "room," it enters the right ventricle, from which it is then pumped to the lungs. Ejected through the *semilunar valves* into the *pulmonary artery*, the blood passes into the right and left main pulmonary vessels. Within both lungs it receives oxygen and releases carbon dioxide.

Through four *pulmonary veins* enriched blood then enters the left *atrium*. It mixes thoroughly in the atrium, necessary because some parts of the lung aerated the blood better than others. Flowing through the *mitral* or *bicuspid* valve, blood then passes into the left ventricle. This contains the thickest muscular wall; it is the strongest portion of the heart. The left ventricle contracts simultaneously with the right, each time ejecting an equal amount of blood. As systole occurs the blood is pushed with great pressure into the aorta through its *semilunar valve*. The mitral valve closes at this time (*systole*) to prevent regurgitation of blood into the atrium. This forceful contraction of the left ventricle produces what we call the "systolic blood pressure."

Blood pressure is the arterial pressure, measured in millimeters of mercury (mm Hg), attained when the heart pumps forcibly. The maximum pressure seen with each contraction is called *systolic pressure*, and is usually written above a slant line as follows: **120/80**. The lower figure reflects the *diastolic blood pressure*, which measures pressure when the heart is not actively beating. Diastolic pressures are related to the elastic tone of the arterial walls. In the ventricles the diastolic blood pressure drops close to zero, allowing the heart valves to open as blood flows in from the upper chamber.

The rhythm of the heart is controlled by our **pacemaker**, a specialized bit of cardiac tissue located in the right atrium. From this mysterious "spark," an electrical current passes through both atria of the heart, initiating a contraction to force blood into both ventricles. A split second delay through the **A–V node** (*atrio-ventricular node*) allows the heart valves to close. The ventricles contract a split second later, squirting blood into the aorta. Nerves affect our heart's rhythm. The *sympathetic nervous system*, as a rule, speeds up the heart rate and elevates the blood pressure, while *vagal nerve* stimulation (*parasympathetic impulses*) does the opposite.

Working constantly, the heart uses very little oxygen from the blood that flows through it. Coronary arteries exit through tiny orifices behind the semilunar valve leaflets in the aorta. These supply blood to the muscular wall of the heart. Our **coronary** (crown-like) vessels divide into three main branches, the *right main*, the *left anterior descending* and the *left circumflex* arteries. Blood returns from the heart muscle (*myocardium*) to the right atrium via the *coronary sinus*. Dietary **cholesterol** accumulates, producing the characteristic features of coronary heart disease—such as angina pectoris, myocardial infarction, or congestive heart failure. See Chapter Four with respect to details of diagnosis and treatment of these problems.

"Lifelines" to our entire body include the arteries, veins and capillaries. Discovered by William Harvey in the 1600's, our vascular structures vessels act like the arteries of a major city freeway system, delivering blood to every organ. The **aorta** is the largest vessel of the body, leaving the left ventricle like a powerful garden hose. It distributes blood through three large branches to our head and upper extremities, then carries this pipeline of precious enriched fluid to our abdominal organs and legs. As blood reaches a myriad of smaller arteries, tiny sphincter muscles are encountered. This fortuitous function allows for shunting blood to the most needy organs. After a meal, for example, our digestive organs receive the largest share. However, during violent exercise more blood flow goes to the muscles.

The closest contact with body tissues is made in our **capillaries**. Blood cells pass single file through these microscopic vessels, distributing numerous nutrients to the tissues. Excess fluids are then taken up by the lymphatic vessels. Capillaries connect with *venules* which terminate in **veins**. They unite, growing progressively larger, to return blood to the heart. This completes the cycle.

The **lymphatic system** consists of a series of one-way channels that bring tissue fluid (*lymph*) toward the lymph nodes. Here it is filtered, and some toxic materials are processed. The purified lymph fluid re-enters the circulation via the *thoracic duct*, located in the upper chest.

The **spleen** also plays its vital role, acting as a "policeman" to remove damaged cells from the circulation. Many reusable blood elements are processed, conserving iron and amino acids for future use. The spleen, moreover, acts as a reservoir. Blood cells, temporarily sequestered there, can be mobilized in case of infection or any sudden hemorrhage. Unforeseen injury may require its removal. Fortunately, one's survival would be unimpaired. Nevertheless, the spleen is a valuable organ for the entire body.

One more feature of circulation deserves mention. In the developing *fetus* oxygen and nutrients are received from the placenta, then brought via the *umbilical cord* to nourish the growing child. The *umbilical vein* receives this blood and channels it through a liver bypass (called the *ductus venosus*) to the heart. Since the child is encased in amniotic fluid, and thereby unable to breathe, a shunt through the heart is provided. A temporary "hole" in the atrial septum (*foramen ovale*) and the *ductus arteriosis* (connecting the aorta with the pulmonary artery) divert most of the blood into the systemic circulation, rather than into the lungs. Coming up from the bladder are two *umbilical arteries*. They return blood to the placenta through the umbilical cord, and thus keep the cycle going. All three of these shunts close within minutes after birth! Then, the adult pattern of circulation is established, leaving only small remnants of fibrous tissue as a reminder. How wonderfully the Creator has thought of our needs in designing the human circulation!

THE URINARY SYSTEM

It is easy to guess the function of the **urinary system**, namely, the secretion and elimination of *urine*. Most people do not realize, however, how essential these functions are for health and survival. It is important in preventive health care to try to understand how these systems work.

First, there are two **kidneys**. They normally lie behind the abdominal organs, against the muscles near the backbone. The left kidney is slightly larger than the right, located farther above the waistline. Each kidney is encased in a cushion of fat, for protection and which helps to hold it in place. Occasionally a kidney will drop (*renal ptosis*) in the vertical position. This hinders urine drainage, by putting a kink in the ureter. The outer portion of the kidney is the *cortex* (a Latin word, meaning "bark" or "rind"). The inner part is called the *medulla*.

Kidney cells are arranged to form unique functional units called **nephrons**. Each nephron consists of three main parts: a *glomerulus*, a *Bowman's capsule*, and a *collecting tubule*. The glomerulus involves a network of capillaries tucked into a microscopic funnel. The top part of the "funnel" is called the Bowman's capsule. Extending from this is a twisted tubule, which continues like a loop, extending into the medulla (called respectively, the *proximal convoluted tubule*, *loop of Henley*, then the *distal convoluted tubule*). About one million nephrons are located in each kidney!

The kidney nephrons are designed to filter our blood. In the Bowman's capsule we encounter an extensive network of thin membranes, to filter both water and dissolved substances as the blood passes through the capillaries. This filtrate trickles through the convoluted tubules. And, as it does so, a large part of the water is reabsorbed into the capillaries. Dissolved substances, such as glucose and various salts are further reabsorbed, so that nothing is wasted by being lost in the urine. Just before the urine is finally sent to the **bladder**, a final exchange of potassium and hydrogen ions occurs. Various drugs are likewise secreted.

Two hormones, **aldosterone**, a salt-retaining hormone, and **ADH** (*antidiuretic hormone*), influence the reabsorption of salts and water. These are controlled, as mentioned above, by the adrenal glands, the pituitary gland, and the brain.

Urine drains out of the collecting tubules into a "basin," in each kidney called the *renal pelvis*. It then passes through two tiny muscular tubes less than ¼ inch wide, called the *ureter*, into the *urinary bladder*. The bladder contains muscular and elastic fibers well suited to expand and hold varying amounts of urine. When the bladder contains about ½ pint of urine, most people feel the desire to void. Occasionally the kidneys do not secrete enough urine. This may be due to inflammation (*nephritis*). **Anuria** is the absence of urine, usually caused by suppression of kidney function. **Oliguria** (scanty urine) occurs from various causes.

351

To leave the body, our urine passes from the bladder through the *urethra*. This is the lowermost part of the urinary tract. Infection occasionally occurs from germs ascending up the urethra, and develops inflammation of the mucous membrane lining the urinary bladder (*cystitis*).

REPRODUCTION

Truly, we are *"fearfully and wonderfully made!"* To duplicate the human body requires one of the most marvelous systems ever designed. **Reproduction** has as its goal the survival of our human species. Although male and female sexes appear significantly opposite, they do share the common function of reproduction.

The **male reproductive system** consists of a pair of sex glands, a series of ducts, several accessory glands, and the external organs. The latter, called *external genitalia*, consists of the *scrotum* and *penis*. A special kind of erectile tissue composes most of the interior of the penis, becoming engorged with blood and distended during erection. The skin overlying the head, or *glans*, is loosely folded into a double layer called the foreskin (*prepuce*). **Circumcision** involves surgically removing the foreskin, thus preventing its fitting too tightly or causing irritation. This simple surgery is commonly performed in newborn males.

The *testes* are two oval-shaped glands, each one capable of forming millions of male sex cells (*spermatozoa*). Any single sperm cell may join with a female sex cell (*ovum*) to produce a new human being! The testes also secrete a male sex hormone (**testosterone**), of such potency that in a few months at **puberty**, it can transform a little boy into a man. The testes are externally, cradled in a pouch-like structure called the *scrotum*. This provides the variation from body temperature (cooler) necessary to promote the development of healthy sperm. The functions of testosterone are described above in the section on endocrine organs.

The ducts that convey the spermatozoa to the outside are called *vas deferens*. They lead from the testes and their attached *epididymis* to enter the *prostate* gland. The *ejaculatory ducts* pass through the prostate gland to empty the sperm into the urethra. This climactic process is called *ejaculation*. For permanent contraception, a minor operation (called the **bilateral partial vasectomy**) is performed to interrupt the duct leading from the testes and produce sterility.

Two *seminal vesicles*, one *prostate* gland, and two *bulbourethral (Cowper's) glands* are accessory male glands that produce alkaline secretions. These constitute the gelatinous fluid part of the *semen*. Normally, about one teaspoonful of semen is ejaculated at one climax. Each milliliter contains over sixty million sperm! Vasectomy does not usually affect the erection or ejaculation response, but renders a man sterile.

The prostate gland frequently enlarges in older men, compressing the urethra and causing obstruction. This may require surgery. The cause of this *benign prostatic hypertrophy* (BPH) is not known. Suspected lifestyle factors include coffee, and the high fat intake of a meat diet.

The **female reproductive system** has several similar structural designs to that of the male. A pair of sex glands, the *ovaries*, are located within the pelvic cavity. After puberty the ovaries go through cyclic changes each month, during which one ovum is produced. The tissue of each ovary comprises several thousand sacs, called *Graafian follicles*. Within each one of these lies an immature *ovum*. Powerful hormones are produced by the ovaries. **Estrogen** is secreted by the Graafian follicles, while the *corpus luteum* (yellow body) produced late in the monthly cycle secretes chiefly **progesterone**. These are the feminizing hormones that produce characteristic changes at puberty.

The tubes connecting the ovaries to the womb are paired. The *Fallopian tubes* (or *oviducts*) are about four inches in length. Their fluted, expanded ends sweep over the ovum at *ovulation*, attracting the mature ovum toward the location where fertilization can occur. Occasionally, conception takes place in the tube, leading to serious complications (**tubal pregnancy**), and requiring emergency surgery.

The *uterus* is a small organ about the size of a pear, but extremely strong. It is almost entirely smooth muscle, with a small cavity inside where *implantation* of a fertilized egg can occur. During **pregnancy** the uterus will grow many times larger, so that it can accommodate the baby plus a considerable amount of fluid. The upper portion, or *body* of the womb, connects with the mouth, called the *cervix*. The uterus actually functions in three distinct processes—menstruation, pregnancy, and labor. Around the age of thirteen years, a girl will begin having *menstrual periods*. The onset of menstruation is called the time of *menarche*. A cyclic hormonal and physiologic change occurs approximately every twenty eight days for the next thirty years or so. Then it ceases. The change of life at the end of the child–bearing age is called *menopause* or the *climacteric*.

The *vagina* is a hollow perineal cavity, composed largely of smooth muscle lined with mucous membrane. Near the opening of the vaginal outlet are the *Bartholin's glands*, which secrete a lubricating fluid, especially important during sexual intercourse.

The external genital parts of the female are called the *vulva*. The external opening for the urinary tract, the *urethra*, empties here. Above the urethral *meatus* is the *clitoris*, a small bit of erectile tissue, presumably the female counterpart of the penis. The *labia majora* and *labia minora* form the so-called lips, while a perforated membrane guards the entrance of the vagina at the *hymenal ring*. Occasionally, the hymen will lack an opening, producing difficulty in starting the menstrual cycle. The treatment for an **imperforate hymen** involves surgical incision.

The *breasts*, after puberty, consist of fifteen to twenty five divisions, arranged like the spokes of a wheel. Each lobe consists of several *lobules*, with grape-like clusters of secreting cells surrounding the small milk ducts. A dark colored area around the nipples is called the *areola*. Under the hormonal influences (*estrogen*, *progesterone*, and *prolactin*) of pregnancy, the breasts develop their milk glands further to permit nursing, or **lactation**.

As we look at our bodies again, with the poetic Psalmist we have to admire the awesome wisdom of our Creator— *"marvelous are Thy works; and that my soul knoweth right well,"* (Psalm 139:14).

CHAPTER TWENTY–FOUR

SPECIAL

SENSES

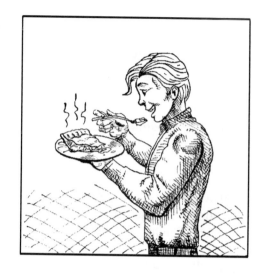

Living in an ever-changing world, we must constantly sense events that may threaten, as well as appreciate the experiences that enrich our lives. Without sense organs to make us aware of danger or enable us to appreciate beauty of our environment, we would be completely helpless. These sensations include touch (*cutaneous*), smell (*olfactory*), taste (*gustatory*), sight (*visual*), hearing (*auditory*), and position (*sensory*). From both clinical and physiologic perspectives this chapter will look at these sense organs, and focus particularly on the eyes and ears.

A sense organ is called a **receptor**. Most receptors are located within the skin or mucous membranes. However, in order to be rightly interpreted, every sensory impulse requires a special pathway to the brain, as well as a sensory *receiver* in the cerebral cortex, where there are sensory areas for each of the senses. Positional location is analyzed for the body through tiny vestibular canals in the ear. Our individual joints, digits, and limbs base their messages on changes in muscle tension. The integration of these impulses occurs in the cerebellum and cerebrum.

Our knowledge of position or location for various parts of our body, without any aid of vision, is called **proprioception**. Closely related to this is our ability to judge the texture of cloth, estimate the weight of objects, and even identify their shape when we are blindfolded. This is called **stereognosis**, a word meaning "solid knowledge." Some examples of skills in which muscle sensitivity is all important are hammering a nail, typing, and playing a musical instrument. Our internal organs are also connected to sensory nerves, which primarily send messages in response to spasm—such as colic, dilatation or stretching of a hollow organ, and irritation by chemicals. Organic sensations arise from stimuli in the internal organs, producing cravings such as hunger and thirst. If these are severe, they produce considerable mental anguish.

The receptors for **smell** are located in the upper part of the nasal cavity. Numerous *olfactory cells* connect with the first cranial nerve, not only to warn us of danger as from breathing poisonous gases, but also to contribute immensely to the pleasure found in a variety of natural scents. The sense of smell is less important in man than in lower animals, but receptors are available for hundreds of different odors. The memory for these is exceptionally keen. Vivid sensations of smell when no stimulus is present (called *olfactory hallucinations*) are a fairly common occurrence in mentally ill patients.

Receptors for our sense of taste are located chiefly on the tongue. There are four basic types of taste buds—**sweet, sour, bitter**, and **salt**. Hundreds of taste buds for sweetness are concentrated on the tip of the tongue. Those for sour sensations are located along the side, while salt taste is distributed around the prominent circumference of the tongue. There are fewer sensors for bitter taste, which primarily serve as a warning for dangerous chemicals, rancidity, or poison. They are located on the base of the tongue near the epiglottis.

HEARING AND THE EAR

Hearing is the sense by which sounds are appreciated. This function is called the "watch dog" of the senses, being the last to disappear when one falls asleep and the first to return when one awakens. This particularly applies to patients in coma or under anesthesia. Two sets of receptors are present within our ears. One set is concerned with hearing, the other with position sense. Both connect with the brain stem through the eighth cranial nerve.

The **ear** consists of three divisions, the external, the middle, and the inner portion. The visible external ear receives the sound waves. This *auricle* or *pinna* comprises cartilage covered with skin. An *auditory canal* extends inward, forward, and downward toward the **eardrum** (*tympanic membrane*). **Cerumen**, a waxy secretion is produced by oil glands in this canal. Excessive amounts may block the ear, causing pressure on the tympanic membrane or hearing loss. Lukewarm water may be used to gently wash out the obstructed ear canal, using an ear syringe or a pulsating device such as the Water Pic. Care must be taken to direct the fluid stream to the *lateral* walls to avoid irritating the drum. Hydrogen peroxide (H_2O_2) can be used similarly as an irrigation solution.

Swimmer's ear is a common complaint in which infection develops in the auditory canal. Caused by excessive moisture, this affliction produces ear pain with a watery drainage. Usually the hearing is unimpaired. *Burrow's solution* (sodium aluminum acetate), hydrogen peroxide, or specially prescribed ear drops can be instilled to relieve pain and counteract infection. Thorough drying after each immersion of a sensitive ear in water is important to prevent this condition, common in the summer swimming season.

The **middle ear** connects with the nasal passageway by the *Eustachian tube*. This provides for the equalization of pressure when one changes altitudes, going up a mountain, or coming down in a pressurized airplane. A small bone called the **hammer** (*malleus*) connects with the eardrum, then transmits the sound vibration through two other bones, the **anvil** and the **stirrup** (called *incus* and *stapes*), to the *oval window*. Occasionally, the middle ear fills with fluid or develops increased pressure due to blockage of the Eustachian tube. A *myringotomy* is a surgical procedure where the eardrum is punctured to equalize pressure while withdrawing fluid. Occasionally tiny tubes are placed through the ear drums of children to maintain drainage of the middle ear. This helps to prevent the recurrent ear infections that follow frequent colds.

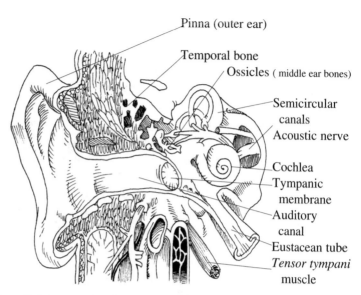

Pinna (outer ear)
Temporal bone
Ossicles (middle ear bones)
Semicircular canals
Acoustic nerve
Cochlea
Tympanic membrane
Auditory canal
Eustacean tube
Tensor tympani muscle

Foreign bodies are common in children's ears. Occasionally, a small beetle or tick will find its way into the external ear canal and attach itself tightly. Irrigation can be attempted after the installation of some oil drops to kill the offending insect, preventing its respiration. However, tiny forceps are needed frequently to remove the offending object. Of importance for direct vision is adequate lighting, and usually the aid of a topical anesthetic. It is extremely important to avoid putting match sticks, bobby pins, and other small objects into the ear canal. Accidental rupture of your eardrum can originate a life-long hearing problem or necessitate an expensive surgical repair.

The **inner ear** consists of the three *semicircular canals* positioned at right angles to each other, which help to maintain our balance. Responding instantly to minute changes in position, this paired organ can create the characteristic dizziness when one spins rapidly. Usually there is a flicker to one side of the eyes (*nystagmus*) associated with this type of problem. Increases of pressure and viral infections of the inner ear can originate acute **labrynthitis**. The syndrome is characterized by a whirling type of dizziness (called *vertigo*) in association with nystagmus, nausea, and extreme discomfort. This annoying condition is usually self-limited. Nevertheless, a special diet and supine position are important aids to healing as the symptoms subside.

The **cochlea** is likewise located deep in the inner ear. This is the actual organ of hearing (called the *Organ of Corti*). It responds to vibrations transmitted through the auditory canal, the ear drum, and the tiny bones (*ossicles*) of the middle ear. Tiny hair cells in the cochlea respond to various frequencies of sound, enabling us to identify a voice on the telephone by a single "hello," or relax to enjoy a beautiful symphony.

Deafness and hearing impairment are increasingly common around the world. There are two types of deafness, one caused by nerve damage, and the *conduction* type related to sound transmission. Older individuals commonly develop hearing impairment due to degeneration of the eighth cranial nerve. This so-called **nerve deafness** (*presbyacousis*) primarily involves the higher frequencies of sound. Thus, a man's voice is easier for older individuals to identify than a woman's, and distinct voices are more readily heard than talking in a group setting. **Conduction deafness** may be of several types. Wax in the ear causes one kind that is easily cured. It obviously is related to blockage of sound transmission via the acoustic canal. Rupture of the eardrum or fluid in the middle ear may also produce conduction deafness, commonly associated with ear infections (*otitis media*). Most cases resolve spontaneously in a few weeks.

Deafness occurring in young people without the presence of ear infection raises the suspicion of **otosclerosis**. This premature hardening of bone in the middle ear stiffens the stapes, preventing vibration of sound at the oval window. An operation to remove the stapes (*stapidectomy*) and replace it with a tiny wire attached to a piece of cartilage restores the hearing for most individuals. Naturally, this delicate surgery must be performed by an expert using the operating microscope.

Hearing aids may be invaluable for those with deafness of congenital or acquired origin. Minute and extremely expensive, the clarity of sound obtained with a hearing aid can enable a deaf individual to communicate once again, being more aware of his or her surroundings or potential danger. Congenital deafness may not be amenable to treatment with hearing aids. Notwithstanding, the affected person can be enrolled in sign language classes or acquire the skill of lip-reading. In actuality, it is my belief that if more people in general were able to communicate via sign language, the better the horizon of possibilities would be for the deaf. Otherwise, they are severely handicapped for life, and frequently unemployable. Most of them are at least of average intelligence and may not only learn skills and trades, but pursue most of the professions open to people with unimpaired hearing.

EYESIGHT

The importance of **vision** to men and women can only be measured by the intense handicap suffered by the **blind**. As everyone knows, the organ of sight is the eye. Sensory vision is carried to the brain through the *optic* or second cranial nerve. The occipital portion of the brain registers these images, recognizes and interprets them in the context of our memory and reason. Looking closely at the eye we see it covered by the *eyelids*, retractable membranes covered with skin and rimmed with tiny hairs, called *eyelashes*. Sensitive reflexes enable these lids to close with a quick blink, protecting the eye against insects and accidents. A thin transparent membrane, the *conjunctiva*, lines the inner portion of the eyelid and the surface of the eye. A thicker transparent window, the *cornea*, protects the visual part of the eye and reflecting light rays slightly, as they enter. Forming the posterior wall of the *anterior chamber* of the eye is the *iris*, usually colored blue, brown, or black, and corresponding to the diaphragm of an ordinary camera.

Light enters through the hole in the center of the iris called the *pupil*. This varies in size according to the intensity of light and usually narrows for distant vision. Drugs such as *atropine* and *adrenalin* can dilate the pupil. *Morphine* and *pilocarpine* will produce pupillary constriction. Light rays are bent, or refracted, by the *lens*. This is a transparent jelly-like substance just behind the pupil. An opaque degenerated lens is called a *cataract*. Light rays pass through the anterior part of the eye and after refraction by the lens are reflected onto the *retina*, where the nerves to the eye enter. Light then passing through a jelly-like substance, the *vitreous humor*.

The retina consists of nerve receptors, millions of them, the *rods* and *cones*. Cones are most numerous in the *fovea centralis*, or point of maximum vision. The cones are receptors for color vision. Black and white contrasting blends, required for night vision, are widely distributed across the retina, and are received by the rods. Nerves from the rods and cones constitute the *optic disc*, seen as one looks at the retina. Numerous blood vessels, and the *sclera*, or hard external capsule, complete the globe of the eye.

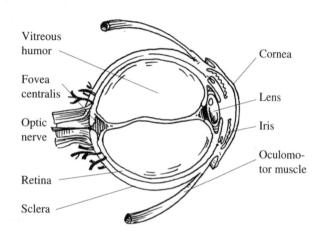

Eye movements are accomplished through fixed muscles innervated by the cranial nerves three, four, and six. These provide for the sensitive parallel motions of the eye ball, giving rise to **binocular vision**, so important in depth perception.

By standard principles of optics, the image projected on the retina is upside down and reversed left to right. Individuals having an eyeball too long will focus the image in front of the retina, producing *myopia* or **nearsightedness**. If the eyeball is too short, the image focuses behind the eye, making vision **farsighted** and requiring a positive lens for correction. This is called *hyperopia*. As one grows older the lens loses its elasticity or hardens, just as one's arteries harden with age. This condition is termed *presbyopia* or "old sight." Elderly people often wear bifocals, which means part of the glass lens is for distant vision and the remainder for near vision.

CATARACT

A **cataract** is an opacity in the lens, and is usually found in older people. Congenital tendency to cataract formation may be evident at birth or a much earlier age. Traumatic injury to the lens can cause this also. More commonly we see a cataract developing in diabetics or merely occurring as a degenerative condition in old age. When a cataract begins to blur one's vision or obscure the entrance of light, it is time for surgery. A trained ophthalmologist can remove the lens, often under local anesthesia, and subsequently fit the patient with contact lenses or glasses. Artificial lens implants are being used more and more in conjunction with cataract removal.

Most comprehensive physical examinations include visualization of the retina. An *opthalmoscope* is a special set of lenses, lighted to observe the retina through the pupil. In a darkened room or with special eye drops, the pupil can be seen with evaluation of many common diseases made possible. High blood pressure and diabetes mellitus produce characteristic changes in the back of the eye. This guides the physician in treatment.

TIPS ON SELECTING GLASSES

When a person's vision has been impaired to the place where corrective lenses are required, an appointment should be made with an ophthalmologist (eye specialist) or optometrist. Both types of doctors are equipped with the instruments necessary to **refract** the eye. Careful evaluation of the vision is performed, along with special tests for *color blindness, astigmatism*, or other eye diseases. The **eye chart** helps to determine the extent of impairment. Normal vision is described as 20/20, meaning that a normal healthy eye will see the letters clearly at 20 feet. On the other hand, 20/40 vision means that your eye sees at 20 feet what another healthy person should see at 40 feet. The large "E" on most eye charts is set for 20/200 vision. Some unfortunate individuals can barely see hand motion. If this cannot be corrected with glasses, they are considered legally blind. Complete **blindness** exists when no light or motion at all can be detected. Of course blind people may become extremely perceptive with their other senses— especially the hearing, touch, and smell. Some have been those talented musicians and gifted authors who overcame the severe handicap of blindness to make their contribution to society. The noted hymn writer, Fanny Crosby, is one outstanding example.

When your prescription for lenses has been written, the selection of your own personal glasses comes next. Be prudent and avoid cut rate chain stores when purchasing eye glasses. Otherwise, the *exact* prescription may not be filled. If a person cannot obtain an exact set of glasses for his or her individual need, try another oculist. The extra time and expense will be worth it. Suitability of the eye glasses themselves should be primary, with the choice of frames a second consideration. As a rule. hardened plastic is more durable and resistant to breakage than glass. However, this material is vulnerable to scratching and must be carefully cared for.

Sunglasses are fashionable. However, they're often used when unnecessary. Some of the cheaper ones permit ultraviolet rays to pass through their lenses. This may damage the eye, whose pupil is dilated because of the decreased light created by the dark glasses. Avoid this type of glass, if possible. Dark green and gray glasses should normally be selected, to filter out ultraviolet light with the visible rays. Amber glasses may be helpful when snow glare is a problem. All sunglasses should be shatterproof, especially if used in athletics or a type of work where flying objects are likely. The special precautions recommended for working around grinding wheels, welding equipment, or other industrial devices should always be observed.

CARE OF THE SENSES

Care of your five senses includes more than physical protection. It has truly been said that the eyes, ears, and other senses are the *"avenues to the soul."* As such, they should be carefully guarded lest your **character** become warped through contact with much evil. Frequent hearing or seeing of violence, immorality, and crime makes powerful impressions on everyone, especially our youth. More importantly, our senses, if carefully preserved, can be channels of communication with our **Creator**. This opens the mind to dimensions of thought, aspirations of holy living, and an exciting hope of total communication that, begun here, that can be freely realized only in eternity. How wisely it was said, *"I have heard of thee by the hearing of the ear: but now mine eye seeth thee,"* (Job 42:5)!

CHAPTER TWENTY–FIVE

THE

GOLDEN

YEARS

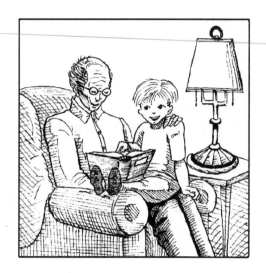

Today's society is growing rapidly in the over sixty–five population. More than twenty three million Americans have passed retirement age. Every day an additional 5,000 men and women join this elite group. While only 3,600 seniors die each day, we see the addition of 1,400 elderly every single day. Our average length of life is now seventy two. However, the figure is likely to rise as social and medical forces combine to increase numerically the individuals who reach old age. There exists already a sizable group of "old, old" people, those over seventy five. And, it is no longer rare for senior citizens to have a parent still living.

The **quality of life** for many old people has greatly improved. The 5,000 newcomers celebrating their 65th birthday each day are, as a rule, relatively healthy and vigorous, increasingly well educated, better off economically, active politically, and seeking new ways of self-fulfillment. In general, they are reaping the benefits of a longer life span, and truly enjoying their leisure years. Collectively, they have exploded the stereotype of the older person as unproductive, institutionalized, unable to adapt, sickly, frail, forgetful, confused, and senile. Most of the elderly, in fact, live at home. Only 5% live in institutions or nursing homes.

Often older people are looked upon as being in the tranquil and inactive phase of their life span. Actually, old age can be as full of **stress** as adolescence. Although the aged are a hardy group of survivors, they are also a vulnerable group. They get sick more often than younger people, and their lives are burdened with many new problems that they must confront and handle.

The elderly are not a homogeneous class, any more than are children. Their reactions to stress run a wide gamut. Some seek it; others avoid it. Some are undermined by the aging process; others are resistant. Some exaggerate its significance, others minimize. Nonetheless, regardless of their wide range of responses, stress of some kind or other is experienced to some degree by most of our elderly friends.

In general these stresses are more taxing when people grow older, than when they were youthful. Because of numerous physiologic changes of aging, a little bit of stress can go a long way toward causing illness. After a stressful experience, the prolonged autonomic arousal takes longer for the body to return to basal hormone and nervous levels. There is moreover a strong social component to these reactions. For example, a life-long investment or family relationship may be threatened, such as the loss of a loved one, the family home, or a cherished career. Given these stresses, what is really remarkable is the strength and capacity to deal with them that is displayed by so many aged individuals.

SLOWING THE AGING PROCESS

Aging is not a disease. Nevertheless, as the years pass, major changes in the body become apparent. Chronic health conditions develop, and mortality increases. Simultaneous with these changes, stress frequently builds up. Actually, the process of aging takes place more gradually, throughout our entire life. According to some specialists, there is a steady decline of about 1% per year in adult functional capacities of the numerous organ systems. This decline takes its toll by reducing the quality of life in the elderly. Hearing and visual impairment are high on the list of chronic conditions that plague them. Sensations of taste and smell may likewise diminish, detracting from their enjoyment of life. Sleep problems frequently develop. And these can affect the elderly individual's capacity to function normally during the day.

Breathing efficiency substantially diminishes, while muscle strength deteriorates. There is a gradual replacement of muscle cells by fatty and fibrous tissues. Our hormones protecting immunity responses decrease. Those hormones that remain do not do the job as adequately as before. The efficiency of mechanisms that control posture and locomotion may be impaired. As a result, older people fall more often, and are decidedly at greater risk of fractures. Additionally. the quality (hardness) of bone declines, especially in women, so that breaks are more likely to occur. Fractures, furthermore, take longer to mend.

On top of these "normal" functional changes, there are pathological changes due to disease. High blood pressure, coronary heart disease, pulmonary disease, allergic reactions, abnormal functioning of the gastrointestinal tract, arthritis, and many other degenerative conditions increase with age. All too often, they lead to chronic disability. These diseases and disabilities are stressful in themselves. They seriously challenge a senior's ability to cope.

As we look at the factors that promote aging, it becomes apparent that time plays a major role. The Scriptural picture of Moses is fascinating to contemplate. At the venerable age of 120, *"his eye was not dim, nor his natural force abated,"* (Deut. 34:7). This shows the remarkable influence of his communion with God, a lifestyle of outdoor living, together with a simple diet. All these factors helped in promoting this superb level of health.

Studies of the Hunzas, living high in the Himalaya Mountains have similarly shown the importance of active outdoor exercise, fresh air, pure water, and a simple diet in retarding the aging process. It is not unusual in that land of tall mountain peaks to see octogenarians still working in their fields, climbing the steep mountains paths to and from their gardens. Women and men not uncommonly reach one hundred years of age. Many live even longer. Other populations in southern Russia and Vilcambamba, Peru likewise testify to the significance of a simple lifestyle in their ability to live a long, fruitful, and productive life.

As a rule, these distinguished people who live to a ripe old age are content with their ultra-simple lifestyle. Their diet is ungarnished, largely vegetarian, with varied combinations of fruits, grains, nuts, and vegetables. Traditionally, they are simply prepared. These people use a minimum of refined modern foods, such as sugar and free fats. These, as you know, have been shown to accelerate the progress of degenerative diseases. Outdoor living is the norm. Their chosen pastoral, rural life is lower in stress, though seeming primitive by Western standards. Habits such as tobacco smoking and alcohol imbibing are rare, for their pleasures are found in a traditional, family centered, social life that brings both satisfaction and peace of mind.

Many of these healthy populations of centenarians continue active physically, taking their daily walk, working in flower beds, or cultivating fruits and vegetables. Memories are well preserved, with a keen sense of humor. Many enjoy telling stories that span many decades of history, giving a rich insight to the culture of a people who have learned how to live.

MIDDLE AGED FOR LIFE

Researchers of biological aging have found that one sign of good aging is the quality of each person's attitude toward the past. People living in nursing homes, especially, have a time perspective primarily concerned with the past. Perhaps this reflects their lack of sense of future outlook for themselves. The elderly invalid's escape to the past may produce less stress than facing the next inevitable step, death. In contrast, reviewing the past but not dwelling on it, can play an important role in adapting healthfully to old age. One esteemed author has said it well, *"We have nothing to fear for the future, except as we shall forget the way the Lord has led us and teaching in our past history."* (Ellen G. White, *Life Sketches,* page 195.)

There is a great capacity for growth in most older people. However, it is too often buried in the sad stereotype of the elderly as being very rigid. Rigidity is not a function of age. Rather, it is part of one's own personality structure. The capacity for curiosity, creativity, surprise, and change does not **invariably** decline with age. In fact, the desire to change and grow can be heightened by the realization that life is drawing to a close.

Many elderly folk will experience a substantial loss of independence. Having a determining role in the scheme of things is important for our mental health. By exercising creatively the brain, this decision making power may even help protect against senility and eventual mental deterioration. One key to keeping older people independently involved in the decision-making process affecting their own lives and affairs is a well preserved, strong family tie. In many situations, the elderly are apart from their family, but maintain regular contact through daily visits or phone calls. The majority of our senior population in the U.S.A. live near at least one child, and see their grandchildren regularly.

Most older Americans prefer to be independent of their families. And, they frequently achieve this until they can no longer manage for themselves. Then, they expect their children to come to their aid. Not only are such expectations realistic, but they are usually fulfilled. Eight percent of the older persons receiving home care get it from family members. The older and sicker the individual, the more likely he or she will have to live with a child. This in harmony with the 5th Commandment given on Sinai: *"Honour thy father and thy mother: that thy days may be long upon the land which the Lord thy God giveth thee."* (Exodus 20: 12).

Although **independence** is a highly desired goal, capacities and desires for it vary widely among older people. One indomitable person will be able to maintain his or her own home for decades. However, a fearful, timid neighbor may have to move to a more protective setting. Thus, the older individuals have as many variations in their needs, desires, and abilities to find fulfillment as do people of any age.

One very **basic need** that each senior citizen expresses is the continued desire to be productive. Helping to maintain his or her home, contributing to the family's financial support, sponsoring charity projects in churches or social agencies—all these bring joy to those who have spent a lifetime serving others. How good it is when a person who has accumulated some wealth, a retirement income, or a valuable property can have the satisfaction of seeing it used for the good of their church, the welfare of beloved family members, or to advance missionary enterprises at home or abroad.

The years of middle age are usually considered most productive ones. Nonetheless, those who retire early often do their best work at that time. Being free from prior distractions, and with the accumulated wisdom and knowledge of many experiences, these senior citizens frequently prove valuable as statesmen, counselors, authors, and guides to the younger generation. Creativity and rugged individuality may characterize the senior citizen, who has well earned the respect of both their family and the surrounding community. Still vigorous and active in mind, these valuable members of society, both men and women, may with proper care of their health and cultivation of the spirit exemplify our vision of "being middle aged for life."

HEALTH PROBLEMS OF THE ELDERLY

One of the greatest threats that our elderly friends face is the possibility of premature senility, sometimes called **Alzheimer's disease**. It is the only total disability that cannot be coped with in some creative way. Senility virtually marks the early "death" of our organ of personality, the forebrain. Senile people lose their individuality; their behavior becomes progressively disorganized.

Fortunately, most senior citizens never become senile. However, a substantial minority, about 30% of those over the age of 80, show evidence of forgetfulness and confusion. This, nonetheless, usually constitutes an unoffending side effect of the normal slowing down that comes with age. Many diseases occur at younger ages, but in the elderly apparently minor illnesses sometimes produce symptoms of disorientation.

Physicians sometimes fail to realize that older people sometimes react differently to their manifestation of disease than do younger people. Neglecting to recognize the peculiarities of older people, including their sensitivity to certain drugs, their noncompliance with therapy, or the way they sometimes mask symptoms such as pain and fever, may lead to misinterpretation by the patient's family doctor. This could deprive an elderly patient of care that would restore him or her to optimally useful life. As many as 10 to 20% of the three million elderly diagnosed as senile are in actuality grossly mislabeled. They suffer, not from dementia—progressive loss of memory and brain function—but rather from conditions that could be treated, if properly diagnosed and managed.

For example, some old men and women who appear confused may simply be dehydrated, since the sensation of thirst diminishes with age. Other conditions which cause brain dysfunction include metabolic diseases, such as diabetes and thyroid problems, nutritional deficiencies caused by faulty diets, and discrete physical illnesses, such as anemia, brain tumors, or kidney failure.

Depression in the elderly individual is easily misdiagnosed as senility because of the similarity of symptoms— poor memory, confusion, and a somber melancholia. The elderly are more prone to depression because of their multiple and irreversible losses, the social isolation, and feelings of uselessness that characterize too many lives. In fact, depression is one of the most common indicators of stress among the elderly.

Providing practical alternatives to loneliness can ameliorate much depression in the aging person. A residence in the child's home, meaningful worship experiences, being included in the social activities of the family, these can bring the elderly relative back to the mainstream of really living. The inadvertent misuse of drugs may cause mental instability and depressive side effects. People over sixty-five use 25% of all medications prescribed, yet many physicians are unaware that the elderly have a lowered tolerance to drugs. It is possible for some of the thirteen different drugs customarily taken per year by the average senior citizen, to interact adversely with each other. Often the best treatment a physician can offer is simply to decrease or halt entirely the use of these chemical agents.

Aging is characterized by a multitude of losses—loss of vigor, loss of life-long career, eventual loss of a spouse of many years, death of good friends, etc. These multiple losses can produce major stress, and are a common basis for depression. Consider the conflict that retirement evokes. After decades of deriving (ideally) great satisfaction from work, most men and an increasing number of women are eligible to retire by the age of sixty-five. It is usually difficult to give up that older familiar occupational role for a new, seemingly lesser one. Having or acquiring a hobby offers a wonderful safeguard to the joys of retirement. Enjoying helping in the neighborhood, caring for lawn and garden, using skills in sewing, arts, or craftsmanship can with minimal expenditure of finances— and even the possibility of a supplemental income— bring joy and satisfaction to the retiree. Individuals who are affected by the emotional impact of retirement often complain about headaches, loss of sleep, irritability, gastrointestinal symptoms, and nervousness. Anticipating these retirement years and preparing for them psychologically will make the ultimate adjustment easier.

One patient, an active white-haired lady in her early eighties, told me that she had determined years ago what she was going to do as she reached this old age. When in her forties she looked around and noticed that many elderly individuals were always welcome in their children's home, sought after as counselors by friends, and generally welcomed wherever they went. Others, on the other hand, were not so welcome, for they had acquired characteristics that made them a trial to their family. A sour disposition, chronic complaining, and ill temper had developed through the years, decreasing their acceptance in their children's homes. My patient determined then, as a middle-aged woman, to cultivate those characteristics that would make the elderly welcome. Finally, in her eighties, this goal was realized.

The loss of a lifelong companion is one of the greatest stresses faced by the elderly. While widowhood is not usually anticipated, as is retirement, women are more prepared for it than are men. Widowhood for men is initially much more disruptive and disturbing. Many men have relied upon their wives for meeting people, and maintaining continuing relationships with friends. Moreover, during the senior years, most older men live with a wife. Only one-third of older women live with a husband. Yet, all may achieve if they will, the spirit of contentment so conductive to peace of mind. *"Thou will keep him in perfect peace, whose mind is stayed on thee: because he trusteth in thee."* (Isaiah 26:3).

SIMPLE TREATMENTS FOR COMMON SYMPTOMS

We have already discussed many emotional problems affecting older people. Depression, worry, fear, and loneliness often have specific causes. These can be remedied with a determined will and a strong faith in God. There are, besides, physical symptoms that express themselves more commonly in senior citizens. These may involve nearly any system in the body. Most commonly, they affect the cardiovascular, gastrointestinal, and urinary systems.

Pain seems to be a not uncommon companion of the senior citizen. Chapter Two presents many causes and treatments of pain patterns. However, some appear more commonly in older individuals. **Arthritis** in the spine can produce chronic pain. This is particularly common in the neck, and may lead to degeneration of the bones, with formation of spurs that could compress one of the spinal nerves. Headaches are regularly caused by these arthritic manifestations. The symptoms may be aggravated by certain positions. The application of a cervical pillow shaped like a bolster, and the use of intermittent neck traction, heat, or massage gives considerable relief to such patients. Often with aging comes a shortened height, the bones gradually losing their calcium and mineral content as the spine settles. There may be some bowing of the upper back or a twisting of the spine into an "S" configuration *(scoliosis)*. This frequently makes it more difficult to ambulate, carry heavy loads, and may later even create difficulty in walking. Careful posture is important, as well as caution in working around the house to prevent accidents and falls.

Arthritis affects the joints of the feet and hands, or the large articulations in the hips, knees, or elbows. Arthritic degeneration is usually of the type characterized in Chapter Five as *degenerative joint disease.* First, the cartilage wears out. Then, the resultant rubbing of two non-padded bones together creates a painful response, frequently associated with weather changes. Many aged sufferers from this so-called "rheumatism" can predict accurately an approaching storm, because the aching in their joints seems to track barometric changes.

If possible, the arthritic individual should be encouraged to take warm tub baths, or use heating pads and moist hot compresses to relieve the local joint pain. Clothing the extremities adequately will help to prevent painful suffering, particularly in women, who seem more intolerant to cold. Especially, keep the knees, ankles, and feet warm, while protecting equally in colder weather the upper extremities. This includes wearing warm gloves.

Common cardiovascular symptoms that frequently affect the older patient are palpitations, dizziness, fainting spells, and periodic shortness of breath. **Congestive heart failure** causes most of these manifestations. It is commonly caused by arteriosclerosis. **Angina pectoris** may appear with minimal activity if the disease is particularly advanced. **Heart attacks** are not uncommon in the elderly, producing characteristic changes in the electrocardiogram and carrying risk of sudden death. Frequently, the heart attack lacks the crushing chest pain that characterizes a massive heart attack in a younger individual, thus making it harder to diagnose. Blood pressure tends to rise with advancing age, paralleling a progressive hardening of the arteries. Chapter Four outlines several symptoms and their rational treatment approaches whenever heart disease is suspected.

The **appetite** may decrease in older individuals. Quite often, this is linked with depression. Loneliness or physical handicaps makes the healthful preparation of food more challenging. Profound weight loss sometimes occurs. As always when the causes are elusive, medical investigation should exclude other causes, such as silently developing tumors, heart disease, or a side effect of medication.

Constipation appears frequently in the elderly. Declining physical activity and a failure to drink adequate amounts of water are common causes. The diet may be too refined, due to the person's inability to prepare a variety of natural foods. On the other hand, he or she may lack sufficient teeth to permit thorough mastication. Laxative abuse is common; using enemas, herbal laxatives, and over–the–counter medicines becomes a way of life. Nevertheless, this substitutes poorly for a proper natural diet, including plenty of fiber, drinking an abundance of water, and exercising in the out–of–doors. All this takes time, but it will yield great dividends.

Foot care may pose a problem. Arthritis in the larger joints makes it difficult to reach your feet to properly clean and trim the nails, or care for painful callouses. Shrinkage (atrophy) of subcutaneous tissue may make bony prominences prone to rub on loose-fitting shoes. I recommend the use of a flat foot file, made either of pumice or metal. Get one with a sturdy handle that is easy to grasp by an older individual. File the callouses and corns, and wear protective moleskin pads to decrease the foot trauma that makes walking painful.

With the increased wrinkling of aging skin, the subcutaneous tissue is lost. Then, the risk of circulatory impairment becomes another health hazard, almost exclusively seen in bedfast older patients. **Decubitus ulcers**, or "bed sores," can be painfully debilitating. They are occasionally found in nursing home patients, especially where inadequate care is given. Prolonged pressure over a bony prominence, usually the hip bones, the sacrum, or the heels breaks down the skin to invite infection. Decubitus ulcers grow rapidly as infection undermines the adjacent tissue, even extending to the bone. Meticulously cleanse such ulcers with hydrogen peroxide or a disinfectant soap. Then, follow this with hygienic protective measures to promote recovery. Pad the susceptible part with sheepskin, foam rubber, and frequently shift the patient's position. These home nursing routines are important to prevent pressure over vulnerable areas of skin breakdown. Pack deeper ulcers with granulated sugar, and wash it out after four to six hours. Change the dressing several times a day to stimulate the formation of granulation tissue and decrease the multiplication of germs. The sugar concentrate prohibits germ multiplication while gradually cleaning up infected areas. Special enzymes may also help to clean the area. These are marketed in an ointment base (such as *Elase*). On the other hand, they can be compounded from papaya or fig preparations containing similar protein dissolving ingredients (*papain* and *ficin*, respectively).

Increased bruising may present a problem, as well as slow healing abrasions. Protect the elbows and forearms with long-sleeved pajamas, or wear special pads over the elbows, heels, or knees. This is definitely advisable in debilitated patients to lessen the likelihood of skin trauma. It can really hurt.

Urinary symptoms may predominate. Incontinence is the most common and distressing. It is discouraging to have to wear a diaper or other protection in order to prevent involuntary urine leakage. This occurs often in older women as the bladder's muscle tone relaxes, or in men as a complication of prostate surgery. Careful evaluation by urologist may be necessary. Be sure to test the urine for possible infection when there is any difficulty in urination. Infection does not always produce the symptoms of burning, frequency, and urgency so typical in younger people. Many senior citizens therefore carry a bladder infection without knowledge that these infecting germs are harbored there. Usually, all one needs to do is increase the fluid intake, drinking ten to twelve glasses of water daily. Consider using supplements of Buchu tea, cranberry juice, or Vitamin C (two grams/day) to combat the resistant bacteria causing infection.

Although many disease conditions occur in our aging population, their clinical courses and treatment are not significantly different from those at other ages. Specific chapters dealing with each type of disease and body system can be consulted (see Table of Contents) to better understand the meaning of symptoms and help find the simplest remedy that may be employed right at home. Periodic medical consultations may be required to pinpoint the diagnosis and provide a needed laboratory diagnosis. Although aging is inevitable, sickness is not. With proper attention to the laws of health and strict obedience to their principles, the sunset years can be full of glory—ever changing, always beautiful. *"The hoary head is a crown of glory, if it be found in the way of righteousness."* (Proverbs 16:31).

CHAPTER TWENTY-SIX

OVERCOMING

UNHEALTHFUL

HABITS

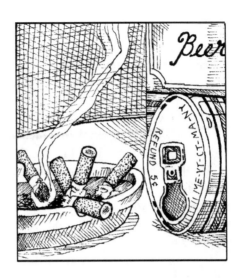

All of us are creatures of habit. From earliest childhood we have repeated many actions, until distinct habits are fixed in our lifestyle. These make up the character of a man or woman. Some habits are good, while others are obviously harmful. A few habits are destructive to society, as well as to the individual. Remember now, *there can be change without improvement; but there can be no improvement without change.* It is for specific aid in this facet of getting well that I focus on some current habits in the American lifestyle. May the information gained in this chapter bring temperance, sobriety, and peace of mind to any reader who is troubled in mind, or enslaved to some poison.

ALCOHOL

Knowledge of chemical alcohol by science and industry is only about 100 years old. However, the production of fermented beverages goes back to antiquity. As early as 2,300 B.C., the patriarch Noah overindulged. Alcohol was the sad downfall of two priests, Nadab and Abihu, during the time of the exodus. About 1,000 B.C. the wise king, Solomon, said, *"Wine is a mocker, strong drink is raging: and whosoever is deceived is not wise"* (Proverbs 20:1).

In the process of fermentation, starches and sugars are converted by yeast enzymes into ethyl alcohol and carbon dioxide. Grain is fermented to produce **beer**, which usually contains 4 to 8% alcohol. Grape juice is the major source of fermented wine, which is 6 to 8% alcohol. This is called **wine** (Hebrew—*yayin*; Greek—*oinos*) in the Bible. When sugar is mingled with the grape juice, fermentation continues further, producing a 14% concentration of alcohol in the wine (sometimes called "strong drink" in the Old Testament,

Hebrew—*shekar*). Enzymes in most types of yeast are naturally inhibited by this much alcohol. To produce liquors with higher than 14% alcohol (maximum fermentation), distillation must occur, or pure alcohol may be added.

By definition, alcohol is classified with organic chemical compounds, containing carbon, oxygen, and hydrogen. Several different alcohols are known. **Methanol** (CH_3OH) is wood alcohol, a very toxic poison to the body, producing blindness when ingested. **Ethyl alcohol**, or ethanol, (C_2H_5OH) is the so-called beverage alcohol, produced by the fermentation of grain. **Isopropyl alcohol** (C_3H_7OH) is used as a disinfectant (called *rubbing alcohol*). More complex alcohols are all highly toxic. Adding oxygen to ethyl alcohol can produce antifreeze (*ethylene glycol*). This is also harmful to the body. Glycerol, the molecule backbone of fats, and many waxes is closely related chemically to ordinary alcohol.

To understand better the naming of alcoholic beverages, let's consider their origins. By grain fermentation one obtains beer (4 to 8% alcohol), and ale (14% alcohol); distillation produces whiskey, gin, and vodka (40 to 50% alcohol). It was the custom in olden days to *prove* that the amount of alcohol on their label was correct by igniting it. Fifty percent alcohol will burn with a light blue flame. Thus, one hundred "proof" whiskey contains 50% alcohol.

Fermentation of fruit juice produces wine, as mentioned above, and brandy (30 to 50% alcohol, after distillation). Since the government tax is very high on ethyl alcohol, it is "denatured" for use in laboratories. This is accomplished by the addition of a bitter alkaloid or foul-smelling substance (*pyridine*), rendering it unfit to drink.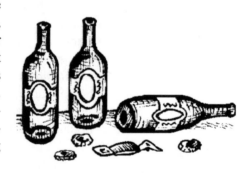

Unlike food nutrients, alcohol can be absorbed directly from the stomach into the blood. Approximately 20% of that ingested enters the body in this way. The remainder is absorbed into the small intestine. The simultaneous ingestion of food decreases this absorption rate. Only a small amount, less than 5% of the ingested alcohol is excreted in the urine or expired air. Ninety percent of this toxin must be removed from the body by chemical oxidation. This is done by a liver enzyme called *alcohol dehydrogenase*. The rate of oxidation varies in individuals. Ordinarily about ten to fifteen ml. of alcohol can be oxidized per hour in the liver, a rate which is relatively constant. This reaction gradually decreases the alcohol blood level after ingestion. Oxidation of alcohol produces seven calories of heat energy per gram, however, this is of practically no nutritional value.

The level of alcohol in the blood can be measured. The legal limit for defining intoxication is 0.1% in most states. This can be reached by the drinking of four to five "shots" of whiskey, six cans of beer, or the same number of glasses of wine. The difference of concentration in these various beverages accounts for the fact that approximately the same number of any alcoholic drink can produce equivalent intoxication.

A number of diseases are associated with alcohol use. Attacks of **gout** occur when the alcohol consumption increases blood *lactic acid*, which in turn suppresses the secretion of uric acid by the kidney. Alcohol–induced increases in liver enzymes may cause fatty change of that vital organ, particularly when alcohol intake is combined with an inadequate diet. There is an increased secretion of zinc and magnesium in the urine of drinkers, tending toward liver damage, nerve impairment, and eventual psychosis. The "**empty calories**" obtained from alcoholic beverages contribute toward obesity in many, and malnutrition in other individuals. Cardiac damage, with sudden rhythm disturbances, has recently been associated with the heavy, chronic use of alcohol.

If all we had to do in medicine was study the chemistry of alcohol, the challenge would interest many. However, we are left with the stark realization that alcohol is destroying more than health! Much of our present erosion of moral values, the decline in governmental integrity, increasing tension in international relations, deterioration of the family unit, and growing statistics of suicide, most can be traced directly to alcohol consumption. The risk of becoming an alcoholic is currently thought to be about 5.6%, or 1 in 18, for all who drink. However, this figure is rising. Today, over ten million people in the United States are classed as *alcoholics*. Eight million more signify their dependence on this substance, demonstrating the disruption to their lives and families with divorce, delinquency and death.

Mortality rates among alcoholics increase annually. Alcoholism is the 10th leading cause of death in California, number six among those aged 35-54. In general, life expectancy of an alcoholic is 10-12 years less than the national average. Information from our National Institute of Mental Health shows a steady trend toward increased alcohol-related admissions to state mental hospitals. One in seven inmates in such hospitals is an alcoholic—an 18% rise in the last ten years! This is definitely serious.

Looking at **crimes** and accidents, we again see alcohol taking its toll. Nearly half of the arrests made each year are for drunkenness, public intoxication, or disorderly conduct related to alcohol. The cost of alcohol-triggered crime runs into the millions. Industries pay also, with a price tag over $4,000,000,000 (four billion dollars) annually. Four to five percent of most company employees are involved in problem-drinking, irrespective of their income level. Increased absenteeism results, as well as decreased work performance, and the gradual loss of special industrial skills.

The number of problem drinkers among **women** and **teenagers** increases rapidly. According to a recent survey, 68% of American adults use alcoholic beverages—77% men and 60% women. Twelve percent of all adults are heavy drinkers.

Motor vehicle accidents markedly increase under the influence of alcohol. Approximately 50% of vehicle fatalities have been associated with alcohol. All too often, innocent people are thus murdered. Pedestrians as well as motorists are affected. One large insurance company (Preferred Risk Mutual) even gives preferential rates on auto insurance to nondrinkers. Household accidents are affected, with 14% of the male and 20% of our female deaths by home accidents associated with alcohol. Such diverse causes as drug overdose, motor exhaust, fires, falls, drowning, and exposure to cold may appear on the death certificate. Nonetheless, alcohol is often the real culprit.

However, more serious than all we have mentioned above are **alcohol's effects on the nervous system of man.** Dr. Cyril Courville has thoroughly documented many forms of long-term damage associated with drinking. Permanent shrinkage of the brain, with actual loss in its volume as well as functional disorders have been described. Studies by Dr. Melvin Kniseley at the University of South Carolina showed how this brain destruction takes place. As beverage alcohol ingestion increases, the blood flow through small vessels begins to stagnate. Clumping of blood cells then occurs, with sludging and decreased oxygen delivery to vital areas. Doctor Kniseley demonstrated how one drinking bout could irreversibly damage *hundreds* of brain cells. How many can we afford to lose?

Not only does alcohol injure adults and teenagers, but the unborn child is affected. The **fetal alcohol syndrome** is receiving increased attention in current medical literature. This syndrome is characterized by growth retardation, mental retardation, with a characteristic facial appearance that the child carries for life. A pregnant woman who drinks alcoholic beverages is, without question, jeopardizing the social success, intellectual growth, and physical prowess of her offspring.

All of this information should lead people to choose the path of total abstinence. Yet, our problem of alcoholism looms ever higher. Millions of teenagers are caught in its clutches, seeking a vain escape from the pressures of real life. Millions of dollars are spent for research each year, following the alcoholic around, checking his or her whims and fancies, and studying their environment. Then we watch this growing army of over ten million alcoholics increase, only to eventually drop by the wayside. Most of these research studies center on the *effects* of alcohol consumption. Some focus on *rehabilitation*. Notwithstanding, we believe it obvious that two things are required to produce an alcoholic, the **drink** and the **drinker**.

Perhaps we should focus more on the harmful beverages. This concept is right in harmony with most dedicated temperance advocates, who have known for years that "alcohol makes alcoholics." Actually, the problem is like a jigsaw puzzle, where **all** pieces need to fit together to make a perfect picture.

Fortunately, more efforts are being made each year to rehabilitate the *victims* of intemperance. In seeking to cure alcoholism, let's first consider the **physical** dimension of man. Usually, in attempting to change the alcoholic's life pattern, we first must give attention to his or her physical needs.

Improper eating habits have too often set the "stage" for compulsive drinking. Therefore, proper **nutrition** is fundamental to a successful transition from habitual intoxication to sobriety.

374

One beneficial effect of improved nutrition appears when vitamins and minerals are replenished. The liver rapidly responds, with healing and regeneration of its tissues. Disease of the nerves is frequently related to a alcohol-induced deficiency in **B complex** vitamins. One study, for example, showed how laboratory animals (white rats) who were given only white bread voluntarily drank much more alcohol than those who were on a whole grain cereal ration. Similar studies at Loma Linda University's School of Nutrition demonstrated that voluntary alcohol drinking of laboratory rats is accelerated on a diet of "junk food," a menu similar to that of the average U.S.A. teenager. With heavy dietary priority on sugar, spices, fried foods, and pastries, a rapid increase of alcohol consumption was observed. When coffee was added to the diet, the drinking behavior reached alarming proportions, showing caffeine to be a powerful stimulant for thirst of alcohol.

Rich diets tend similarly to create a desire for strong drink. An overabundance of meats, sweet confections, and excessively salty foods all tend to promote the abnormal thirst for alcohol, especially in susceptible individuals. To rehabilitate an alcoholic, then, the diet must be of the most simple kind. It must provide maximum nourishment to the system with a superior content of natural nutrients. Whole grains, rich in the B–complex vitamins, with naturally prepared vegetables and fruits, contain these elements. Also, the necessary trace minerals help foster a calmness to the nervous system. This serenity decreases any abnormal stimulation to the animal passions, thereby lessening an innate propensity toward alcoholism.

Exercise is extremely vital for the alcoholic. His or her occupation should be satisfying and steady, contributing directly toward eventual financial independence. Preferably, the occupation should be out–of–doors, where an abundance of pure air and sunshine can be obtained.

Adequate rest at night and frequent periods of recreation are beneficial. Mental attitudes can be distorted, with unnatural physical cravings stimulated, by excessive fatigue. Unless these habits are soon corrected, exhaustion will eventually sabotage the nervous system. Thus, many physiologic factors are related to the all–too–frequent falls from sobriety that plague each victim of alcoholism.

Secondly, but much more primary, are the **mental** factors. Temperance advocates for many decades have encouraged alcohol users to sign a *pledge of total abstinence*. This document has proved a safeguard to many in times of sudden temptation. The true force of our **will power** must be understood by any person struggling with temptation. The will is the governing power in the nature of man—the power of decision, of choice. **Everything depends on the right action of the will.** Notwithstanding, this power of choice must be exercised in order to grow strong. Through the proper use of your will power, an entire change may be make in the life.

Many view alcohol dependency as a learned behavior pattern. In order to overcome its clutches, your will must be enlisted to make a strong effort to form better health habits. The "conditioned response" to drinking must be replaced, never again allowed to predominate over more desirable behaviors.

Social aspects of alcoholism create enormous problems. The apostle Paul said, *"none of us liveth to himself,"* (Romans 14:7). We are gregarious beings, meant to live in communities. Sadly, our culture still fosters social drinking, and has thus set the stage for alcoholism.

The role of hospitality is significant. In some social circles, a guest who does not drink is considered out of place, simply not a part of the social group. Party hosts play their roles, pressing drinks upon each guest. One who does not participate is regarded as stingy, and runs the real risk of becoming a target of malicious gossip. Thus, dubious social factors that encourage alcohol abuse must first be curtailed, and drinking behavior de-emphasized. Then our society may improve in its efforts to combat the growing trend toward alcoholism.

Thirst is a normal physiologic reaction. Usually it indicates a need for water. If this most precious beverage is preferentially used as a thirst quencher, with fruit juices or herb teas as alternates, satisfactory host-guest relationships can continue, while sensible sobriety survives.

We must never overlook the powerful forces of commercial interests in aggravating the problem of alcoholism. Consistent propaganda bombards our minds from billboards, TV, radio, and magazines, all appealing to the weaknesses of humanity. Advertisers hold alcohol up as great and grand, while hiding the inevitable emptiness, poverty, and disease that follow. The entire brewing industry devotes millions of dollars to promoting their beverages. They do this, not as benefactors of the human race, but, like a *wolf in sheep's clothing*, to its destruction. Liquor peddlers have purely commercial interests in mind. Legislators tend to shift the emphasis, and allow continued promotion and sale of alcohol poisons. Even now liquor is making inroads into schools and churches, corrupting our unguarded, uninformed, unsuspecting youth.

Freudian psychology must carry its share of the blame. Sigmund Freud's doctrine teaches that in childhood nothing is to be restrained or denied. Every whim or wish is to be met. Thus, we see modern society "doing its own thing." Humanism's scholarly breakdown of moral values paved the way for a new type of liberation, falsely termed *freedom*. It is **not** just "your own business" what you do when drinking behavior disrupts the home, causes accidents, increases crime, and puts people into the hospital, as well as the local morgue.

This brings me to one of the most basic aspects of alcohol and a costly clue to successful rehabilitation. No lasting or strong impression can make our world decent through intellectual power alone. Conscience, heart, and soul must be enlisted if your life will be channeled in the way of salvation. **Alcoholics Anonymous** recognizes the importance of this spiritual dimension. Of their twelve steps, the first one states, *"We have come to believe that a power greater than ourselves could restore us to sanity."* The second step follows, *"We sought through prayer and meditation to improve our contact with God as we under-*

stood Him, praying for knowledge of His will for us and the power to carry it out."

Therefore, while we give first attention to the physical condition, providing wholesome food, clean clothing, and an opportunity to work, we must never neglect the **spiritual power** found in personal prayer. Open your Bible and read the promises of God to each struggling one. This will bring power like *leaves from the tree of life.* As you choose to serve God and give Him your will, He will work in us *"to will and to do according to His good pleasure,"* (Philippians 2:13). Thus, your whole nature may be brought under the control of God, the One who always has your best good in mind.

Little by little the alcoholic becomes restored in health. Next, his or her regained sense of self-respect will lead them to work for others. This ministry should be encouraged. In association with experienced, God-fearing servants, the rehabilitated one may help in lifting others from the pit of destruction where they themselves were rescued. Some of the redeemed will stand nearest to the throne of God in the final days, loving their Savior the most because they have been forgiven most.

TOBACCO

No generation has received more scientific light on the use of tobacco than ours. When the first Surgeon General's report, *Smoking and Health*, came off the presses, Americans realized that the mounting research pointed a long accusing finger at the substance called tobacco. Nevertheless, in spite of the over 100,000 doctors who quit smoking and the numerous adults who gave up the habit in response, a new threat now emerges.

For two decades since 1964 the pernicious smoking habit has risen sharply among girls. Furthermore, tobacco addiction remains virtually at the same level among women. They have really "come a long way"! Surgeon General Richmond's 1979 report revealed 100,000 children twelve years old or younger smoking, with six million teen puffers under the age of twenty. Unfortunately, women become hooked more readily than men; and they are finding it harder to quit.

Because of these facts a recent H.E.W. (Department of Health, Education & Welfare) secretary called smoking a "national tragedy." All modern scientific data simply echoes the hundred-year-old assertion of Ellen G. White, a prominent temperance lecturer, who declared, *"Tobacco is a slow, insidious, but most malignant poison,"* (see *The Ministry of Healing*, page 327). That warning was decades ahead of modern medical research worldwide.

The fight for clean air was spurred on by research in the 1970's. Scientists discovered that **side-stream smoke** rising from each cigarette when the smoker is not puffing contains a heavy concentration of poisonous substances. Thus, the thoughtless smoker's gift to his or her immediate environment is about like automobile exhaust in a closed garage. High concentrations of **carbon monoxide** pollute the *passive smoker's* blood when he or she sits or works in an unventilated room blue with smoke. Alas, this could be your living room, a conference room, an automobile, or even your bedroom. It does not just apply to the local bar.

Carbon monoxide (CO) is one of the three leading killers found in tobacco smoke. It ties up the vital hemoglobin in our red blood cells, inhibiting their ability to carry oxygen. Carbon monoxide, moreover, injures the delicate lining of coronary arteries, opening "holes" in their *endothelial* lining cells, thereby permitting cholesterol to enter. Low levels of CO can disturb our senses, including vigilance, color discrimination, peripheral vision, and the complex processing of information. These proficiencies are crucial for driving, flying, and really living.

Children of smoking parents are really in for trouble. Pneumonia and bronchitis during the first year of life appear twice as commonly in children, if both parents smoke. Even the baby's risk of sudden infant death increases. Additionally, the example of parents is sadly tarnished by the smoking image projected. "Like father, like son" is more than a trite cliche.

Lung cancer is the leading killer in smokers, caused principally by chemical *carcinogens*, substances which produce cancer. *Benz-0-pyrine* and numerous similarly potent chemicals are inhaled in the mainstream smoke. Involuntary (second-hand) smokers are affected, too. Because the acceptance of female smokers has matured, lung cancer in women is five times greater today than in 1964, and is still rising. Some analysts predicted that if modern "liberated" women continued this trend, lung cancer would become the number one malignant killer for them, as it has been for men. That prediction is now fulfilled.

Unfortunately, surgery and other high-priced healing measures still fail to save people from death. Only 30% of those who get lung cancer survive even one year. Five years later less than 10% are still alive. The longer you smoke, the more you smoke, and the more you inhale, the worse becomes your cancer risk. Using more than one pack per day will give any smoker **ten times the risk of lung cancer**, compared to the nonsmoker!

Moreover, on its way to your lungs, tobacco smoke goes through the *larynx*, or voice box. As a result, there is three times more cancer of the larynx among smoking women, even when they smoke filter tips. But if a woman smokes more than one pack per day, this risk jumps to twenty-one times more!

Babies born to smoking mothers weigh about one–half pound less than the average full-term infant. The nicotine poison in tobacco constricts the delicate uterine arteries, supplying nutrients to her womb. Smaller chests and

378

smaller heads are seen in these tiny "smokers of the womb." Mental retardation in such children lasts for years. Damage becomes most severe in the unfortunate children born to mothers that have smoked the most. Stunted height, retarded growth, and decreased learning ability all appear in the offspring of smoking mothers. In animal studies, even subsequent generations have been affected by maternal tobacco use.

Scientists calculate that smoking kills more than 346,000 people per year in the U.S.A. alone! Sixty-five percent of these deaths come from heart attacks and strokes. This means one funeral every minute, ten hours per day, all year round. Tobacco's chemicals, carbon monoxide and nicotine, are both poisonous to the heart and major arteries. Blood pressure rises, pulse rate increases, and the calcification of cholesterol plaques advances rapidly. When alcohol is combined with tobacco the calamity increases. Smoking just one cigarette makes some of your blood cells (*platelets*) sticky. Clots form more readily in heart (*coronary*) and brain arteries.

Thus, current evidence shows tobacco smoking as a major world health problem, not only for men and women, but for unborn children, and for the rest of us who cannot avoid the smoker's poisonous breath. Tobacco smoking is a horrible habit, as well as a powerful addiction. Fortunately, for the smoker who wants to quit, there is a better plan.

Most addicted smokers know that they would be better off if they could kick the habit. Some pause to wonder, "Should I taper off or stop cold turkey?" For several reasons, it is best to quit immediately. Quitting, actually, is not as hard as you might think. Over forty million Americans have done it already. Here is a simple program to make it easier:

First, determine to quit. Then, **stop all at once**. It is much easier on your system to have a few rough days and be through with it, than to drag the quit-smoking torture out for weeks and months. Set a goal of ten days to completely restructure your life. The *ten day plan* worked wonders for Daniel.

When a person quits smoking the hardest part comes during the first three days. However, by the end of the fifth day, most individuals find the craving just about gone. Repeat often the words, **"I choose not to smoke."** Firmly maintain your decision from morning till night. Be sure you really mean it. Many people discover with the hourly repetition of this decision, a growing positive resistance develops to the physical craving for tobacco.

Remember the effect of **will power** on your mind and body. Therefore, use the power of choice to strengthen your resolution. Through a proper use of your will, you can gradually bring other habits under the control of your newly enlightened reason. Claim divine help every day. Besides, pray for heaven's power; for this victory is God's best plan for you, too.

Water will help you in flushing out the poisons. Drink at least 6-8 glasses of water, especially between meals. Remember, take no alcoholic beverage, absolutely nothing that could weaken your will power. Try drinking a glass or two of hot lemon water upon arising each morning. You can make it with lemon juice (bottled) or squeeze one or two teaspoonful into a glass of hot water. Then drink another glassful now and then throughout the day. Warm tub baths also will help you relax.

The **cold mitten friction** is a powerful natural stimulant that helps soothe jangled nerves. It will really speed up your circulation. After taking a warm to hot shower, turn on the cold water. Immediately rub your skin briskly with a wash cloth until it glows. As blood vessels on the surface dilate, a healthy pink skin color predominates. This tonic effect will make you feel wide awake and stimulated, without triggering the craving for another smoke.

Adequate **rest** becomes important, as well as a regular relaxed time for meals. Conserve your nervous energy, and retire early. Fatigue, in many ways, is an enemy to the will power.

Stop-smoking meals should be simple. A **fruit diet** for a day or two is wonderful for cleansing the system. Fruits, grains, vegetables, and nuts may be used abundantly after that, but **nothing between meals**. Avoid highly spiced foods, fried or rich foods, too. Condiments should be bypassed, such as hot sauce, mustard, black pepper, chili, and horse-radish. If it's *"hot when it is cold,"* please avoid it. Give your body a chance to readjust to the new diet. Increased amounts of **B–complex vitamins**, particularly thiamine, will help keep your nerves calm. Be sure to start every day with a good **breakfast**. After meals take a walk. **Exercise** is a wonderful tranquilizer.

Avoid sedatives and stimulants in order to build up your nervous reserve. Skim milk, buttermilk, fruit juices, and water should be your main beverages. **Do not drink any alcohol, coffee, or cola drinks!** Caffeine can trigger an explosive craving for the very tobacco that you are trying to quit! An long-established habit pattern, moreover, may link your cup of coffee with a cigarette, sabotaging the whole stop-smoking plan.

Special tablets and smoker's aids are highly advertised. While some people receive supposed benefits, others find them a waste of money. Group therapies in live-in stop-smoking programs are usually the most successful.

Finally, here is my most important advice when kicking the tobacco habit. **Get help from God!** Make Him your partner. Ask, and you will receive. Our heavenly Father has assured us of His power to aid in overcoming *any* defiling habit. Never hesitate to ask for strength. But, as you ask, **believe** that you will receive it, and you will have your request. As the "irresistible urge" comes, pause and say, **"I choose not to smoke."** Then get a drink of water, take some deep breaths, and breathe a prayer. The craving will gradually lessen.

Maintain these simple habits for a lifetime, if you want to really succeed. Many become careless in their habits of eating, drinking, working, and sleeping. Then they find their will power drifting into inactivity. If your guard drops, the enemy may sneak right in. Your job now is to **establish the habit of *not* smoking** just as firmly, or more so, as before when you had the smoking habit. It may take time. But with God's help, a determined will, and the simple measures mentioned above, you will succeed.

DRUG ADDICTION

Recent changes have occurred in the types of people who use drugs. Addiction at one time was considered limited to the slums, and affecting principally our lower socioeconomic classes. Nowadays, all classes of people are included— university students, the children of wealthy parents, even "good" people coming from religious homes. All drug addicts, however, have certain basic characteristics. Primarily, they are unstable, impulsive, often emotionally disturbed. Their antisocial behavior is the outgrowth of a fundamental character defect— where purpose in life, respect for patents, and love for their fellow men was deficient. They are often demanding, defensive, and self-satisfied. We will look at several types of drugs abused today. But first, let us consider the hallmarks of addiction.

Drug **addiction** is definitely a chemical dependency. There is usually a **physical dependence** on the addicting drug, with physiologic **withdrawal** effects when the drug is not available. **Tolerance** develops in the user's body. Then, the consumer needs an increased dose regularly in order to obtain the same desired effect. A **compulsion** to continue the use of the intoxicating agent is seen. There is obvious physical, mental, and social **harm** to the individual from the use of addicting agents. A **mental dependency** may also be present.

Opium and its derivatives, most of which come from the Middle East and the Orient, are the most heavily used addicting drugs. Opium's derivative compounds, such as **morphine**, are among the most highly addicting substances known to man. Synthetic "relatives" have been prepared in laboratories. Some were initially used by physicians to relieve the pain of surgery or terminal illness, as their addicting potential was not recognized when they were first developed. **Heroin** finds widespread use by urban addicts. It is illegal, of course; and heavy penalties are attached to its use. Notwithstanding, heroin flourishes in most large cities, and not only in the ghettos.

The user of heroin may often have "needle tracks," small puncture marks, usually over a vein on the arm or leg. Abscesses or boils frequently develop at the site of injections. Contamination of shared needles used to inject these depressant drugs may produce blood poisoning (septicemia), infection of the heart valves (*endocarditis*), **hepatitis**, and the frightening possibility of **AIDS** (*HIV*). The death rate from these infections is very high.

A person abusing narcotics will usually have a pallid complexion. Careful scrutiny of the eyes will reveal "pin point" pupils. A craving for sweets and liquid foods is sometimes seen.

The cost of **heroin** addiction is enormous. Several hundred dollars a day may be required to support the habit. Illicit money is frequently obtained by stolen goods or through prostitution. Drug abuse costs society millions of dollars every day.

The rehabilitation of a narcotic addict is extremely difficult. Confinement and isolation are usually necessary. The **withdrawal syndrome** is painful, with abdominal cramps, tremors, nausea and vomiting. There is rapid change of mood, with violent behavior at times. During this detoxification period, which peaks within 24 hours and fades over five to seven days, there is a watery discharge from the eyes and nose and profuse perspiration, as well as painful abdominal symptoms. Fortunately, the withdrawal of heroin or morphine seldom threatens life. Nevertheless, this syndrome often drives the addict back to his or her source of the nearest "fix." Because of the medical difficulty in rehabilitating addicts permanently, our government instituted maintenance programs supplying a "legal" drug, *Methadone,* in carefully supervised centers. This is, however, merely a substitution of one addiction for another. The total rehabilitation of an addict—spiritually, physically, and mentally—can be obtained only when he or she is off all drugs and the lifestyle is changed.

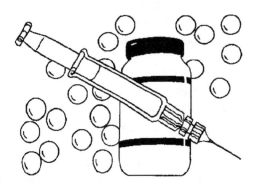

Another class of commonly used depressant drugs is the **barbiturate** compounds. These are all dangerous prescription drugs, and are usually prescribed as sleeping pills. They depress the central nervous system. Most barbiturates are highly addictive. Marketed in red, yellow, and blue capsules, and as colorful (rainbow) combination drugs—Nembutal, Seconal, etc. —barbiturates cause rapid drowsiness and eventual sleep. Overdosage with barbiturates, particularly in combination with alcohol, is a common method of high–society suicide.

Any sudden withdrawal of barbiturates from an addict can be hazardous. The person will feel better in twelve to sixteen hours, but later may develop tremors and twitching behavior. Severe convulsions could occur up to the third day during detoxification. Rarely, rapid barbiturate withdrawal has caused sudden death!

Barbiturate addicts are *mentally* "hooked," psychologically dependent, as well as addicted physically. The body rapidly builds up tolerance, as it does with heroin. Then, increased doses are required for the same effect. The best safeguard against barbiturate addiction is the avoidance of sleeping pills entirely. However, when addiction has occurred, the dosage should be tapered slowly to avoid seizures.

We turn now to several **stimulant drugs**, commonly termed "uppers." **Amphetamines** are the most dangerous stimulants, and are too often prescribed as diet pills. They all stimulate the central nervous system. The hapless user of amphetamines is usually overactive, unusually talkative, frequently argumentative. After taking an amphetamine a person is temporarily unable to eat. He or she has no appetite, and seldom can lie down and rest. Unusual behavior appears as the inhibitions are released. There may be mental confusion, unpredictable and irrational behavior, or even violence. Severe fatigue develops in the overstimulated body, destroying reserves of nervous energy. This depletion makes the user extremely vulnerable to disease.

Psychological dependence upon amphetamines is common. Users regularly return to stimulant abuse, some becoming so uncomfortable that they are unable to manage without their "upper."

One stimulant is customarily injected. **Methamphetamine**, nicknamed "speed," is usually given intravenously. During a so-called "run," the user is in tremendous danger to themselves and their associates. He or she becomes extremely confused, and their behavior irrational and unpredictable. Violence is common, with acute paranoia. Some abusers collect weapons, because they are convinced that people are plotting their death. A "speed freak" may suddenly believe that he or she must "kill before being killed." Visual changes (*hallucinations*) cause people and objects to loom up immediately before the user, then disappear, and alarmingly reappear. "Speed" aggravates any heart condition. It can cause strokes. All amphetamines are harmful to the circulation, increasing the heart rate, as well as the blood pressure.

The "come down" or "crashing" occurs when the abuser stops taking injections. Usually this is unintentional, resulting from his or her exhausting all reserves of energy. He or she then goes into hallucinations, and a deep sleep or coma that lasts from 18 to 48 hours! Profound depression and extreme fatigue will make him or her susceptible to numerous infectious diseases.

Another popular and powerful stimulant is **cocaine**. Its effects upon the body and mind may possibly exceed those of "speed." Cocaine is an extremely hazardous drug, classified a narcotic by law. It is taken in various ways. Some individuals "snort" the cocaine. This can destroy the delicate lining inside the nose. Addiction rapidly occurs; and mental stability is lost.

Recently, a new cheaper type of cocaine appeared. In the crystalline forms, called "crack" and "ice," cocaine can be smoked (*vaporized*) or snorted. Much harm to young people has resulted from the illicit use of cocaine. Drug cartels and hardened criminals make millions from their victims, then discard their prey like broken glass. Citizen groups, government, and churches must do all they can to stop this criminal distribution of cocaine in all its forms.

Some drugs are taken to disorganize the mind. These are called **hallucinogens**. **LSD** is a common one, "blowing the mind" with a very destructive and dangerous "trip." Many hallucinogenic plants and synthetic chemicals are also abused, including **STP**, **peyote** (*mescaline*), and certain species of seeds. Both auditory and visual hallucinations occur, with changes in the level of consciousness. The user of LSD has very unpredictable and irrational behavior. The suddenly disoriented mind may panic. Physical harm results from the bizarre behavior evoked. Some victims have looked at the sun and gone blind. Others have committed suicide under the severe mental changes of a bad "acid trip."

Certain unfortunate sufferers have become psychotic, even permanently insane. Typical abusers can emerge with severely altered personalities. Recurrence, called "flashbacks," may occur up to three years after the last use of LSD! The effects of LSD type drugs can last for extended periods, the so-called "freak out." A terrifying drug experience, "the bummer," may occur. During this "bad trip," the LSD abuser sometimes believes that their face is melting, that they are dying, or already dead, or that suicide has resulted. Obviously LSD is a route to someplace worse than nowhere, an extremely dangerous substance that should *never* be used.

Birth defects have resulted in offspring of parents who took LSD. This is true as well for other mind-affecting drugs. The chromosomes are damaged. The poor child may be mentally retarded, physically deformed, and destined to a life of hardship, just because of some foolishness in a reckless youth.

The use of **marijuana** was briefly discussed in Chapter 18. For completeness, now, I will give an overview of its mind-altering effects. The intoxicant in marijuana is called **THC** *(tetrahydrocannabinol)*. It is a very unpredictable and hazardous drug. **Hashish** is the marijuana plant's *resin* (powder). It causes severe harm to both mind and body. In a person under the influence of any marijuana product, THC disorganizes and confuses many parts of the central nervous system.

The user of marijuana—nicknamed "grass," "pot," or "weed" —may have dilated pupils. The eyes appear large and wide. Dark glasses are often worn to hide their dilated, blood-shot appearance, and also to combat the excessive sensitivity to sunlight. The marijuana abuser exhibits a craving for sweet foods and liquids. Emotional extremes may appear, from drowsiness and depression to anxiety or even hysteria. A false sense of well-being may result, even in the face of real danger. One may develop a very talkative disposition, and be much more vulnerable to suggestion. Thus, the abuse of marijuana often paves the way for the first narcotic drug experience.

Marijuana products have a heavy, musty odor. This odor clings to the user, their clothing, and the surroundings. Typically, the self–achievement level of a marijuana abuser will rapidly decline. School dropouts are common among those who smoke "pot." It is solemn to contemplate how much our society is possibly being shaped today by minds altered by marijuana. Fortunately, its sale is still illegal.

Intravenous injection of marijuana causes nausea and bloody diarrhea. A high fever usually develops, with hemorrhage, shock, or even coma. The withdrawal of marijuana use, however, does not produce any specific syndrome. For this reason it is not considered addicting. Nevertheless, marijuana certainly can produce psychological dependency. This terrible distortion of reality is one of its principal objections. Real life is so much better.

HOW TO OVERCOME

The first prerequisite to overcoming any of these drug habits is **personal determination**. You must want help before you can ever receive it. Desires for health, peace of mind, and a successful future are right in so far as they go. But without the decision of the WILL all such dreams will be to no avail. Since character and even life are endangered by the use of stimulants, the only safe course is to **touch not, taste not, handle not.**

Anyone who attempts to leave off these drugs will for a time feel a loss, and perhaps will suffer without them. Notwithstanding, by persistence and time, a person can overcome the craving and cease to feel the lack. Nature will require a little time to recover from the abuse she has suffered. But, give her a chance. Your body will again rally and perform nobly and well. Health can be restored in most cases.

Provide a diet of wholesome food, with simple, nonstimulating meals, free of spices, coffee, tea, and excessive sugar. On occasion, a period of fasting with the use of fruit and plain cereals will aid the recovery of damaged mental powers. An abundant intake of water will flush out the system and assist in the elimination of impurities.

Steam baths and hot sweating treatments are helpful to aid in the excretion of poisons. Heavy smokers, for example, when wrapped in a sheet and sweated in the steam bath, can find yellow stains on the wrapping. A characteristically unpleasant tobacco odor comes right out of their pores! The skin, the kidneys, and the liver can all be assisted by the proper use of water, externally and internally, to detoxify poisons and excrete impurities.

Proper diet and a determined will, however, **must** be linked with the supernatural healing power of God! Without heaven's help in resisting temptation, our determinations and promises are like ropes of sand. Here is a precious scripture promise from the Lord: *"There hath no temptation taken you but such as is common to man: but God is faithful, who will not suffer you to be tempted above that ye are able; but will with the temptation also make a way of escape, that ye may be able to bear it,"* (I Corinthians 10:13).

Yes, friend, there is power in prayer, and strength in the Word. These Bible promises can be like leaves from the tree of life, which are *"for the healing of the nations,"* (Revelation 22: 2). This higher experience is possible, as my next chapter will show.

385

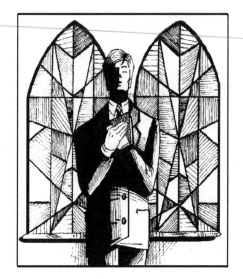

CHAPTER TWENTY-SEVEN

HEALTH

OF

THE

SOUL

Our modern society is riddled with great unrest. Newspapers are filled with accounts of violence, civil war, international intrigue, and mounting economic pressures. The precious yet elusive gift of peace is sought everywhere, but in vain. Some look for peace in a pill or a drug. Others look for it in a bottle of alcohol. Some search vainly through the whole world traveling. Modern man hopes to be happy in a merry–go–round of hedonistic pleasure. Growing groups of Eastern worshipers seek peace through meditation and Oriental religions. Meanwhile, so-called intellectuals delve into the depth of modern psychology, looking for philosophic answers.

The sacred Scriptures present for our solace a *"peace of God, which passeth all understanding."* (Philippians 4: 7). This experience we desperately need, heaven's forgiveness and peace and love in the soul. Money cannot buy it; intellect cannot procure it; wisdom cannot attain to it. We can *never* hope by our own efforts to secure this eternal perfect peace. But it can become yours, offered as a gift *"without money and without price,"* (Isaiah 55: 1).

Jesus himself promised, *"What things soever ye desire, when ye pray, believe that ye receive them, and ye shall have them."* (Mark 11: 24). This tremendous transaction contains but one condition, that we pray according to the will of God. It is our daily privilege to go to Jesus and be cleansed. He has promised to make us His children, and thus enable us to live a holy life. So we may ask for these blessings, then believe that we will receive them. Next, as the healed paralytic did, we must thank God that we have received the proffered gift.

THE POWER OF PRAYER

Through our daily deeper communion with God, the Christian receives a never-failing source of strength. It is more than a trite euphemism, "the family that prays together, stays together." The loyal family of God does likewise. There must be close communication, daily dialog. **Prayer**, by one writer's definition, is the opening of the heart to God, as to a friend. Of course, it is not necessary to make known to God *what* we are. Nevertheless, prayer enables us to receive **Him**. It is our *key* in the hand of faith that unlocks heaven's storehouse. The best prayer example for us was set by our Saviour, who in His humanity found prayer power both a necessity and a privilege. There was comfort and joy in close communion with His Father. The same experience may be ours.

There are several **conditions** that our all-wise Heavenly Father looks to see manifested in His children. One condition is that we *feel our need* of help form Him. Those who hunger and thirst after righteousness may be confident that they will be filled. The human heart must be opened to the spirit's influence or God's blessing cannot be received (see Matthew 5: 6; and E.G. White, *Steps to Christ*, page 95).

If unconfessed sins are harbored in our proud hearts, the Lord cannot hear us. Meanwhile, the prayer of a humble penitent one is *always* accepted. As soon as known wrongs are righted, we may believe and know that God will answer our petition. It is **not** the merit of man that commends us to the favor of God. Rather, the grace of our Lord Jesus Christ and His atoning blood provides the merit that cleanses us from all sin. (I John 1:7).

Another factor in the powerful prayer life is **faith**. *"He that cometh to God must believe that He is, and that He is a rewarder of them that diligently seek Him."* (Hebrews 11: 6). We must learn to take the Lord at His word! Some people when they do not receive immediately the very things that they asked for, or who discover that prolonged delay tries their faith, then commence to doubt God. We are *so* short-sighted as humans. Sometimes we even ask for things that would be no help to us. Then, our heavenly Father, in love, answers our feeble prayers by giving us that which would be for our **higher** good. It would be presumption to claim that earnest prayer will *always* be answered in the very way we desire. Our great and powerful God is too wise to err, and too compassionate to withhold any good thing from those who are His friends.

If we dwell in fear, listening to our own doubts, perplexity will only increase. We must come to God feeling helpless and dependent, as we really are. When in humble, trusting faith we make known our wants to Him. He will permit divine light to shine in our hearts. It is a high privilege to thus be brought in connection with the mind of the Infinite.

A **humble spirit** must be cultivated if we are to receive the full blessing of God. In the Lord's Prayer we all learned to say *"forgive us our debts, as we forgive our debtors."* (Matthew 6: 12). A **forgiving spirit** must be cherished and cultivated if we expect our prayers to be heard. Just as we expect to be forgiven, should we also forgive others.

Perseverance is also required. We are to *"continue in prayer"* (Colossians 4: 2), to *"pray without ceasing."* (I Thessalonians 5: 17). This priceless unbroken union of the soul with God can then be maintained, so that life from God flows vibrantly into our daily lives. With this spiritual *recharging*, our deepened love and desire to serve flows out to others and back to God.

Although public prayer has its proper place, it is in the "closet" of secret communion that we receive the most help from God. Free from surrounding influences, the needy soul can commune in a way that calmly and humbly, yet fervently, claims Divine rays of light to strengthen and sustain. *"God is our refuge and strength, a very present help in trouble."* (Psalm 46: 1).

Spending a "quiet time" for communion each morning, any person who fears God may go about his or her daily labor, *assured* that help will come when it is needed most. There is no time or place, moreover, when it is inappropriate to send up a petition to God. In crowded streets, on planes and trains and buses, in the classroom, or in a clinic or hospital we may petition God and plead for heavenly guidance. This *closet of communion* may be found wherever we are. Our heart's door should be open continually, the invitation going up that Christ Jesus may come in and abide as a heavenly Guest. Thus, although a tainted and corrupt atmosphere may surround us, we need not breathe its spiritual "smog," but we can reside in the pure air of heaven. Like Enoch, we may "walk with God."

TRUST

Our Divine Savior asked the poignant question, *"When the Son of Man cometh, shall He find faith on the earth?"* (Luke 18: 8). The sick were frequently challenged by the words, *"According to your faith, be it unto you."* There is definitely an abundant demand for such simple trust in God today. Instead of choosing our own way, **faith** leads us to choose God's way, believing that He loves us and knows best what is for our *good*. In place of our ignorance, we accept His wisdom; in place of our weakness, His strength; in place of our sinfulness, His righteousness. Truth, uprightness, and purity have been pointed out as secrets of life's success. It is faith that puts us in possession of these principles. (Ellen G. White, *Education,* pg. 253).

Faith grows by exercise just as our muscles do. As we take for our guide book the Word of God, and claim His promises, that seed of faith that God has given will increase. In order to strengthen our faith we must often bring it into contact with God's Word.

Evidence for such power inherent in the Sacred Word was found at creation. *"He spake, and it was done; He commanded, and it stood fast."* (Psalm 33: 9). The apostle Paul, speaking of this marvelous creative power declared, *"For God, who commanded the light to shine out of darkness, hath shined in our hearts, to give the light of the knowledge of the glory of God in the face of Jesus*

Christ." (II Corinthians 4: 6). It was this type of faith, true trust in God, that sustained ancient patriarchs like Enoch and Noah. Faith brought wisdom to statesmen like Joseph and Daniel. It led the apostle Paul to live a life of sacrifice for the Gospel, and faith in God inspired numerous reformers during the Middle Ages.

Notwithstanding, God's children need to trust in small things as well as the great affairs of life. From a human viewpoint, life is an untried path. In our deeper experiences, we each walk alone. How important it is, then, to hear and know the voice of God, to sense His presence constantly. Such childlike trust was illustrated by a friend who encountered a fierce tornado. Filled with fear, she huddled in the bathroom, piling pillows and blankets over herself in flimsy defense. The little four year old, sensing her mother's growing apprehension, came close to her side and whispered, "Mommy, this storm is really upsetting me! Let's talk to Jesus and ask Him to help us." As the mother gratefully responded to her child's simple trust, a peace came in to banish all fear. The storm soon passed without damage.

The abiding sense of God's presence helps also to shield us from temptation. It was this realization that protected Joseph amid the temptations of Egypt. His reply to the temptress was firm, *"How then can I do this great wickedness, and sin against God?"* (Genesis 39: 9). The invincible shield of faith, when cherished, will bring security to each of us. *"Through faith in Christ, every deficiency in character may be supplied, every defilement cleanses, every fault corrected, every excellence developed." "Ye are complete in Him."* (EGWhite, *Education*, p. 257; Colossians 2: 10).

"An intensity such as never before was seen is taking possession of the world. In amusement, in money-making, in the contest for power, in the very struggle for existence, there is a terrible force that engrosses body and mind, and soul. In the midst of this maddening rush, God is speaking. He bids us come apart and commune with Him. "Be still and know that I am God." Ps. 46:10.

"Many, even in their seasons of devotion, fail of receiving the blessing of real communion with God. They are in too great haste. With hurried steps they press through the circle of Christ's loving presence, pausing perhaps for a moment within the sacred precincts, but not waiting for counsel. They have no time to remain with the divine Teacher. With their burdens they return to their work.

"These workers can never attain the highest success until they learn the secret of strength. They must give themselves time to think, to pray, to wait upon God for a renewal of physical, mental, and spiritual power. They need the uplifting influence of His Spirit. Receiving this, they will be quickened by fresh life. The wearied frame and tired brain will be refreshed, the burdened heart will be lightened." (Ibid., p. 260, 261).

I CHALLENGE YOU TO TRY IT AND SEE.

GOOD FOOD FOR THE MIND

The wise man Solomon wrote of "many books" and said, "Much study is a weariness of the flesh." (Ecclesiastes 12: 12). A German saying puts it this way, *"The good is the enemy of the best."* We know of thousands who spend their leisure hours watching TV, of others who feed their mind from the pages of trivial or trashy literature. Cheap novels, like the frogs of Egypt, are covering the land. Other friends, non-discriminating though sincere, spend countless hours with sensational religious fiction or the latest gospel rock cassettes, occupying precious time that could be better spent with the Word of God.

The prophet Isaiah pointed forward to the faithful servant who "stoppeth his ears from hearing of blood, and shutteth his eyes from seeing evil." To these Heaven's promise is, *"Thine eyes shall see the king in His beauty."* (Isaiah 33:15-17). It seems paradoxical, but no less true, that those who are really seeking the wisdom from God must become practically "fools" in the sinful knowledge of this age in order to be wise. We should shut our eyes from much of the modern media, that we may see and know no evil. We should close our ears, lest we hear that which is evil, and obtain that knowledge which stains the purity of thought and act. It was from the tree of knowledge of good and evil that Eve first ate. Then she shared the forbidden fruit with Adam. Seeking to be wise, the serpent's way, they lost their home in the beautiful garden of Eden. By only one foolish act, they passed on a heritage of sin and death to all mankind (Romans 5: 12).

A person whose spirit is receptive cannot read a single passage from the Bible without gaining some helpful thought. The most valuable teachings, however, are not gained by occasional or disconnected study. Many Scriptural treasures lie beneath the surface, and can be obtained only by diligent research and continuous effort. As one searches out and gathers up these truths "here a little, and there a little" (Isaiah 28:10) the message of the Bible will be found to fit perfectly. The Gospels supplement each other. The prophecies explain one another. Truths are built like a building, each part dependent on the other, the final structure so complete that no other mind than that of the Infinite could have fashioned it.

The study of the Word of God also brings mental power. At any age— childhood to adult—the Bible is more effective as a means of intellectual training than all other books combined. God can teach us more in one moment by His Spirit than all the great men of the earth. The beauty of Bible poetry, the power of the promises, the dignified simplicity of God's requirements and the sublime inspiration of its biographies cannot but expand and strengthen the mind. As we study God's Word with a sincere and teachable spirit, there is room for infinite development of the mind and soul.

Some question whether science can be harmonized with the Bible. They point to the many conflicting theories among the scientists today, and are led to question God's Word. Nevertheless, true science brings from her research nothing that, rightly understood, conflicts with divine revelation. The book of nature and the written word each shed light upon the other. They make us acquainted with God by teaching us of His working in nature (see Nehemiah 9: 6; Job 26: 7-14).

God's power is, moreover, exercised in upholding the objects of His creation. (Col.1:17). It is not because of a mechanism set in motion long ago that the pulse beats and breath follows breath. *"In Him we live, and move, and have our being."* (Acts 17:28). Furthermore, a truth even more marvelous, is that the Hand that sustains the world in space, the Hand that holds the planets in their orderly arrangement, is the Hand that was nailed to the cross for you and me. (*Ibid.* p. 132). Under the direction of our all–knowing Creator, we shall, by studying His works, be enabled to think His thoughts after Him. And, by meditating on Christ, we can be changed into His likeness (II Corinthians 3: 18).

ACTIVITIES TO LIFT THE SPIRIT

Christ declared of His mission in life, *"My meat is to do the will of Him that sent me, and to finish his work."* (John 4:34). As the Son of Man He came to dwell with us *"as He that serveth"* (Luke 22:27). Most of the time that Jesus walked this earth, He was helping others. Faithfully working at the carpenter's bench during His youth, He brought cheer and presented a radiant spirit to all who passed by. Later, when taking up His life ministry, He spent more time ministering to the sick than preaching the Gospel. His example is to be ours.

Deeds of kindness and unselfish service are twice a blessing, benefiting both the giver and the receiver of the kindness. *"The consciousness of right doing is one of the best medicines for diseased bodies and minds. When the mind is free and happy from a sense of duty well done and the satisfaction of giving happiness to others, this cheering, uplifting influence brings new life to the whole being."* (see E. G. White, *Ministry of Healing,* page 257).

It is for lack of this spirit in many believers that love has waned and faith grown dim. "If you will go to work as Christ designs that His disciples shall, and win souls for Him, you will feel the need of a deeper experience and a greater knowledge in divine things, and will hunger and thirst after righteousness. You will plead with God, and your faith will be strengthened, and your soul will drink deeper drafts at the well of salvation. Encountering opposition and trials will drive you to the Bible and prayer. You will grow in grace and the knowledge of Christ, and will develop a rich experience.

"The spirit of unselfish labor for others gives depth, stability, and Christlike loveliness to the character, and brings peace and happiness to its possessor... Those who thus exercise the Christian graces will grow and will become strong to work for God." (White, *Steps to Christ,* p. 80). This unselfish service for the good of others is the most sure way to work out your own

salvation, remembering that, *"It is God which worketh in you both to will and to do of His good pleasure,"* (Philippians 2: 13).

The 58th chapter of Isaiah contains heaven's prescription for sickness of the body or soul. If we desire health, and the true joy of life, we must put into practice the rules given in this Scripture. More than once I have seen this illustrated in my own experience and that of others, the **Law of Benevolence** bringing its sure result in a renewal of strength, health, and inner peace. Meditate often on this Bible chapter.

Thousands of people today are seeking a life of respectable convention-ality for themselves and for their children. Although professing to be Christians, they lack the self-sacrificing spirit of the Master. Thus they reject the only training that imparts a fitness for participation with Christ in His glory, the fellowship of **service**. This training gives strength and nobility to the character and a deeper sympathy with Jesus, who sacrificed and suffered for us. (I Peter 2:21).

In the soul touched by the Saviour's love there is begotten a desire to work for Him. Love and loyalty to Christ are reflected in true service, bringing a wonderful fellowship with our Master, and making us coworkers with heavenly angels. As we cooperate with them, we receive the benefit of their education, providing an experience that far transcends any university course the world can offer!

Now, touched with sympathy for our fellow men, whether they be stricken with poverty, afflicted with sickness, or ignorant of God, we can go forth to labor for souls. As we work hand in hand with the Light of the world, we will find privilege where others see only hardship, order in apparent confusion, and success in what appears to be failure. By faith, we see God at work and rejoice with the privilege of being His helping hand.

It is my desire that you, dear reader, by partaking of these promises, and by sharing in the Master's service, may *personally* experience this peace that passes all understanding. Motivated by love (read I Corinthians 13) and in response to God's marvelous grace (Ephesians 2: 8,9), you, my friend, can know God, Whom to know is life eternal (John 17:3). Won't you seek Him now?

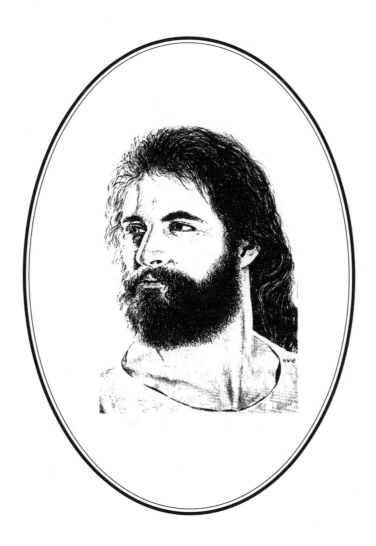

GLOSSARY

Abrasion (ah-bra'zhun). A scraping injury in which the skin or a membrane is denuded.

Acidosis (as'i-do'sis). A pathological condition resulting from an accumulation of acid or loss of base in the body, and characterized by increase in hydrogen ion concentration.

Adrenal glands (ad-re'nal). Two small endocrine glands located one above each kidney.

Aflatoxins (a'flah-tok'sin). Group of toxic substances produced by certain molds which grow on peanuts and cereals and which have toxic and carcinogenic effects in many animal species.

Alimentary canal (al-e-men'tar-e). The continuous tract from mouth to anus through which food moves during the process of digestion.

Alkalosis (al'kah-lo'sis). A pathological condition resulting from accumulation of base or loss of acid in the body and characterized by a decrease in hydrogen ion in the body.

Allergen (al'er-jen). Any substance capable of inducing allergy.

Alveoli (al-ve'o-li). Very small air sacs in lung tissue through which oxygen and carbon dioxide are exchanged.

Amino acids (a-me'no as'ids). Organic compounds containing nitrogen known as the building blocks of the protein molecule.

Amylase (am'i-las). A pancreatic or salivary enzyme that digests starch.

Amylose (am'i-los). The straight chain soluble form of starch.

Anterior chamber. Frontal space in the eyeball; bounded by cornea, iris, and lens.

Antibodies (an'ti-bod-es). Substances built up by lymphoid tissue as defensive response to invasion by organism, foreign proteins, etc.

Anticoagulant (an'ti-ko-ag'-u-lant). A substance that inhibits or prevents blood coagulation by interfering with the clotting mechanism.

Antioxidant (an'ti-ok'se-dant). A substance that prevents or delays oxidation. Often applied to vitamin E.

Anus (a'nus). Terminal portion of the intestinal tract, about 1"-1½" long.

Aorta (a-or'tah). Largest artery in the body; arises from the heart and courses down the body trunk.

Aortic valve. Fibrous tissue flaps or leaflets which open and close between the left ventricle and the aorta. Valve closure prevents backflow (reflux) of blood.

Appendix (ah-pen'diks). Blind, wormlike pouch normally found at the cecum. Has no known role in digestion.

Aqueous humor (a'kwe-us hu'mor). Watery, transparent fluid found in the anterior and posterior chambers of the eye; helps maintain conical shape of the front of the globe and assists in focusing light rays on the retina.

Arteries (ar'ter-es). Elastic, extensive vessels which carry blood in the direction away from the heart.

Arteriole (ar-te're-ol). A very small artery.

Articular cartilage (ar-tik'u-lar kar'ti-lij). A special type of dense connective tissue which covers bone surfaces in a joint.

Articulation (ar-tik-u-la'shun). Junction of two or more bones; a joint.

Ascorbic acid (a-skor'bik). Vitamin C, deficiency of which is a causative factor in scurvy.

Aspergillus flavus (as'per-jil'us fla-vus). A group of molds found on corn, peanuts, and certain grains when improperly dried and stored; source of aflatoxin.

Ataxia (ah-tak'se-ah). Failure of muscular coordination; irregularity of muscular action.

Atrium; auricle (a'tre-um; aw're-kl). One of the two upper chambers of the heart (right and left).

Auditory canal (aw'di-to-re). Channel for entry of sound from outside; extends to the eardrum.

Auditory ossicles (aw'di-to-re os'si-kls). Three small bones of the middle ear which vibrate and conduct sound.

Avitaminosis (a-vi'ta-min-o'sis). A condition due to the lack or the deficiency of a vitamin in the diet, or to lack of absorption or utilization of it.

Axilla (ak-sil'ah). Armpit.

Axillary (ak'si-lar-e). Pertaining to the armpit.

Bicuspid valve (bi-kus'pid). The two-leaflet heart valve between the left upper and left lower chambers. The bicuspid valve is also called the mitral valve.

Bile. Fluid secreted by the liver, stored in the gall bladder, and emptied into the small intestine where it assists in absorption of fats.

Biotin (bi'o-tin). A member of the vitamin B complex.

Bladder (blad'der). Hollow muscular organ which serves as the reservoir for urine.

Blood. Fluid which circulates throughout the body, carrying nutrients to cells and removing wastes from cells. Arterial blood contains a heavy concentration of oxygen while venous blood contains carbon dioxide in large amounts.

Blood capillary (kap'i-lar-e). A microscopic vessel through which blood travels from arteriole to venule.

Bone. An individual part of the skeleton; osseous tissue.

Bony orbit. Rounded socket in the cranium in which the eyeball is partially sunk.

Bone shaft. The body (diaphysis) of a long bone.

Botulism (bot'u-lizm). Poisoning from the toxin produced by the organism *Clostridium botulinum*. The toxin has a selective action on the nervous system.

Bronchial tubes; bronchi (brong'ke-al; brong'-ki). Branches of the right and left main stem passageways extending from the trachea.

Calciferol (kal-sif'er-ol). Vitamin D_2, produced by irradiating ergosterol.

Calcification (kal'si-fi-ka'shun). Process by which organic tissue becomes hardened by a deposit of calcium salts.

Calcitonin (kal'si-to'nin). A hormone secreted by the thyroid gland which participates with parathyroid hormone in the regulation of calcium ions in the blood.

Calcium (kal'se-um). An element which occurs naturally in all body tissues and fluids such as bones, teeth, and blood.

Capillaries (kap'i-lar-es). Minute blood vessels which connect the smallest units of arteries (arterioles) with the smallest veins (venules).

Carbon dioxide (CO_2). Odorless, colorless gas produced in tissue cells as a by-product of metabolism. CO_2 is excreted by the lungs.

Carotene (kar'o-ten). A yellow pigment which exists in several forms; alpha, beta, and gamma carotene are provitamins which may be converted in vitamin A in the body.

Carotid arteries (kah-rot'id). Vessels which provide the major supply to the head and neck.

Cartilage (kar'ti-lij). Relatively hard, dense connective tissue which serves to cushion jolts and bumps.

Casein (ka'se-in). The principal protein of milk, the basis of cheese.

Cecum (se'kum). First portion of the large intestine. The ileum joins the cecum at a right angle, and the appendix is attached to the cecum.

Cervical os (ser'vi-kl os). Opening in the cervix (lower end) of the uterus.

Cheilosis (ki-lo'sis). A condition marked by lesions on the lips and cracks at the angles of the mouth.

Cholesterol (ko-les'ter-ol). The most common member of the sterol group, defined below. It is a precursor of vitamin D and closely related to several hormones in the body. It constitutes a large part of the most frequently occurring type of gallstones, and occurs in atheroma of the arteries.

Choline (ko'len). A component of lecithin. Necessary for fat transport in the body. Prevents the accumulation of fat in the liver.

Chylomicrons (ki'lo-mi'krons). Particles of emulsified lipoproteins containing primarily triglycerides from dietary fat and very little protein.

Chyme. Semiliquid material resulting from action of digestive juices on food in the stomach.

Chymotrypsin (ki'mo-trip'sin). One of the proteolytic enzymes of the pancreatic juice.

Circulatory. Pertaining to movement through a circuitous route with return to origin.

Clostridium (klos-trid'e-um). A bacterium, *C. perfringens* (and other species) a cause of gangrene.

Cochlea (kok'le-ah). Spiral canal hollowed out of the temporal bone; shaped like a snail shell and located in the anterior portion of the inner ear.

Collagen (kol'a-jen). The main protein constituent of connective tissue and of the organic substance of bones; changed into gelatin by boiling.

Colon (ko'lon). Second portion of the large intestine which is subdivided into four sections: ascending colon, transverse colon, descending colon, and sigmoid colon.

Congenital (kon-jen'i-tal). Existing at or before birth.

Conjunctiva (kon-junk-ti'vah). Mucous membrane which lines the eyelids and covers the anterior surface of the globe except for the cornea.

Connective tissue. Tissue which supports and connects other body tissues; usually contains both collagen and elastic fibers.

Cornea (kor'ne-ah). Transparent frontal layer of the eyeball.

Cranium (kra'ne-um). Skull bones which encase the brain.

cretinism (kre'tin-izm). A chronic condition due to congenital lack of thyroid secretion.

Crystalline lens (kris'tal-lin). That part of the eye which, in addition to the cornea, refracts light rays and focuses them on the retina.

Cyanocobalamin (si'ah-no-ko-bal'ah-men). Vitamin B_{12}, a dark red compound containing cobalt and a cyanide group.

Cyclamate (si'kla-mat). Sodium or calcium cyclamate, known as Sucaryl, used as an artificial sweetener. Use prohibited by FDA.

Dehydration (de'hi-dra'shun). Removal of water from food or tissue; or the condition that results from undue loss of water.

Dermis (der'mis). Deep layer of skin; also called corium.

Diabetes (di-ah-be'tez). A condition in which cells of the pancreas called islets of Langerhans fail to produce enough insulin for proper metabolism of sugars and starches.

Diaphragm (di'ah-fram). The musculomembranous "partition" between the chest cavity and abdominal cavity which acts as a bellows in breathing.

Diaphysis (di-af'i-sis). Shaft of a long bone.

Digestion (di-jest'yun). Process by which ingested food is converted for absorption and use as nutrients for body cells.

Digestive system (di-jest'iv). The group of structures concerned with the process of digestion (alimentary canal and accessory organs).

Disaccharides (di-sak'ah-ri-das). An enzyme which hydrolyzes disaccharides.

Disaccharide (di-sak'a-rid). Any one of the sugars which yields two monosaccharides on hydrolysis.

DNA, deoxyribonucleic acid (de-ok'se-ri'bo-nu-kle'ik). Found in the nucleus of living cells; functions in the transfer of genetic characteristics.

Ductless gland. A gland without excretory ducts or channels.

Duodenum (du-o-de'num). First portion of small intestine, about 10" long, extending from the *stomach* to the *jejunum*.

Elastic fibers. Tissue fibrils capable of expansion and contraction.

Electrolyte (e-lek'tro-lit). The ionized form of an element. Common electrolytes in the body are sodium, potassium, and chloride.

Electrolyte balance. Distribution of acids, bases, and salts in tissue cells, fluids, and blood plasma which helps maintain normal **pH** and control the passage of water between cell membranes.

Elimination (e-lim-i-na'shun). Movement of bowels to expel waste products from the body.

Endemic (en-dem'ik). A disease of low morbidity that is constantly present in a human community.

Endocrine gland. An organ which secretes hormones directly into the circulatory system to influence and regulate numerous body processes.

Endometrium (en-do-me'tre-um). Lining of the uterus.

Enzyme (en'zim). A substance, usually protein in nature and formed in living cells, which brings about chemical changes.

Epidermis (ep-i-der'mis). External layer of skin.

Epididymis (ep-i-did'i-mis) (pl. -mides). Small but lengthy convoluted tube which begins at its attachment to the testis and ends in the vas deferens.

Epiglottis (ep-i-glot'is). "Lid" which covers and closes the larynx during swallowing to prevent entry of food into lungs.

Epinephrine (ep'i-nef'rin). A hormone secreted by the adrenal medulla and released predominantly in response to hypoglycemia.

Epiphysis (e-pif'i-sis). Two ends of a long bone.

Equilibrium (e-kwi-lib're-um). Balance.

Ergosterol (er-gos'ter-ol). A sterol found in plant and in animal tissues which, on exposure to ultraviolet light, is converted into vitamin D. (See *sterol*).

Esophagus (e-sof'ah-gus). Tube-like passageway which connects pharynx to stomach.

Eustachian tube (u-sta'ki-an). Conduit 3-4 cm long from middle ear to pharnyx.

Evaporation (e-vap-o-ra'shun). Conversion of a liquid to a vapor.

Excretory (eks'kre-to-re). Pertaining to discharge of waste products from the body.

Exhale (eks-hale'). To expel air from the lungs.

External ear. Pinna and external auditory canal.

Fallopian tube (fal-lo'pe-an). Tubal passageway in which the egg travels from the ovary to the uterus.

Fatty acids (fat' as'ids). The organic acids which combine with glycerol to form fat.

Femur (fe'mur). Long bone of the thigh which extends from hip to knee.

Fertilization (fer-ti-li-za'shun). Union of ovum and spermatozoon.

Folic acid (fo'lic as'id). A vitamin of the B complex group, known also as pteroylglutamic acid or folacin.

Galactose (gah-lak'tos). A monosaccharide derived from lactose by hydrolysis.

Gastric (gas'trik). Pertaining to the stomach.

Genes (jens). Units of hereditary DNA, carried by chromosomes.

Genitals; genitalia (jen'i-tals, jen-i-ta'le-ah). Organs of reproduction.

Gliadin (gli'a-din). One of the proteins found in the gluten of cereal grains.

Globe. Eyeball.

Glucose (gloo'kos). One form of sugar, a product of starch metabolism in the body.

Gluten (gloo'ten;-t'n). A protein found in many cereal grains.

Glycogen (gli-ko-jen). A carbohydrate, similar in composition to the amylopectin form of starch. In this form, carbohydrate is stored in the liver and the muscles.

Gonads (gon'ads). Glands which produce sex hormones and germ cells necessary for reproduction.

Hair cells. The final sensory receptors of sound.

Hair follicles (fol'li-kls). Glands in the dermal layer of skin which produce hairs.

Heart. Powerful, muscular organ which pumps blood to all parts of the body.

Homogenized (ho-moj'e-nizd). Made homogeneous. Usually applied to dispersing milk fat in such fine globules that cream will not rise to the top.

Hormone (hor'mon). Chemical substance produced and secreted by an endocrine gland.

Hormones (hor'mons). Complex chemical substances which profoundly affect organ and body growth, development, and activities. The ovaries and testes produce hormones.

Hydrogenation (hi'dro-jen-a'shun). The process of introducing hydrogen into a compound, as when oils are hydrogenated to produce solid fats.

Hymen (hi'men). Membranous tissue fold which partially covers the external opening of the vagina.

Hypercalcemia (hi-'per-kal-se'me-ah). An excess of calcium in the blood.

Hypercholestermia (hi'per-kal-se'me-ah). Excess of cholesterol in the blood.

Hyperglycemia (hi'per-gli-se'me-a). An increase in the blood sugar level above normal.

Hyperplasia (hi'per-pla'zhe-a). Increase in number of normal cells in normal arrangement in a tissue.

Hypertrophy (hi-per'tro-fe). Increase in cell size.

Hypervitaminosis (hi'per'vi'ta-min-o'sis). A condition due to an excess of one or more vitamins.

Hypocalcemia (hi'po-kal-se'me-a). Abnormally low blood calcium.

Hypoglycemia (hi'po'gli'se'me-a). A decrease in the blood sugar level below normal.

Hypoproteinemia (hi'po-pro'te-in-e'me-a). A decrease in the normal quantity of serum protein in the blood.

Iatrogenic (i'atro'jen'ik). Resulting from the activity of physicians.

Idiopathic (id'i-o-path'ik). Self-originated; occurring without known cause.

Incus (ing'kus). One of the three auditory ossicles; also called anvil due to its shape.

Inhale (in-hale'). To take air into the lungs.

Insulin (in'su-lin). Substance produced by an area of the pancreas.

Internal ear. Vestibule, semicircular canals, and cochlea; contains end organs of sound perception and equilibration.

Involuntary muscle. A muscle not subject to control by human will.

Iris. Colored membrane of the eye which separates the anterior and posterior chambers; contracts and dilates to regulate entrance of light rays.

Islets of Langerhans (lahng'er-hanz). Group of cells of the pancreas which secrete insulin.

Joint. Articulation.

Joint capsule. The fibrous sheath which encloses articular bone surfaces.

Ketosis (ke-to'sis). A condition in which there is an accumulation in the body of the ketone bodies as a result of incomplete oxidation of the fatty acids.

Kidney. Large bean-shaped gland located at each upper side of the posterior abdominal cavity. Kidneys extract wastes from blood, from urine, and discharge it continuously into the ureters.

Kneecap. Patella.

Kwashiorkor (kwa-shi-or'ker). A severe protein-calorie deficiency disease occurring in small children. Endemic in many parts of the world.

Labia majora (la'be-a majo'ra). Two outer borders of raised, fleshy tissue extending from the mons pubis down past the vaginal opening.

Labia minora (la'be-a mi-no'ra). Two inner borders of tissue between the labia majora and the vaginal opening.

Lacrimal ducts and glands (lak'ri-mal). System of ducts and glands which secretes and conducts tears.

Larynx (lar'inks). The organ of voice.

Lecithin (les'i-thin). A phospholipid containing glycerol, fatty acids, phosphoric acid, and choline.

Ligament (lig'ah-ment). Band of exceptionally strong, flexible connective tissue which joins articular bone surfaces.

Linoleic acid (lin'o-le'ik as'id). A polyunsaturated fatty acid essential for nutrition.

Lipase (li'pas; lip'as). An enzyme that digests fat.

Lipid (lip'id), **lipoid** (lip'oid). Fat or fatlike substances.

Lipoprotein (lip'o-pro'te-in). Combination of a protein with a fat, found in both animal and plant tissues.

Lobe. The major divisions of a lung.

Locomotion (loko-mo'shun). Process of moving about.

Lung. Major organ of respiration; consists of spongy, porous, elastic tissue.

Lymph (limf). Substance continuously formed by filtration from tissue fluids.

Lymph nodes. Small bodies of lymphoid tissue arranged in chains to filter lymph and help prevent the spread of infection.

Lymphatic duct (lim-fat'ik). One of two large vessels which empty lymph collected in various parts of the body into the venous bloodstream.

Lymphocyte (lim'fo-site). A particular type of white blood cell which is formed in the reticular (net-like) tissue of lymph glands.

Lysosomes (li'so-soms). Membranous structures in cytoplasm which contain hydrolytic enzymes.

Lysozyme (li'so-zim). Enzyme that digests certain high molecular weight carbohydrates and some gram-positive bacteria.

Malabsorption syndrome (mal'absorp'shun). A group of symptoms which result from the inability to digest or absorb food in the intestinal tract.

Malleus (mal'e-us). One of the three auditory ossicles; hammer- shaped.

Mammary glands (mam'er-e). Breasts.

Marasmus (ma-raz'mus). Wasting and emaciation, especially in infants due to underfeeding or disease.

Medulla (me-dul'lah). The middle, inmost part.

Melanin (mel'ah-nin). The dark amorphous pigment of the skin, hair and certain other tissues which derives from tyrosine metabolism.

Menstruation (men-stroo-a'shun). Normal uterine bleeding which usually occurs monthly as the endometrium is shed by the non- pregnant female.

Metabolism (me-tab'o-lizm). The physical and chemical processes by which ingested food and fluids are converted to energy or body tissues.

Middle ear. Extends from eardrum to oval window; contains auditory ossicles.

Mitochondria (mit'o-kon'dre-ah). Small granules or rod-shaped structures in the cell.

Mitral valve (mi'tral). Fibrous tissue leaflets which open and close between the left upper and left lower heart chambers. Closure prevents reflux blood.

Monosaccharide (mon'o-sak'a-rid). A simple sugar which cannot be decomposed by hydrolysis.

Mono-unsaturated (mon'o-un-sat'u-rated). An organic compound such as a fatty acid in which two carbon atoms are united by a double bond.

Motor nerves. Nerves which activate muscles and glands by conducting impulses away from the center (brain); efferent nerves.

Mucous membrane (mu'kus). Thin layer of smooth tissue which lines many cavities and has special ability to secrete a slimy fluid called mucus.

Muscle. Groups of special cells (muscle fibers) with the ability to contract or shorten.

Muscle insertion. Point of attachment of skeletal muscle to bone most moved by its contraction.

Myelin (mi'e-lin). The fat-like substance forming a sheath around certain nerve fibers.

Nasopharnx (na-zo-far'inks). Upper part of the back of the throat where the nasal cavity opens into the pharynx.

Neutropenia (nu'tro-pe'ne-ah). A decrease in the number of neutrophilic leucocytes in the blood.

Niacin (ni'a-sin). A member of the vitamin B complex, formerly known as nicotinic acid. An antipellagra factor.

Nutrient (nu'tre-ent). An organic or inorganic substance in food which is digested and absorbed in the gastrointestinal tract and utilized in intermediary metabolism.

Occipital lobe (ok-sip'i-tal). Posterior section of the brain.

Olfactory receptors (ol-fak'to-re). Nerves in the upper part of the nasal cavity concerned with the sense of smell.

Optic nerve (op'tik). Second cranial nerve with special sense of sight.

Organ of Corti. The hair cells (final sensory receptors of sound) located in the inner ear.

Osteomalacia (os'te-o-ma-la'she-a). Softening of the bone due to loss of calcium. Occurs chiefly in adults.

Osteoporosis (os'te-o-po-ro'sis). Abnormal porousness or rarefaction of bone due to failure of the osteoblasts to lay down bone matrix, and occurring when resorption dominates over mineral deposition.

Oval window. Division between middle and inner ear.

Ovarian follicles (o-va're-an fol'li-kls). Blisterlike formations on the ovary which rupture when they ripen and release the egg cell of reproduction in the female.

Ovaries (o'vah-res). The two sex glands in the female which produce egg cells for reproduction.

Ovulation (ahv-u-la'shun). Discharge of the egg from the ovary.

Ovum (o'vum). Female egg cell of reproduction.

Oxygen (ok'si-jen). Gaseous element found in free air; essential to life of human tissue cells.

Oxygenated (ok'si-je-na-ted). Saturated with oxygen.

Pancreas (pan'kre-as). A gland which is both endocrine and exocrine; located behind the stomach, the pancreas produces secretions concerned with digestion.

Pantothenic acid (pan'to-then'ik). A member of the vitamin B complex.

Parathyroid glands (par-ah-thi'roid). Two pairs of small endocrine glands usually attached to the back of the thyroid gland.

Pelvis (pel'vis). Bony structure surrounding the pelvic cavity.

Peptide (pep'tid). A compound of two or more amino acids containing one or more peptide bonds. Peptides are formed as intermediary products of protein digestion.

Periosteum (per-e-os'te-um). Double layer of connective tissue which covers bone except at joints; inner layer can make new bone.

Pesticide (pes'ti-sid). A poison used to destroy pests of any sort. The term includes fungicides, insecticides, and rodenticides.

Pharynx (far'inks). Area in the back of the throat located between mouth and nose and upper end of the esophagus.

Phenylketonuria (PKU) (fen'il-ke-ton-nu're-ah). An inborn error of the metabolism of phenylalanine; phenylpyruvic acid appears in the urine.

Phospholipid (fos'fo-lip'id). A fat in which one fatty acid is replaced by phosphorus and a nitrogenous compound.

Photosynthesis (fo'to-sin'the-sis). Formation of carbohydrate from carbon dioxide and water in the chlorophyll tissue of plants under the influence of light.

Pinna (pin'nah). Auricular appendage; portion of external ear visible at sides of the head.

Pituitary gland (pi-tu'i-tar-e). The "master" gland of the body, so-called because of the many ways it controls and influences organs and body processes.

Plasma (plaz'mah). Fluid portion of blood in which cells are suspended.

Pleura (ploor'ah). Membranous sac which encloses the lungs and lines the chest cavity. *Parietal* pleura lines the chest cavity and *visceral* pleura adheres closely to the lungs.

Polysaccharide (pol'e-sak'ah-rid). A complex carbohydrate which contains more then ten molecules of monosaccharides combined with each other.

Polyunsaturated (pol'e-un-sat'u-rat'ed). An organic compound such as a fatty acid in which there is more than one double bond.

Pregnancy (preg'nan-ce). Condition in which the fertilized egg normally is implanted in the uterine lining, grows and develops for about 9 months until the infant is capable of living in the outside environment.

Prophylaxis (pro'fi-lak'sis). Preventive treatment.

Prostate (pros'tate). Gland in the male which surrounds the bladder neck and contributes secretions to seminal fluid.

Proteinuria (pro'te-i-nu're-a). Presence of protein in the urine.

Ptyalin (ti'a-lin). The starch-splitting enzyme amylase of saliva.

Puberty (pu'ber-te). Onset of sexual maturity; appearance of adult secondary sex characteristics.

Pulmonary artery (pul'mo-ner-e). Vessel which carries venous blood from right lower heart chamber to the lung for oxygenation.

Pulmonary valve. Fibrous tissue leaflets which open and close between the right ventricle and pulmonary artery, preventing backflow of blood.

Pulmonary vein. Vessel which returns oxygenated blood from the lung to the left upper heart chamber.

Pupil. Opening at the center of the iris.

Purine(s) (pu'ren). A nonprotein heterocyclic nitrogenous base. End products of nucleoprotein metabolism.

Pyridoxine (pi'ri-dok'sin). Vitamin B_6, a member of the vitamin B complex.

Red blood cells. Erthrocytes which are the iron and oxygen- bearing cells of the blood.

Reproduction (re-pro-duk'shun). Process of creating new life by fusion of male spermatozoon with female ovum.

Respiration (res-pi-ra'shun). Inspiration and expiration of air via the lungs.

Reticuloendothelial system (re-tik'u-lo-en'do-the'le'al). Group of cells, except leukocytes, with phagocytic properties.

Retina (ret'i-nah). The "seeing" membrane lining the inside of the posterior eye where images are focused by the lens and cornea then transmitted to the brain via the optic nerve.

Rhodopsin (ro-dop'sin). Visual purple, formed in the rods of the retina by combining the protein opsin and vitamin A aldehyde.

Riboflavin (ri'bo-fla'vin). Heat-stable factor of B complex, sometimes called vitamin B_2.

Ribonucleic acid (RNA) (ri-bo-nu'kle-ik). A nucleic acid replicated from DNA and found in cytoplasm.

Round window. Membrane through which sound waves escape after passing hair cells.

Sclera (skle'ra). The white outer coat of the eye which extends from the optic nerve to the cornea.

Scrotum (skro'tum). Two-compartment pouch of tissue located externally on the male body; contains the testes.

Sebaceous glands (se-ba'shus). Oil-secreting glands.

Semen (se'men). Thick white fluid which contains sperm and other secretions; discharged by the male during sexual intercourse.

Semicircular canals. Three bony canals of the inner ear.

Seminal vesicle (ves'i-kl). Two small pouches attached to the bladder which join with the seminal ducts to form the ejaculatory ducts.

Sensory perception. Recognition of sensation such as pain, touch, pressure, and heat.

Sensory receptors. Rods and cones in the retinal layer which are stimulated by light rays to conduct nerve impulses to the brain via the optic nerve.

Serum globulin (glob'u-lin). A protein constituent of blood plasma associated with antibodies and immune substances.

Skeletal muscle. Muscle which is connected to bone.

Skeleton. Bony framework of the body.

Skin appendages (ah-pen'di-jes). Hairs, nails, sweat glands, oil glands and ducts.

Smooth muscle. Involuntary muscle tissue which lacks cross- striations on microscopic exam; found in areas such as the gastrointestinal tract, respiratory tract, and uterus.

Sperm; spermatozoon (sper-mah-tozo'on) (pl. -zoa). Male germ cell.

Spermatic cord (sper-ma'tik). Tubal passageway by which the testis is suspended in the scrotum.

Spinal cord. The major pathway for transmission of nerve impulses between the brain and all parts of the body. The spinal cord extends about 18" from the base of the brain down the spinal canal.

Spleen. A large lymphoid organ located in the left upper abdomen behind the stomach. The spleen plays a role in the production, storage, and destruction of blood cells, and in lymphocyte production.

Staples (sta'pez). One of the three auditory ossicles; stirrup- shaped.

Steatorrhea (ste'a-to-re'a). Presence of an excess of fat in the stools.

Striated muscle (stri'a-ted). Muscle which has cross-striations on microscopic exam; found in skeletal muscles.

Synovial membrane (si-no've-al). Lining of the joint capsule.

Synthesis (sin'the-sis). The process of building up a chemical compound.

Tendon (ten'don). Fibrous tissue structure which serves to connect muscle to bone and other parts.

Testes (tes'tes) (sing. -is). The two glands situated in the male scrotum which produce sperm.

Thiamine (thi'am-in). Vitamin B_1 Antineuritic factor, member of the B complex.

Thoracic (tho-ras'ik). Pertaining to the chest.

Thymus (thi'mus). A gland located in the neck and upper chest which is thought to play a role in the immune mechanism of the body.

Thyroid gland (thi'roid). An endocrine gland located in the anterior neck at the trachea. Secretions of the thyroid gland are important in certain metabolic processes.

Thyrotoxicosis (thi'ro-tok'si-ko'sis). A morbid condition resulting from overactivity of the thyroid gland.

Tocopherol (to-kof'er-ol). An alcohol-like substance, several forms of which have vitamin E activity.

Toxin (tok'sin). A "poisonous" substance; one capable of damaging body cells.

Trachea (tra'ke-ah). Passageway for air between larynx and bronchi.

Trichinosis (trik'i-no'sis). A disease due to infection with trichinae—parasites found in raw pork.

Tricuspid valve (tri-kus'pid). Valve with three fibrous tissue leaflets which open and close between the right upper and right lower chambers of the heart to prevent backflow of blood.

Trigone of bladder (tri'gon). A triangular area at the base of the urinary bladder.

Tularemia (too'la-re'me-ah). A disease of rodents, resembling plague, which is transmitted by the bites of flies, fleas, ticks, and lice and may be acquired by man through handling of infected animals.

Tympanic membrane (tim-pan'ik). Eardrum.

Urea (u-re'a). The chief nitrogenous end product of protein metabolism in the body.

Ureter (u-re'ter; u're-ter). One of two small diameter tubes extending from the kidney to the bladder; conveys urine.

Urethra (u-re'thrah). Passageway which extends from the urinary bladder to the body exterior for the elimination of urine.

Urinate (u'ri-nate). To empty the urinary bladder.

Urine (u'rin). Waste-containing liquid produced by the kidneys, stored in the bladder, and eliminated through the urethra.

Uterus (u'ter-us). The womb, a muscular organ in which the fertilized ovum is implanted and develops.

Vagina (vah-ji'nah). Passageway for infant birth.

Vas deferens (vas def'er-ens). The excretory duct of the testis; also called ductus deferens.

Vascular (vas'ku-lar). Pertaining to vessels.

Vein. Vessel which carries blood in the direction toward the heart.

Ventricle (ven'tri-kl). One of the two (right and left) lower chambers of the heart.

Venule. A very small vein.

Vertebral column (ver'te-bral). Series of bones or vertebrae which make up the bony spine.

Viscera (vis'er-ah). Internal organs within the chest, abdominal and pelvic cavities.

Vitreous humor (vit're-us). Transparent substance of raw eggwhite consistency which fills the posterior cavity of the eyeball. Vitreous also is called the hyaloid.

Vocal cords (vo'kal cords). Fibrous, elastic ligaments in the larynx which function to produce voice.

Voluntary muscle. Muscle under control of the conscious will.

Voluntary nervous system. Nerves which act in response to human will.

Vulva (vul'vah). External genitalia of the female.

Wernicke-Korsakoff syndrome (ver'ni-ke-kor-sak'of). A psychosis which is usually based on chronic alcoholism, probably due to prolonged thiamine deficiency.

White blood cells. Principally three types of corpuscles (cells) normally present in blood—lymphocytes, monocytes, and granulocytes.

Xerophthalmia (ze'rof-thal'mi-a). A dry and lusterless condition of the conjunctiva of the eyes resulting from a vitamin A deficiency.

Zein (ze'in). A protein obtained from corn.

DIRECTORY

of

HEALTH & HEALING CENTERS

Black Hills Health Center

Box 19
Hermosa, SD 75544
(605) 255-4101

Eden Valley Lifestyle Center

6263 N. County Rd. #29
Loveland, CO 80538
(303) 669-7730

Hartland Health Center

Box 1
Rapidan, VA 22733
(703) 672-3100

Living Springs Lifestyle Center

12 Living Springs Lane
Putnam Valley, NY 10579
(914) 526-2800

Poland Spring Health Institute

RFD 1, Box 4300
Poland Spring, ME 04274
(207) 998-2894

Uchee Pines Institute

30 Uchee Pines Road
Seale, AL 36875
(205) 855-4764

Weimar Health Center

P.O. Box 486
Weimar, CA 95736
(916) 637-4111

Wildwood Lifestyle Center & Hospital

P.O. Box 129
Wildwood, GA 30757
(706) 820-1493

COMPOSITION OF FOODS

Food and Description	Wt. Gm.	Approximate Measure	Food Energy K.Cal.	Protein Gm.	Fat Gm.	Carbohydrate Total Gm.	Fiber Gm.	Water Gm.	Ca Mg.	P Mg.	Fe Mg.	Vita-min A I.U.	Thiamine Mg.	Riboflavin Mg.	Niacin Mg.	Ascorbic Acid Mg.
Acerola (West Indian cherry) raw	100	1 c.	28	Tr.	Tr.	7	0.4	92	12	11	0.2	—	0.02	0.06	0.4	1,300†
Almonds, salted	15	12-15	94	3	9	3	0.4	1	35	75	0.7	0	0.04	0.14	0.5	Tr.
Apples:																
Raw, pared	100	medium	54	Tr.	Tr.	14	0.6	85	6	10	0.3	40	0.03	0.02	0.1	2
Apple juice, bottled or canned . . .	250	1 c.	120	Tr.	0	30	—	220	15	22	1.5	—	0.03	0.05	0.3	3
Apple sauce, canned:																
Unsweetened	100	½ c. scant	41	Tr.	Tr.	11	0.6	88	4	5	0.5	40	0.02	0.01	Tr.	1
Sweetened	100	½ c. scant	91	Tr.	Tr.	24	0.5	76	4	5	0.5	40	0.02	0.01	Tr.	1
Apricots:																
Raw	100	3 medium	51	1	Tr.	13	0.6	85	17	23	0.5	2,700	0.03	0.04	0.6	10
Canned: Solids and liquid water pack	100	½ c. scant	38	1	Tr.	10	0.4	89	12	16	0.3	1,830	0.02	0.02	0.4	4
Dried, sulfured uncooked	100	20 large or 30 sm. halves	260	5	Tr.	67	3.0	25	67	108	5.5	10,900	0.01	0.16	3.3	12

Asparagus:															
Fresh, cooked	100	6-7 spears	20	2	Tr.	4	0.7	94	21	50	0.6	900	0.16	0.18	1.4	26
Frozen, cooked	100		22	3	Tr.	4	0.8	92	22	67	1.1	780	0.16	0.14	1.1	26
Avocados, raw commercial varieties	100	½ peeled	167	2	16	6	1.6	74	10	42	0.6	290	0.11	0.20	1.6	14
Bananas, raw	100	1 small	85	1	Tr.	22	0.5	76	8	26	0.7	190	0.05	0.06	0.7	10
Barley, pearled, light uncooked	100	½ c.	349	8	1	79	0.5	11	16	189	2.0	0	0.12	0.05	3.1	0
Beans, common or kidney:																
Red kidney, canned or cooked, solids and liquids	100	½ c. scant	90	6	Tr.	16	0.9	76	29	109	1.8	0	0.05	0.04	0.6	—
Beans, Lima:																
Fresh, cooked	100	⅔ c.	111	8	Tr.	20	1.8	71	47	121	2.5	280	0.18	0.10	1.3	17
Frozen, cooked	100	⅔ c.	99	6	Tr.	19	1.6	74	20	90	1.7	230	0.07	0.05	1.0	17
Beans:																
Snap green:																
Cooked, fresh or frozen	100	¾ c.	25	2	Tr.	5	1.0	92	50	37	0.6	540	0.07	0.09	0.5	12
Canned, drained solids	100	¾ c.	24	1	Tr.	5	1.0	92	45	25	1.5	470	0.03	0.05	0.3	4
Wax or yellow:																
Canned, drained solids	100	½ c.	22	1	Tr.	5	1.0	93	50	37	0.6	230	0.07	0.09	0.5	13

Tr. (trace) is used to indicate values that would round to zero with the number of decimal places carried to this table. Thus Tr. means 0.4 Gm. or less of protein, fat, carbohydrate or water.

† Value for fully ripe fruit. Av. for firm ripe is 1,900; Av. for partially ripe is 2,500.

COMPOSITION OF FOODS (Continued)

Food and Description	Wt. Gm.	Approximate Measure	Food Energy K Cal.	Protein Gm.	Fat Gm.	Carbohydrate Total Gm.	Fiber Gm.	Water Gm.	Ca Mg.	P Mg.	Fe Mg.	Vitamin A I.U.	Thiamine Mg.	Riboflavin Mg.	Niacin Mg.	Ascorbic Acid Mg.
Bean Sprouts, mung, raw	100	1 c.	35	4	Tr.	7	0.7	89	19	64	1.3	20	0.13	0.13	0.8	19
Beets, cooked, drained	100	½ c.	32	1	Tr.	7	0.8	91	14	23	0.5	20	0.03	0.04	0.3	6
Beet greens, cooked	100	⅔ c.	18	2	Tr.	3	1.1	94	99†	25	1.9	5,100	0.07	0.15	0.3	15
Blackberries: including dewberries, boysenberries																
Raw	100	⅔ c.	58	1	1	13	4.2	85	32	19	0.9	200	0.03	0.04	0.4	21
Canned, solids and liquids: Water pack	100	½ c. scant	40	1	1	9	2.8	89	22	13	0.6	140	0.02	0.02	0.2	7
Blueberries:																
Raw	100	⅔ c.	62	1	1	15	1.5	83	15	13	1.0	100	0.03	0.06	0.5	14
Frozen without sugar	100	⅔ c.	55	1	Tr.	14	1.5	85	10	13	0.8	70	0.03	0.06	0.5	7
Canned, solids and liquids: Water pack	100	½ c. scant	39	Tr.	Tr.	10	1.0	89	10	9	0.7	40	0.01	0.01	0.2	7
Bran (breakfast cereal, almost wholly bran)	28	1 oz.	95	3	1	21	2.0	1	24	350	2.9	0	0.11	0.09	5.0	0

Food	Grams	Measure														
Brazil nuts, shelled	100	⅔ c.	654	14	67	11	3.1	5	186	693	3.4	Tr.	0.96	0.12	1.6	0
Breads:																
Boston brown (Enr)	100	2 sl.	211	6	1	46	0.7	45	90	160	1.9	—	0.11	0.06	1.2	0
French or Vienna	100	3.5 oz.	290	9	3	55	0.2	31	43	85	2.2	0	0.28	0.22	2.5	Tr.
Italian (Enriched)	100	3.5 oz.	276	9	1	56	0.2	32	17	77	2.2	0	0.29	0.20	2.6	0
Raisin	23	1 sl.	60	2	1	13	Tr.	7	16	20	0.3	Tr.	0.01	0.02	0.2	0
Rye (⅓ rye, ⅔ wh)	100	4 sl.	243	9	1	52	0.4	36	75	147	1.6	0	0.18	0.07	1.4	0
Whole wheat	23	1 sl.	56	2	1	11	0.4	9	23	53	0.6	Tr.	0.06	0.03	0.6	Tr.
Broccoli, flower stalks, fresh or frozen	100	⅔ c.	32	4	Tr.	6	1.5	89	103	78	1.1	2,500	0.10	0.23	0.9	113
cooked	100	⅔ c.	26	3	Tr.	5	1.5	91	88	62	0.8	2,500	0.09	0.20	0.8	90
Brussels sprouts, fresh or frozen, cooked	100	¾ c.	36	4	Tr.	6	1.6	88	32	72	1.1	520	0.08	0.14	0.8	87
Buckwheat flour, light	100	1 c. sifted	347	6	1	80	0.5	12	11	88	1.0	0	0.08	0.04	0.4	0
Butter	14	1 tbsp.	100	Tr.	11	Tr.	0.0	2	3	2	0.0	460‡	—	—	—	0
Buttermilk, cultured (made from skim milk)	100	½ c. scant	36	4	Tr.	5	0.0	91	121	95	Tr.	Tr.	0.04	0.18	0.1	1

‡ Year-round average.

COMPOSITION OF FOODS (Continued)

Food and Description	Wt. Gm.	Approximate Measure	Food Energy K Cal	Protein Gm.	Fat Gm.	Carbohydrate Total Gm.	Fiber Gm.	Water Gm.	Ca Mg.	P Mg.	Fe Mg.	Vitamin A I.U.	Thiamine Mg.	Riboflavin Mg.	Niacin Mg.	Ascorbic Acid Mg.
Cabbage:																
Raw	100	wedge 3½ x 4½ in.	24	1	Tr.	5	0.8	92	49	29	0.4	130	0.05	0.05	0.3	47§
Cooked (short time)	100	1⅔ c.	20	1	Tr.	4	0.8	94	44	20	0.3	130	0.04	0.04	0.3	33
Cabbage, celery or Chinese,																
raw	100	1 c., 1-in. pieces	14	1	Tr.	3	0.6	95	43	40	0.6	150	0.05	0.04	0.6	25
Cantaloupe (raw)		5" dia	30	1	Tr.	8	0.3	91	14	16	0.4	3,400	0.04	0.03	0.6	33
Carrots (raw)	100	2 carrots	42	1	Tr.	10	1.0	88	37	36	0.7	11,000	0.06	0.05	0.6	8
(cooked)	100	⅔ c.	31	1	Tr.	7	1.0	92	33	31	0.6	10,500	0.05	0.05	0.5	6
Cashew nuts (cooked)	28	1 oz.	168	5	14	9	0.4	1	11	112	1.1	30	0.13	0.08	0.5	0
Cauliflower (raw)	100	1 c.	27	3	Tr.	5	0.9	91	25	56	1.1	60	0.11	0.10	0.7	78
(cooked)	100	1 c.	22	2	Tr.	4	0.9	93	21	42	0.7	60	0.09	0.08	0.6	55
Celery (raw)	100	2 lg. stalk	17	1	Tr.	4	0.6	94	39	28	0.3	240	0.03	0.03	0.3	9
(cooked)	100	¾ c.	14	1	Tr.	3	0.6	95	31	22	0.2	230	0.02	0.03	0.3	6

Food															
Chard (leaves-cook)	100	⅔ c.	18	2	Tr.	3	0.7	94	73	24	1.8	5,400	0.04	0.11	0.4	16
Cherries (sour-raw)	100	1 c.	58	1	Tr.	14	0.2	84	22	19	0.4	1,000	0.05	0.06	0.4	10
(sweet-raw)	100	⅔ c.	70	1	Tr.	17	0.4	80	22	19	0.4	110	0.05	0.06	0.4	10
Chickpeas (dry)	100	½ c.	360	21	5	61	5.3	11	150	331	6.9	50	0.31	0.15	2.0	—
Coconut (fresh)	100	1 c. shred.	346	4	35	9	4.0	51	13	95	1.7	0	0.05	0.02	0.5	3
Coleslaw (Fr. dressg)	100	¾ c.	95	1	7	8	0.7	84	42	26	0.4	110	0.04	0.04	0.3	29
Collards (cooked)	100	½ c.	33	4	1	5	1.0	90	188	52	0.8	7,800	0.11	0.20	1.2	76
Corn (sweet-cooked)	100	1 sm. ear	91	3	1	21	0.7	74	3	89	0.6	400†	0.11	0.10	1.4	9
(canned-cream)	100	½ c.	82	2	1	20	1.0	76	3	56	0.6	330†	0.03	0.05	1.0	5
Corn bread (whole cn)	100	2 muffins	215	7	6	35	0.6	49	141	216	1.7	130†	0.15	0.18	0.8	0
Corn Flakes (w/iron)	28	1 c.	108	2	Tr.	24	0.2	1	5	13	0.4	0	0.12	0.02	0.6	0
Corn grits (Enr-ckd)	100	½ c.	51	1	Tr.	11	0.1	87	1	10	0.3	Tr.	0.04	0.03	0.4	0
Cowpeas (cooked)	100	⅔ c.	108	8	1	18	1.8	72	24	146	2.1	350	0.30	0.11	1.4	17
Crackers (Graham)	14	2 med.	55	1	1	10	0.1	1	3	28	0.3	0	0.04	0.02	0.2	0

§ Freshly harvested av. 51 Mg.; stored av. 42 Mg.

411

COMPOSITION OF FOODS (Continued)

Food and Description	Wt. Gm.	Approximate Measure	Food Energy K Cal.	Protein Gm.	Fat Gm.	Carbohydrate Total Gm.	Carbohydrate Fiber Gm.	Water Gm.	Minerals Ca Mg.	Minerals P Mg.	Minerals Fe Mg.	Vitamins Vitamin A I.U.	Vitamins Thiamine Mg.	Vitamins Riboflavin Mg.	Vitamins Niacin Mg.	Vitamins Ascorbic Acid Mg.
Cranberries (raw)	100	1 c.	46	Tr.	1	11	1.4	88	14	11	0.5	40	0.03	0.02	0.1	11
(Juice-cocktail)	100	½ c.	65	Tr.	Tr.	17	Tr.	83	5	3	0.3	Tr.	0.01	0.01	Tr.	40†
Cucumbers (raw)	100	⅓-8'' cu.	14	1	Tr.	3	0.3	96	17	18	0.3	Tr.	0.03	0.04	0.2	11
Currants (raw)	100	1 c.	50	1	Tr.	12	3.4	86	32	23	1.0	120	0.04	0.05	0.1	41
Dandelion greens (ck)	100	½ c.	33	2	1	6	1.3	90	140	42	1.8	11,700	0.13	0.16	—	18
Dates (fresh/dried)	100	½ c. ptd	274	2	1	73	2.4	23	59	63	3.0	50	0.09	0.10	2.2	0
Eggplant (boiled)	100	3.5 oz.	19	1	Tr.	4	0.9	94	11	21	0.6	10	0.05	0.04	0.5	3
Eggs (whole)	50	1 med.	81	7	6	Tr.	0.0	38	27	102	1.2	590	0.05	0.15	Tr.	0
Farina (enr-cooked)	100	½ c.	43	1	Tr.	9	0.0	89	60	13	5.0	0	0.05	0.03	0.4	0
Fats (Vegetable)	12.5	1 Tbsp.	110	0	13	0	0.0	0	0	0	0.0	0	0.00	0.00	0	0

Food																
Figs (raw)	100	3 small	80	1	Tr.	20	1.2	78	35	22	0.6	80	0.06	0.05	0.4	2
(dried)	100	5 figs	274	4	1	69	5.6	23	126	77	3.0	80	0.10	0.10	0.7	0
Filberts or hazelnuts	100		634	13	62	13	3.0	6	209	337	3.4	—	0.46	—	0.9	Tr.
Fig bars	25	1 lg.	88	1	1	19	0.4	3	17	17	0.3	0	0.01	0.01	0.2	0
Grapefruit (white)	100	½ small	41	1	Tr.	11	0.2	88	16	16	0.4	80	0.04	0.02	0.2	38
(canned with liqd.)	100	½ c.	70	1	Tr.	18	0.2	81	13	14	0.3	10	0.03	0.02	0.2	30
(juice-fresh or fz.)	100	½ c.	41	1	Tr.	10	Tr.	90	10	17	0.1	10	0.04	0.02	0.2	38
Grapes (raw)	100	1 bunch	69	1	1	16	0.6	82	16	12	0.4	100	0.05	0.03	0.3	4
(European type)	100	⅔ c.	67	1	Tr.	17	0.5	82	12	20	0.4	100	0.05	0.03	0.3	4
(Juice-commercial)	100	3.5 oz.	66	Tr.	0	17	—	83	11	12	0.3	—	0.04	0.02	0.2	Tr.
Guavas (raw)	100	1 large	62	1	1	15	5.5	83	23	42	0.9	280	0.05	0.05	1.2	242†
Honey (strained)	21	1 Tbsp.	64	Tr.	0	17	—	4	1	1	0.1	0	Tr.	0.01	Tr.	Tr.
Honeydew melon (raw)	100	1.5 x 7″ Wdg.	33	1	Tr.	8	0.6	91	14	16	0.4	40	0.05	0.03	0.6	23
Kale: Leaves only																
Cooked, fresh	100	1 c.	39	5	1	6	—	87	187	58	1.6	8,300	0.10	0.18	1.6	93
Frozen, boiled, drained	100	1 c.	31	3	1	5	0.9	90	121	48	1.0	8,200	0.06	0.15	0.7	38

† Value for fully ripe fruit. Av. for firm ripe is 1,900; Av. for partially ripe is 2,500.

COMPOSITION OF FOODS (Continued)

Food and Description	Wt. Gm.	Approximate Measure	Food Energy K Cal.	Pro- tein Gm.	Fat Gm.	Carbo- hydrate Total Gm.	Fiber Gm.	Water Gm.	Ca Mg.	P Mg.	Fe Mg.	Vita- min A I.U.	Thia- mine Mg.	Ribo- flavin Mg.	Nia- cin Mg.	Ascorbic Acid Mg.
Kohlrabi:																
Raw	100	¾ c. diced	29	2	Tr.	7	1.1	90	41	51	0.5	20	0.06	0.05	0.2	66
Cooked	100	⅔ c.	24	2	Tr.	7	1.1	92	33	41	0.3	20	0.06	0.03	0.2	43
Lemons, peeled fruit	100	1 medium, 2¾ x 2 in.	27	1	Tr.	8	0.4	90	26	16	0.6	20	0.04	0.02	0.1	53
Lemon juice, fresh and canned, unsweetened	100	½ c. scant	24	Tr.	Tr.	8	0.0	91	7	10	0.2	20	0.03	0.01	0.1	42
Lentils, mature, cooked	100	3½ ozs.	106	8	Tr.	19	1.2	72	25	119	2.1	20	0.07	0.06	0.6	0
Lettuce, crisp, headed	100	¼ head	13	1	Tr.	3	0.6	96	20	22	0.5	330	0.06	0.06	0.3	6
leafy types, Boston, Bibb	100	4 large leaves	14	1	Tr.	3	0.5	95	35	26	2.0	970	0.06	0.06	0.3	8
Limes, peeled fruit	100	2 medium	28	1	Tr.	10	0.5	89	33	18	0.6	10	0.03	0.02	0.2	37
Loganberries, raw	100	⅔ c.	62	1	1	15	3.0	83	35	17	1.2	200	0.03	0.04	0.4	24

Food	Weight (g)	Measure														
Macaroni: Enriched: Cooked,* firm	100	⅔ c. elbow type	148	5	1	30	0.1	64	11	65	1.1	0	0.18	0.10	1.4	0
Mangos, raw	100	½ medium	66	1	Tr.	17	0.9	81	10	13	0.4	4,800	0.05	0.05	1.1	35
Margarine, fortified	14	1 tbsp.	101	Tr.	11	Tr.	0.0	2	3	2	0.0	460	—	—	—	0
Milk, cow: Fluid (pasteurized and raw): Whole	244	1 c.	160	8.5	8.5	12	0.0	212	288	226	0.2	350	0.08	0.42	0.2	2
Nonfat (skim)	246	1 c.	88	8.8	Tr.	13	0.0	224	297	234	0.2	Tr.	0.10	0.44	0.2	2
Milk, goat, fluid	244	1 c.	164	7	10	12	0.0	212	315	259	0.2	390	0.10	0.26	0.7	2
Molasses, cane: First extraction or light	100	⅓ c.	252	—	—	65	—	24	165	45	4.3	—	0.07	0.06	0.2	—
Second extraction or medium	100	⅓ c.	232	—	—	60	—	24	290	69	6.0	—	—	0.12	1.2	—
Third extraction or blackstrap	100	⅓ c.	213	—	—	55	—	24	579	85	11.3	—	0.12	0.18	2.0	—
Muffins, made with enriched wheat flour*	100	2 muffins, 3¾-in. diam.	294	8	10	42	0.1	38	104	151	1.6	100	0.17	0.23	1.4	Tr.
Corn, enriched, ungerminated meal	100		314	7	10	48	0.2	33	105	169	1.7	300	0.20	0.23	1.6	Tr.

* Values are calculated from a recipe.

COMPOSITION OF FOODS (Continued)

Food and Description	Wt. Gm.	Approximate Measure	Food Energy K Cal.	Protein Gm.	Fat Gm.	Carbohydrate Total Gm.	Carbohydrate Fiber Gm.	Water Gm.	Minerals Ca Mg.	Minerals P Mg.	Minerals Fe Mg.	Vitamins Vitamin A I.U.	Vitamins Thiamine Mg.	Vitamins Riboflavin Mg.	Vitamins Niacin Mg.	Vitamins Ascorbic Acid Mg.
Mushrooms,																
cultivated, raw	100	½ c.	28	3	Tr.	4	0.8	90	6	116	0.8	Tr.	0.10	0.46	4.2	3
canned, solids and liquids	100	½ c.	17	2	Tr.	2	0.6	93	6	68	0.5	Tr.	0.02	0.25	2.0	2
Mustard greens:																
Cooked	100	⅔ c.	23	2	Tr.	4	0.9	92	138	32	1.8	5,800	0.08	0.14	0.6	48
Frozen, cooked	100	⅔ c.	20	2	Tr.	3	0.9	93	104	43	1.5	6,000	0.03	0.10	0.4	20
Nectarines, raw	100	1 small	64	1	Tr.	17	0.4	82	4	24	0.5	1,650	—	—	—	3
Oatmeal or rolled oats:																
Cooked*	100	⅔ c.	55	2	1	10	0.2	87	9	57	0.6	0	0.08	0.02	0.1	0
Oils, salad or cooking	100	½ c.	884	0	100	0	0.0	0	0	0	0.0	0	0.00	0.00	0.0	0
	14	1 tbsp.	124	0	14	0	0.0	0	0	0	0.0	0	0.00	0.00	0.0	0
Okra, cooked	100	9 pods	29	2	Tr.	6	1.0	90	92	41	0.5	490	0.13	0.18	0.9	20
Olives, pickled:																
Green	100	16 olives	116	1	13	1	1.3	78	61	17	1.6	300	—	—	—	—
Ripe, Mission	100	10 olives	184	1	20	3	1.5	73	106	17	1.7	70	Tr.	Tr.	—	—

Food															
Onions:															
Mature:															
Raw	100	1 onion, 2½-in. diam.	38	2	9	0.6	89	27	36	0.5	40	0.03	0.04	0.2	10
Cooked, drained	100	½ c.	29	1	7	0.6	92	24	29	0.4	40	0.03	0.03	0.2	7
Young, green, raw bulb and white top	100	12 small, without tops	45	1	11	1.8	88	40	39	0.6	Tr.	0.05	0.04	0.4	25
Oranges, all varieties peeled fruit	100	1 small	49	1	12	0.6	86	41	20	0.4	200	0.10	0.04	0.4	50‡
Orange juice:															
Fresh	100	½ c. scant	45	1	11	0.1	88	11	17	0.2	200	0.09	0.03	0.4	50‡
Canned, unsweetened	100	½ c. scant	48	1	11	0.1	88	10	18	0.4	200	0.07	0.02	0.3	40
Papayas, raw	100	½ c., ½ in. cubes	39	1	10	0.9	89	20	16	0.3	1,750	0.04	0.04	0.3	56
Parsley, common raw	3½	1 tbsp. chopped	1	Tr.	Tr.	Tr.	3	7†	2	0.2	300	Tr.	0.01	0.1	7
Parsnips, cooked	100	⅔ c.	66	2	15	2.0	82	45	62	0.6	30	0.07	0.08	0.1	10
Peaches:															
Raw	100	1 peach, 2½ x 2 in. diam.	38	1	10	0.6	89	8	19	0.5	1,330§	0.02	0.05	1.0	7

* Values are calculated from a recipe.
‡ Year-round average.
† Calcium may not be available because of the presence of oxalic acid.
§ Based on yellow varieties; White types 50 I.U. 100 Gm.

COMPOSITION OF FOODS (Continued)

Food and Description	Wt. Gm.	Approximate Measure	Food Energy K Cal.	Protein Gm.	Fat Gm.	Carbohydrate Total Gm.	Fiber Gm.	Water Gm.	Ca Mg.	P Mg.	Fe Mg.	Vitamin A I.U.	Thiamine Mg.	Riboflavin Mg.	Niacin Mg.	Ascorbic Acid Mg.
Peaches:																
Canned, solids and liquid:																
Water pack	100	½ c. scant	31	Tr.	Tr.	8	0.4	91	4	13	0.3	450	0.01	0.03	0.6	3
Frozen, sliced	100	3½ ozs.	88	Tr.	Tr.	23	0.4	77	4	13	0.5	650	0.01	0.03	0.7	40¶
Dried, sulfured:																
Uncooked	100	⅔ c.	262	3	1	68	3.1	25	48	117	6.0	3,900	0.01	0.19	5.3	18
Peanuts:																
roasted and salted	100	⅔ c.	585	26	50	19	2.4	2	74	401	2.1	0	0.32	0.13	17.2	0
	9	1 tbsp. chopped	52	2	5	2	0.2	Tr.	7	36	0.2	0	0.03	0.01	1.6	0
Peanut butter, made with small am't added fat	15	1 tbsp.	87	4	7	3	0.3	Tr.	10	61	0.3	0	0.02	0.02	2.3	0
Pears:																
Raw, including skin	100	1 med. pear, 2½ x 2 in.	61	1	Tr.	15	1.4	83	8	11	0.3	20	0.02	0.04	0.1	4
Canned, solids and liquid:																
Water pack	100	½ c. scant	32	Tr.	Tr.	8	0.7	91	5	7	0.2	Tr.	0.01	0.02	0.1	1

¶ Ascorbic acid added in processing.

Food	Weight (g)	Measure														
Peas, greens: Immature:																
Cooked fresh or frozen	100	⅔ c. drained	72	5	Tr.	12	2.0	82	22	93	1.9	610	0.27	0.10	2.0	16
Canned:																
Solids and liquid	100	½ c. scant	66	4	Tr.	13	1.5	83	20	66	1.7	450	0.09	0.05	0.9	9
Pecans, shelled	100	1 c. halves	687	9	71	15	2.3	3	73	289	2.4	130	0.86	0.13	0.9	2
	7½	1 tbsp. chopped	51	1	5	1	0.2	Tr.	5	22	0.2	10	0.06	0.01	0.1	Tr.
Peppers, green:																
Raw	100	1 large	22	1	Tr.	5	1.4	93	9	22	0.7	420	0.08	0.08	0.5	128
Persimmons, Japanese, raw	100	1 medium	77	1	Tr.	20	1.6	79	6	26	0.3	2,710	0.03	0.02	Tr.	11
Pickles:																
Dill, cucumber	100	1 large	11	1	Tr.	2	0.5	93	26	21	1.0	100	Tr.	0.02	Tr.	6
Sweet, cucumber or mixed	100	½ c.	146	1	Tr.	37	—	61	12	16	1.2	90	Tr.	0.02	Tr.	6
Pies:*		⅙ of 9-in. pie														
Apple	160		410	3	18	61	0.6	76	1	35	0.5	48	0.03	0.03	0.6	2
Blueberry	160		387	4	17	56	1.1	82	18	37	1.0	48	0.03	0.03	0.5	5
Cherry	160		418	4	18	62	0.2	74	22	40	0.5	705	0.03	0.03	0.8	Tr.
Pecan	160		668	8	37	82	0.8	31	75	165	4.5	256	0.25	0.11	0.5	Tr.
Pumpkin	150		317	6	17	37	0.8	94	76	104	0.8	3,700	0.04	0.15	0.8	Tr.
Pimientos, canned																
solid and liquid	38	1 medium	10	Tr.	Tr.	2	0.2	35	3	6	0.6	875	0.01	0.02	0.1	36

* Values are calculated from a recipe.

COMPOSITION OF FOODS (Continued)

Food and Description	Wt. Gm.	Approximate Measure	Food Energy K.Cal.	Protein Gm.	Fat Gm.	Carbohydrate Total Gm.	Fiber Gm.	Water Gm.	Ca Mg.	P Mg.	Fe Mg.	Vita-min A I.U.	Thiamine Mg.	Riboflavin Mg.	Niacin Mg.	Ascorbic Acid Mg.
Pineapple:																
Raw	100	¾ c. diced or 1 med. slice	52	Tr.	Tr.	14	0.4	85	17	8	0.5	70	0.09	0.03	0.2	17
Canned, solids and liquid in juice	100	1 med. slice	58	Tr.	Tr.	15	0.3	84	16	8	0.4	60	0.10	0.03	0.3	10
Pineapple juice, canned unsweetened	100	½ c. scant	55	Tr.	Tr.	14	0.1	86	15	9	0.3	50	0.05	0.02	0.2	9
Pine nuts:																
Piñon	100	3½ ozs.	635	13	61	21	1.1	3	12	604	5.2	30	1.28	0.23	4.5	Tr.
Pistachio nuts	100	3½ ozs.	594	19	54	19	1.9	5	131	500	7.3	230	0.67	—	1.4	0
Plantain, raw, baking banana	100	1 small	119	1	Tr.	31	0.4	66	7	30	0.7	—	0.06	0.04	0.6	14
Plums:																
All, excluding prunes, raw	100	2 medium	48	1	Tr.	12	0.6	87	12	18	0.5	250	0.03	0.03	0.5	6
Italian prunes, canned, syrup pack, solids and liquid	100	½ c. scant or 3 med. prunes	83	Tr.	Tr.	22	0.3	77	9	10	0.9	1,210	0.02	0.02	0.4	2

Food	Gm	Measure														
Popcorn, popped	14	1 c.	54	2	1	10	0.3	1	2	39	0.4	0	—	0.02	0.3	0
Potatoes:																
Baked in skin	100	1 med.	93	3	Tr.	21	0.6	75	9	65	0.7	Tr.	0.10	0.04	1.7	20‡
Boiled, pared before cooking	100	1 med.	65	2	Tr.	15	0.5	83	6	48	0.5	Tr.	0.09	0.03	1.2	16
Prunes:																
Dried, softenized uncooked	100	⅔ c. medium	255	2	1	67	1.6	28	51	79	3.9	1,600	0.09	0.17	1.6	3
Cooked, no sugar added	100	6 prunes, 2 tbsp. juice	119	1	Tr.	31	0.8	66	24	37	1.8	750	0.03	0.07	0.7	1
Prune juice, canned	100	½ c. scant	77	Tr.	0	19	—	80	14	20	4.1	—	0.01	0.01	0.4	2
Pumpkin, canned	100	⅞ c.	33	1	Tr.	8	1.2	90	25	26	0.4	6,400	0.03	0.05	0.6	5
Radishes, raw	40	4 small	7	Tr.	Tr.	1	0.1	37	12	12	0.4	Tr.	0.01	0.01	0.1	10
Raisins, natural dried, seedless (unbleached)	10	1 tbsp.	29	Tr.	Tr.	8	0.1	2	6	10	0.3	Tr.	0.01	0.01	Tr.	Tr.
Raspberries:																
Black, raw	100	¾ c.	73	2	1	16	5.1	81	30	22	0.9	0	0.03	0.09	0.9	18
Red, raw	100	¾ c.	57	1	1	14	3.0	84	22	22	0.9	130	0.03	0.09	0.9	25

‡ Year-round average. Recently dug potatoes contain about 24 mg. of ascorbic acid per 100 Gm. The value is only half as high after 3 months of storage and about one-third as high when potatoes have been stored as long as 6 months.

COMPOSITION OF FOODS (Continued)

Food and Description	Wt. Gm.	Approximate Measure	Food Energy K Cal.	Protein Gm.	Fat Gm.	Carbohydrate Total Gm.	Carbohydrate Fiber Gm.	Water Gm.	Minerals Ca Mg.	Minerals P Mg.	Minerals Fe Mg.	Vitamins Vitamin A I.U.	Vitamins Thiamine Mg.	Vitamins Riboflavin Mg.	Vitamins Niacin Mg.	Vitamins Ascorbic Acid Mg.
Rhubarb, stems only:																
Raw	100	¾ c. diced	16	1	Tr.	4	0.7	95	96†	18	0.8	100	0.03	0.07	0.3	9
Rice:																
Brown, cooked	100	⅔ c.	119	3	1	26	0.3	70	12	73	0.5	0	0.09	0.02	1.4	0
Precooked, instant, cooked	100	⅔ c.	109	2	Tr.	24	0.1	73	3	19	0.8	0	0.13§	0.01	1.0§	0
Rutabagas, boiled, drained	100	⅔ c. diced	35	1	Tr.	8	1.4	91	59	31	0.3	550	0.06	0.06	0.8	26
Rye wafers or "Swedish health bread" or Rye Krisp	13	2 wafers 1⅞ x 3½ in.	43	2	Tr.	10	0.3	1	6	52	0.6	0	0.04	0.03	0.2	0
Sauerkraut, canned, drained solids	100	⅔ c.	18	1	Tr.	4	0.7	93	36	18	0.5	50	0.03	0.04	0.2	14
Soups:																
Celery, cream of	100	⅖ c.	69	3	4	6	0.2	86	81	63	0.3	160	0.02	0.11	0.3	1
Mushroom, cream of	100	⅖ c.	88	3	6	7	0.1	83	78	69	0.2	100	0.02	0.14	0.3	Tr.
Onion	100	⅖ c.	27	2	1	2	0.2	93	12	11	0.2	Tr.	Tr.	0.01	Tr.	—
Pea (green), made with water	100	⅖ c.	53	2	1	9	0.4	86	18	46	0.4	140	0.02	0.02	0.4	3
Tomato, with water	100	⅖ c.	36	1	1	6	0.2	91	6	14	0.3	410	0.02	0.02	0.5	5

Food	Grams	Measure	Calories	Protein (g)	Fat (g)	Carbohydrate (g)	Fiber (g)	Water (g)	Calcium (mg)	Phosphorus (mg)	Iron (mg)	Vitamin A (I.U.)	Thiamine (mg)	Riboflavin (mg)	Niacin (mg)	Ascorbic Acid (mg)
Soybeans, canned immature, boiled	100	3½ ozs.	103	9	5	7	1.4	77	67	114	2.8	340	0.06	—		2
Soybean Products:																
Soybean milk, fluid	100	½ c. scant	33	3	2	2	0.0	92	21	48	0.8	40	0.08	0.03	0.2	0
Soybean curd (Tofu)	100	3½ ozs.	72	8	4	2	0.1	85	128	126	1.9	0	0.06	0.03	0.1	0
Soy sauce	15	1 tbsp.	10	1	Tr.	1	0.0	10	12	16	0.7	0	Tr.	0.04	0.1	0
Soybean sprouts, cooked boiled, drained	100	1 c.	38	5	1	4	0.8	89	43	50	0.7	80	0.16	0.15	0.7	4
Spinach:																
Raw	100	3½ ozs.	26	3	Tr.	4	0.6	91	93¶	51	3.1	8,100	0.10	0.20	0.6	51
Cooked	100	½ c. packed	23	3	Tr.	4	0.6	91	93¶	38	2.2	8,100	0.07	0.14	0.5	28
Squash:																
Summer: Cooked, diced, fresh or frozen	100	½ c.	15	1	Tr.	3	0.6	95	25	25	0.4	440	0.05	0.08	0.8	11
Winter: Baked	100	3½ ozs.	63	2	Tr.	15	1.8	86	28	48	0.8	4,200	0.05	0.13	0.7	13
Boiled, mashed	100	½ c.	38	2	Tr.	9	1.4	89	19	32	0.5	3,500	0.04	0.10	0.4	8
Starch, pure (including arrowroot, corn, etc.)	8	1 tbsp.	29	0	0	7	Tr.	1	0	0	0.0	0	0.00	0.00	0.0	0

† Calcium may not be available because of the presence of oxalic acid. ¶ Calcium may not be available because of presence of oxalic acid.

§ Based on minimum levels of enrichment specified in standard of identity, F.D.A., for iron, thiamine, riboflavin and niacin.

COMPOSITION OF FOODS (Continued)

Food and Description	Wt. Gm.	Approximate Measure	Food Energy K Cal.	Protein Gm.	Fat Gm.	Carbohydrate Total Gm.	Fiber Gm.	Water Gm.	Ca Mg.	P Mg.	Fe Mg.	Vitamin A I.U.	Thiamine Mg.	Riboflavin Mg.	Niacin Mg.	Ascorbic Acid Mg.
Strawberries:																
Raw	100	⅔ c.	37	1	1	8	1.4	90	21	21	1.0	60	0.03	0.07	0.6	59
Sweet potatoes:																
Baked in skin	100	1 small	141	2	1	33	0.9	64	40	58	0.9	8,100	0.09	0.07	0.7	22
Boiled in skin	100	½ medium	114	2	Tr.	26	0.7	71	32	47	0.7	7,900	0.09	0.06	0.6	17
Tangerines (including other Mandarin type oranges)	100	1 medium	46	1	Tr.	11	0.5	87	40	18	0.4	420	0.06	0.02	0.1	31
Tapioca, cream pudding	100	½ c.	134	5	5	17	0.0	72	105	109	0.4	290	0.04	0.18	0.1	1
Tomatoes:																
Raw	100	1 small	22	1	Tr.	5	0.5	94	13	27	0.5	900	0.06	0.04	0.7	23
Canned or cooked	100	½ c.	23	1	Tr.	5	0.4	94	6	19	0.5	900	0.05	0.03	0.7	20
Tomato juice, canned	100	½ c. scant	19	1	Tr.	4	0.2	94	7	18	0.9	800	0.05	0.03	0.8	16
Tortillas	30	1 tortilla	63	2	Tr.	13	0.3	8	35	57	0.3	0	0.03	0.07	0.6	—

Food	gm	Approximate measure														
Turnips:																
Raw	100	¾ c. diced	30	1	Tr.	7	0.9	92	39	30	0.5	Tr.	0.04	0.07	0.6	36
Cooked, boiled, drained	100	⅔ c. diced	23	1	Tr.	5	0.9	94	35	24	0.4	Tr.	0.04	0.05	0.3	22
Turnip greens, boiled in small amount of water, short time	100	⅔ c.	20	2	Tr.	4	0.7	93	184	37	1.1	6,300	0.15	0.24	0.6	69
Waffles, made with enriched flour*, egg and milk	100	2 small waffles, 4½ x 5½ x ½ in	279	9	10	38	0.1	41	113	173	1.7	330	0.17	0.25	1.3	Tr.
Walnuts, Persian or English	100	1 c. of halves	651	15	64	16	2.1	4	99	380	3.1	30	0.33	0.13	0.9	2
	8	1 tbsp. chopped	52	1	5	1	0.2	Tr.	8	31	0.2	Tr.	0.03	0.01	0.1	Tr.
Watermelons	100	3½ oz. portion	26	1	Tr.	6	0.3	92	7	10	0.5	590	0.03	0.03	0.2	7
Wheat flours:																
Whole (from hard wheat)	100	1 c. scant	333	13	0	71	2.3	12	41	372	3.3	0	0.55	0.12	4.3	0
Patent: All purpose or family flour: Enriched	100	1 c. scant	364	11	1	76	0.3	12	16	87	2.9†	0	0.44	0.26	3.5	0
Wheat products:																
Germ, commercially milled	100	3½ ozs., 1 c.	363	27	11	47	2.5	12	72	1,118	9.4	0	2.01	0.68	4.2	0
Rolled, cooked*	100	½ c. scant	75	2	Tr.	17	0.5	80	8	76	0.7	0	0.07	0.03	0.9	0

* Values are calculated from a recipe.

† Based on the minimum level of enrichment specified under the Food, Drug and Cosmetic Act.

COMPOSITION OF FOODS (Continued)

Food and Description	Wt. Gm.	Approximate Measure	Food Energy K Cal.	Protein Gm.	Fat Gm.	Carbohydrate Total Gm.	Carbohydrate Fiber Gm.	Water Gm.	Minerals Ca Mg.	Minerals P Mg.	Minerals Fe Mg.	Vitamins Vitamin A I.U.	Vitamins Thiamine Mg.	Vitamins Riboflavin Mg.	Vitamins Niacin Mg.	Vitamins Ascorbic Acid Mg.
Wheat products: Shredded, plain	30	1 large biscuit, 4 x 2¼ in.	107	3	1	24	0.7	2	13	117	1.0	0	0.07	0.03	1.3	0
Wheat and malted barley cereal quick cooking, cooked	100	½ c. scant	65	2	Tr.	13	0.2	84	9	59	0.4	0	0.05	0.01	—	0
Wild rice, parched, raw	100	⅔ c.	353	14	1	75	1.0	9	19	339	—	0	0.45	0.63	6.2	0
Yeast: Dried, brewer's	8	1 tbsp.	22	3	Tr.	3	0.1	1	16	141	1.4	0	1.24	0.35	3.0	0
Yogurt, from partially skimmed milk	246	1 c.	123	8	4	13	0.0	218	295	230	Tr.	170	0.10	0.43	0.2	2

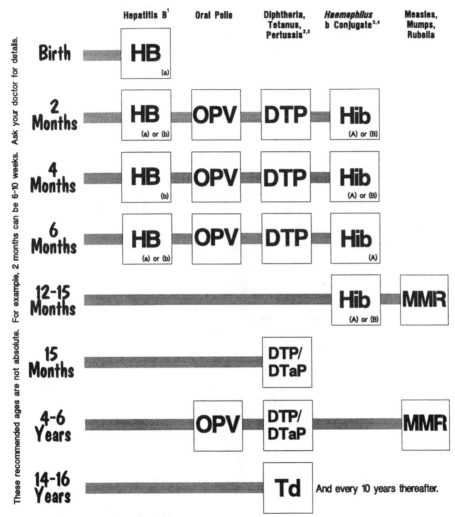

ACIP Recommended Immunization Schedule

(All recommended vaccines may be given simultaneously.) 11/93

	Hepatitis B[1]	Oral Polio	Diphtheria, Tetanus, Pertussis[2,3]	*Haemophilus* b Conjugate[3,4]	Measles, Mumps, Rubella
Birth	**HB** (a)				
2 Months	**HB** (a) or (b)	**OPV**	**DTP**	**Hib** (A) or (B)	
4 Months	**HB** (b)	**OPV**	**DTP**	**Hib** (A) or (B)	
6 Months	**HB** (a) or (b)	**OPV**	**DTP**	**Hib** (A)	
12-15 Months				**Hib** (A) or (B)	**MMR**
15 Months			**DTP/ DTaP**		
4-6 Years		**OPV**	**DTP/ DTaP**		**MMR**
14-16 Years			**Td** And every 10 years thereafter.		

(Left margin, vertical text: These recommended ages are not absolute. For example, 2 months can be 6-10 weeks. Ask your doctor for details.)

[1] Hepatitis B vaccine may be given in either of 2 schedules:
   (a) Birth, 1-2 Months, 6-18 Months
   (b) 1-2 Months, 4 Months, 6-18 Months

[2] DTP preparation containing acellular pertussis vaccine (DTaP) is recommended for the 4th and 5th doses, but whole-cell DTP may still be used if DTaP is not available.

[3] Combination DTP/Hib conjugate vaccine may be used when both shots are scheduled simultaneously.

[4] There are 2 schedules for Hib conjugate vaccines:
   (A) HbOC (HibTITER™), PRP-T (ActHIB™), or DTP/HbOC (TETRAMUNE™): 2, 4, 6, & 12-15 Months
   (B) PRP-OMP (PedvaxHIB®): 2, 4, & 12-15 Months

CDC
CENTERS FOR DISEASE CONTROL
AND PREVENTION

APPENDIX 3

Formulas for Skin Remedies
and other Preventive Agents

Many topical agents are in common use for the treatment or prevention of disease. Various classes of these will be listed below to guide in their proper use:

A. ANTISEPTICS

1. **Cresol** (*Lysol*). A potent disinfectant, but one which should never be taken internally.

2. **Hexachlorophene**. This is incorporated in soaps and creams, such as *Phisohex*. It should not be left on the skin or be applied for prolonged periods to a newborn, as brain damage has been reported with its use.

3. **Merbromin** (*Mercurochrome*) and **thimerosal** (*Merthiolate*). These are organic mercury-containing compounds used primarily for disinfecting the skin, and on cuts and abrasions.

4. **Silver Nitrate** ($AgNO_3$). This is used in a 1% solution on the eyes to prevent *ophthalmia neonatorum*.

5. **Tincture of Iodine** (2% iodine). This is a common antiseptic for use on the skin for surgical procedures. It should not replace simple cleansing for cuts and scratches.

6. **Halazone**. 4-8 mg./L of this compound can be used to disinfect small amounts of drinking water.

7. **Hydrogen Peroxide** (H_2O_2). A 3% solution may cleanse a wound by bubbling out foreign material and by oxidizing germs.

8. **Isopropyl alcohol**. A 50% solution is used on the skin for disinfection before injection and for drying purposes.

9. **Benzalkonium chloride** (*Zephiran*). This is an antiseptic solution of the cationic type, used to cleanse minor cuts and abrasions.

B. COUNTERIRRITANTS

Counterirritants may lessen pain by distracting the patient's attention, and redden the skin by producing reflex vasodilation. The basic mechanism is irritation. They produce warmth, but may even cause blisters.

1. **Mustard** plaster has been used in past generations, applied to the chest in bronchitis, or the back in backache.

2. **Methyl Salicylate** may be rubbed over painful joints.

3. **Oil of wintergreen** is used similarly for counterirritation in cases of arthritis.

C. CAUSTIC AGENTS

These are corrosive substances that coagulate protein. They are primarily used to remove granulation tissue, excessive growths, or warts. They may also be used for a styptic effect to stop bleeding.

1. **Silver nitrate** is used on an applicator stick to remove granulation tissue.

2. **Podophyllum** is useful in removing venereal warts. Protection of surrounding normal skin with Vaseline is essential.

3. **Alum** $(Al_2[SO_4]_3)$ was formerly used on canker sores. It has a *styptic* effect.

D. ASTRINGENTS

These agents produce mild coagulation of tissue proteins and are used to dry, harden, and protect the skin.

1. **Zinc oxide** (ZnO). In powder and ointment form this acts as a protective sun screen, also as a drying agent.

2. **Calamine** lotion (contains $ZnCO_3$). This widely used protective helps to relieve itching and is commonly used on insect bites and *poison ivy*.

3. **Compound tincture of benzoin**. This mixture of *benzoic* and *cinnamic* acids with resins and essential oils gives protection to the skin. It is also used in vaporizers and helps to toughen the skin areas sensitive to pressure sores in prolonged bed patients.

4. **Selenium sulfide** lotion (*Selsun*) is used as a detergent lotion and shampoo in dandruff of the scalp (*seborrheic dermatitis*).

5. **Benzoic** and **salicylic** ointment (*Whitfield's ointment*). This contains 12% and 6% of the respective acids. This has been used to treat fungal infection of the skin and tends to cause peeling.

E.   PROTECTIVES

Protectives are agents which smooth, soften, and otherwise protect the skin. They are most used as ingredients in powder, ointments, and dressings.

1. **Poultices** are substances applied as a moist water base dressing. They usually are left on for several hours to hasten the "pointing" in boils. Poultices provide some comfort in relief of pain. Here are a few types:
 a. *Linseed* poultice.
 b. *Cataplasm* of *kaolin* (mud packs).
 c. Oatmeal (*aveno*).
 d. Starch.
 e. Flax seed.
 f. Charcoal.

These various poultices are soothing to the skin and relieve itching. They may be combined with anti-inflammatory agents.

2. **Demulcents** soothe and protect the skin by providing extra surface covering or lubrication. Starch and purified talc (magnesium trisilicate) are used as lubricating powders. They may be useful for diaper rash and oversensitive skin.

3. Flexible **collodion** (*cellulose tetranitrate* in ether and alcohol) can be used to cover sutured areas in babies or on the scalp. It is generally used for protection.

4. **Paraffin**.

F.   EMOLLIENTS

Emollients soften and lubricate the skin and mucous membranes. They are usually ingredients in various ointments.

1. **Theobromine** oil (cocoa butter) is a base commonly used for suppositories.

2. **Olive** oil may be used as an enema.

3. **Liquid petrolatum** (mineral oil) is used for a laxative and a solvent.

4. **Petrolatum** (petroleum jelly) serves as an ointment base and a lubricant.

5. **Lanolin** (hydrous wool fat).

6. **Glycerin**.

G.   ADSORBENTS

A number of chemically inert powders are used internally as protectives to the gastrointestinal tract and *adsorbents*. The latter term implies a surface active property by which noxious substances, such as gases, toxins, and bacteria are attracted to the surface to which they adhere.

1. **Activated charcoal**. An odorless, tasteless, fine black powder that occupies a favored place in the treatment of dyspepsia, flatulence, diarrhea, and dysentery. It is particularly effective in the dry state and is the chief protective agent in modern gas masks. Because of its broad spectrum of adsorptive activity and its rapidity of action, activated charcoal is considered to be the most valuable single agent for the emergency treatment of certain cases of drug poisoning. In such an emergency, the usual dose of 1-8 grams can be approximated by stirring sufficient activated charcoal into water to make a thick soup. (See Chapter 18 for further discussion of the home uses for activated charcoal.)

2. **Magnesium trisilicate**. In addition to its use in antacids, it is an effective gastrointestinal adsorbent. Reacting with a patient's gastric contents it produces the gelatinous *silicon dioxide*, said to protect ulcerated mucosal surfaces and favor healing.

3. **Kaolin**. This hydrated *aluminum sulfate* has long been used in China for the treatment of diarrhea and dysentery. It tends to adsorb bacteria and toxins in the colon and is usually given as a mixture with pectin.

4. **Pectin**. Obtained from the acid extraction of the rind of citrus fruits or from apple. Pectin is widely employed in the treatment of diarrhea. Dissolved in 20 parts of water it forms a colloidal solution. Pectin (1%) is often used in combination with an adsorbent, such as kaolin (20%). However, it may be administered simply and conveniently in the form of ground, raw apple.

These are just a few of the common agents used in the treatment of skin conditions. A wide array of mixtures can be obtained with various herbs in conjunction with some of the above vehicles.

In general, *creams* are used to soothe dry scaly lesions while *ointments*, consisting of an oily rather than a water base, are applied more commonly to moist, weeping lesions. Prolongation of the effect of any topical agent can be obtained by covering with a polyethylene film, such as *Saran Wrap* or wearing a plastic or rubber glove. Prolonged covering of the skin is inadvisable in most cases, because of the maceration that occurs in contact with prolonged moisture.

In treating skin disease remember the importance of **sunlight**, not only to kill germs, but to "tone up" the exposed skin. Bathing with soap and water and frequent changes of clothing also promote a health of our skin that can make visible the well-being we desire to possess.

Selected Fatty Acids and
Cholesterol in Common Foods

Amount in 100 G. Edible Portion

Item and Description	Total Fat G.	Total Saturated Fat G.	Unsaturated Fatty Acids		Cholesterol Mg.
			Oleic G.	Linoleic G.	
Almonds, shelled	54.2	4	36	11	0
Avocado, raw	16.4	3	7	2	0
Bacon, broiled or fried	52.0	17	25	5	100
Beef, edible, raw, chuck	31.4	13	13	1	68
Brazil nuts, shelled	66.9	13	32	17	. .
Butter	81.0	46	27	2	250
Cashew nuts	45.7	8	32	3	. .
Cheese, cottage, creamed	4.2	3	1	Tr.	19
Chicken, raw, edible portion Fryer	7.2	2	2	2	67-88
Chocolate, bitter, cooking	53.0	30	20	1	0
Coconut, shredded, sweetened	39.1	34	3	Tr.	0
Cream, heavy whipping	36.7	23	9	1	133
Custard, baked, milk and egg	5.0	3	2	Tr.	105
Eggs, whole	11.3	3	4	1	504
yolks only	30.6	10	13	2	1,480
Filberts, shelled	62.4	3	34	10	0
Ice cream, 10% fat	10.6	7	4	Tr.	40
Ice milk	5.1	3	2	Tr.	20
Lamb, shoulder, edible portion	23.9	13	9	1	71
Lard	100	38	46	10	75
Liver, pork, raw	3.7	1	1	Tr.	300
Margarine, hydrogenated, all vegetable oil	81.0	18	47	14	0
Milk, whole, cow's	3.7	2	1	Tr.	14
Oils: corn	100	10	28	53	0

Amount in 100 G. Edible Portion

Item and Description	Total Fat G.	Total Saturated Fat G.	Unsaturated Fatty Acids		Cholesterol Mg.
			Oleic G.	Linoleic G.	
cottonseed	100	25	21	50	0
olive	100	11	76	7	0
peanut	100	18	47	29	0
safflower seed	100	8	15	72	0
soybean	100	15	20	52	0
Olives, ripe, Mission type	20.1	2	15	1	0
Peanuts, roasted, shelled	48.7	11	21	14	0
Pecans, shelled	71.2	5	45	14	0
Pistachio nuts, shelled	53.7	5	35	10	0
Popcorn, popped, plain	5.0	1	1	3	0
Potatoes, scalloped, milk and margarine	3.9	2	1	Tr.	6
Potato chips, vegetable oil	39.8	10	8	20	0
Salad dressings made with soybean, cottonseed or corn oil French, commercial	38.9	7	8	20	0
Mayonnaise, with egg	79.9	14	17	40	70
Russian salad dressing	50.8	9	11	26	
Salmon, canned, pink	5.9	2	1	Tr.	35
Tuna fish, canned in oil, drained solids	8.2	3	2	2	65
Turkey, dark meat, cooked	8.3	3	4	2	101
light meat, cooked	3.9	1	2	1	77
Veal, total edible, raw Chuck, medium fat	10.0	5	4	Tr.	70
Walnuts, shelled, black	59.3	4	21	28	0
English type	64.0	4	10	40	0
Wheat germ, commercial	11.5	2	3	6	0

Figures in this table are taken from Table 3, Handbook No. 8. Washington, U.S.D.A., 1963, and from Hardinge, M. G., and Crooks, H.: J. Am. Dietet. A., 34:1065, 1958; Feeley, R. M., Criner, P. E., Watt, B. K.: J. Am. Dietet. A., 61:134, 1972; Anderson, B. A., Kinsella, J. E., Watt, B. K.: J. Am. Dietet. A., 67:35, 1975; Posati, L. P., Kinsella, J. E., Watt, B. K.: J. Am. Dietet. A., 66:482, 1975.

COMMON LABORATORY TESTS AND THEIR NORMAL VALUES

Whole Blood Tests

DETERMINATION	NORMAL VALUES	CLINICAL SIGNIFICANCE
Clotting time	5-10 min.	Prolonged in hemorrhagic disease and in various coagulation factor deficiencies.
Fibrinogen	0.2-0.4 gm./100 ml.	Increased in pregnancy, pneumonia, infections accompanied by leukocytosis, and nephrosis. Decreased in acute yellow atrophy of liver, cirrhosis, typhoid fever, chloroform poisoning, abruptio placentae.
Prothrombin time	70-100% of control	Prolonged in hemorrhagic diseases, and in cirrhosis, hepatitis, and acute toxic necrosis of the liver.
Red blood cell count	Male: 4,600,000-6,200,000 per cu. mm. Female: 4,200,000-5,400,000 per cu. mm.	Increased in severe diarrhea and dehydration, polycythemia, acute poisoning, pulmonary fibrosis. Decreased in all anemias, leukemia, and after hemorrhage, when blood volume has been restored.
Erythrocyte sedimentation rate	Male: 0-9 mm./hr. Female: 0-20 mm./hr.	Increased in tissue destruction, whether inflammatory or degenerative, and during menstruation, pregnancy, and in acute febrile diseases.
Hematocrit	Male: 42-50% Female: 40-48%	Decreased in severe anemias, anemia of pregnancy, acute massive blood loss. Increased in erythrocytosis of any cause, and in dehydration or hemoconcentration associated with shock.
Hemoglobin	Male: 13-16 gm./100 ml. Female: 12-14 gm./100 ml.	Decreased in various anemia, pregnancy, severe or prolonged hemorrhage, and with excessive fluid intake. Increased in polycythemia, chronic obstructive pulmonary diseases, failure of oxygenation because of congestive heart failure, and normally, in people living at high altitudes.

White blood cell count	Total: 5,000-10,000 cu. mm.	Elevated in acute infectious diseases—predominately with bacterial diseases. Eosinophils elevated in allergy, intestinal parasitosis. Elevated in acute leukemia, following menstruation, and following surgery or trauma. Depressed in aplastic anemia, and by toxic agents, such as chemotherapeutic agents used in treating malignancy.
Neutrophils	60-70%	
Eosinophils	1-4%	
Basophils	0-0.5%	
Lymphocytes	20-30%	
Monocytes	2-6%	
Reticulocytes	0.5-1.5% of red cells	Increased with any condition stimulating increased bone marrow activity, i.e., infection, blood loss (acute and chronic), following iron therapy in iron deficiency anemia. Decreased with any condition depressing bone marrow activity, acute leukemia, late stage of severe anemias.
Platelet count	200,000-350,000 per cu. mm.	Increased with chronic leukemia. Decreased in acute leukemia, aplastic anemia, and during cancer chemotherapy.

Blood Chemistries

		(Increased)	**(Decreased)**
Amylase	80-150 units/ml.	Acute pancreatitis Mumps Duodenal ulcer Carcinoma of head of pancreas Prolonged elevation with pseudocyst of pancreas	Chronic pancreatitis Pancreatic fibrosis and atrophy Cirrhosis of liver Acute alcoholism Toxemias of pregnancy
Ascorbic acid (Vitamin C)	0.4-1.5 mg./100 ml.		Rheumatic fever Collagen diseases Deficient vitamin C intake Renal and hepatic disease Congestive heart failure

435

Blood Chemistries (Continued)

DETERMINATION	NORMAL VALUES	CLINICAL SIGNIFICANCE (Increased)	(Decreased)
Bilirubin	Total: 0.1-1.0 mg./100 ml. Direct: 0.1-0.2 mg./100 ml. Indirect: 0.1-0.8 mg./100 ml.	Hemolytic anemia (indirect) Biliary obstruction Hepatocellular damage Pernicious anemia Hemolytic disease of newborn Eclampsia	
Calcium	9-11 mg./100 ml.	Tumor or hyperplasia of parathyroid Hyperparathyroidism Hypervitaminosis D Multiple myeloma Nephritis with uremia	Hypoparathyroidism Diarrhea Celiac disease Rickets Osteomalacia Malnutrition Nephrosis After parathyroidectomy
CO_2 content	Adults: 24-32 mEq./L. Infants: 20-26 mEq./L.	Tetany Respiratory disease Intestinal obstruction Vomiting	Acidosis Diarrhea Nephritis Anesthesia Eclampsia
Carotene, Beta (pro Vitamin A)	100-300 ug./100 ml.	Carotenemia Hypothyroidism Diabetes Hyperlipemia	Malabsorption syndromes Hepatic disease Dietary deficiencies
Chloride	95-105 mEq./L.	Nephritis Urinary obstruction Cardiac decompensation Anemia Ether anesthesia	Diabetes Vomiting Diarrhea Pneumonia Heavy metal poisoning Cushing's syndrome Burns Intestinal obstruction

436

Test	Normal Value		
Cholesterol	150-220 mg./100 ml. (Ideal is 100 + age)	Lipemia Obstructive jaundice Diabetes Hypothyroidism	Pernicious anemia Hemolytic jaundice Hyperthyroidism Severe infection Terminal states of debilitating disease
Creatine phosphokinase (CPK)	Male: 0-20 I.U./L. Female: 0-14 I.U./L.	Myocardial infarction Skeletal muscle diseases	
Creatinine	1-2 mg./100 ml.	Nephritis Chronic renal disease	
Fibrinogen**	0.1-0.4 gm./100 ml.	Pneumonia Acute infections Pregnancy Nephrosis Carcinoma	Cirrhosis Acute toxic necrosis of liver Anemia Typhoid fever Chloroform or phosphorus poisoning Abruptio placentae
Glucose	70-115 mg./100 ml.	Diabetes Nephritis Hyperthyroidism Cerebral lesions Infections Pregnancy Uremia	Hyperinsulinism Hypothyroidism Pernicious vomiting Addison's disease Extensive hepatic damage

437

Blood Chemistries (Continued)

DETERMINATION	NORMAL VALUES	CLINICAL SIGNIFICANCE	
		(Increased)	(Decreased)
Iron	65-150 µg./100 ml.	Pernicious anemia Aplastic anemia Hemolytic anemia Hepatitis Hemochromatosis	Iron deficiency anemia
Iron binding capacity	150-225 µg./100 ml.	Iron deficiency anemia	Chronic infectious diseases
Lactic dehydrogenase (LDH)	60-100 units/ml.	Untreated pernicious anemia Myocardial infarction Pulmonary infarction Liver disease	
Magnesium	1.8-2.2 mEq./L.	Ingestion of epsom salts Parathyroidectomy	Chronic alcoholism Toxemia of pregnancy Severe renal disease
Phosphatase, acid	0-2 units/ml.	Carcinoma of prostate Advanced Paget's disease Hyperparathyroidism	
Phosphatase, alkaline	4-17 units/ml.	Rickets Hyperparathyroidism Liver disease	
Phosphorus, inorganic	3.0-4.5 mg./100 ml.	Chronic nephritis Hypoparathyroidism	Hyperparathyroidism
Potassium	3.5-5.0 mEq./L.	Addison's disease Oliguria Tissue breakdown or hemolysis	Diabetic acidosis Diarrhea Vomiting

Test	Normal Value	Increased	Decreased
Protein, total	6-8 gm./100 ml.	Hemoconcentration Shock Multiple myeloma	Malnutrition Hemorrhage Loss of plasma from burns Proteinuria
Albumin	3.5-5 gm./100 ml.		
Globulin	1.5-3 gm./100 ml.	Chronic infections	
Sodium	135-145 mEq./L.	Hemoconcentration Nephritis Pyloric obstruction	Alkali deficit Addison's disease Myxedema
Triglyceride (fasting)	30-150 mg./100 ml.	Diabetes Hypothyroidism Obesity Hereditary	Low fat diet Exercise
Urea nitrogen	10-20 mg./100 ml.	Acute glomerulonephritis Obstructive uropathy Mercury poisoning Nephrotic syndrome	Severe hepatic failure Pregnancy
Uric acid	1-6 mg./100 ml.	Gouty arthritis Acute leukemia Toxemia of pregnancy	
Vitamin A	0.5-2.0 units/ml.	Hypervitaminosis A	Vitamin A deficiency

Urine Chemistries

Test	Normal Value	Increased	Decreased
Porphobilinogen	Zero	Acute porphyria Liver disease	
Protein	Zero	Nephritis Cardiac failure Mercury poisoning	

Urine Chemistries (Continued)

DETERMINATION	NORMAL VALUES	CLINICAL SIGNIFICANCE	
		(Increased)	(Decreased)
Glucose	Zero	Multiple myeloma Febrile states Hematuria Amyloidosis Diabetes mellitus Pituitary disorders Intracranial pressure Lesion in floor of 4th ventricle	
Vanilmandelic acid (VMA)	0.7-6.8 mg./24 hr.	Pheochromocytoma	
D-Xylose absorption	5-hr. excretion of 16-33% of test dose		Malabsorption syndromes

Cerebrospinal Fluid

DETERMINATION	NORMAL VALUES	CLINICAL SIGNIFICANCE	
Cell count	0-5 mononuclear cells/cu. mm.	Bacterial meningitis syphilis poliomyelitis Encephalitis	
Chloride	100-130 mEq./L.	Uremia	Acute generalized meningitis Tubercular meningitis
Glucose	50-75 mg./100 ml.	Diabetes mellitus Diabetic coma encephalitis Uremia	Acute meningitis Tuberculous meningitis Insulin shock

Protein   15-45 Mg./100 ml.

Acute meningitis
Tubercular meningitis
Syphilis
Poliomyelitis
Guillain-Barré syndrome

Toxicology

Carbon monoxide   0-2%

Ethanol   Zero

Symptoms with over 20% saturation

Maximal level allowable by courts = 0.10%
0.3-0.4% = marked intoxication
0.4-0.5% = alcoholic stupor

Gastric Analysis

Free HCl   0-30 mEq./L.
Total acidity   15-45 mEq./L.

Neuroses
Peptic ulcer
Zollinger-Ellison syndrome

Pernicious anemia
Gastric carcinoma
Chronic atrophic gastritis
Decreases normally with age

441

Exercises for better back care

General Instructions

Your best back support is derived from your own back muscles! Faithful performance of back exercises often avoids the necessity of an external brace or corset. Back muscles can give you all the support needed if you strengthen them by routine performance of prescribed exercises.

Exercises

Follow the exercise routine prescribed by your doctor. Gradually increase the frequency of your exercises as your condition improves, but stop when fatigued. If your muscles are tight, take a warm shower or tub bath before performing your back exercises. Do not be alarmed if you have mild aching after performing exercises. This should diminish as your muscles become stronger.

Exercise on a rug or mat. Put a small pillow under your neck. Wear loose clothing; no shoes. Stop doing any exercise that causes pain until you have checked with your doctor.

Additional Instructions

Helpful hints for a healthy back

Standing and walking

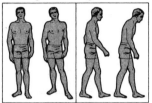

Correct Incorrect   Correct Incorrect

Try to toe straight ahead when walking; put most of your weight on your heels; hold your chest forward and elevate the front of the pelvis as if walking up an incline. Avoid wearing high heels. Stand as if you are trying to touch the ceiling with the top of your head, eyes straight ahead. All the elements of good posture will flow from these simple maneuvers.

Sitting

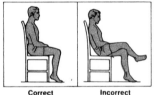

Correct   Incorrect

Sit in a hard-back chair with spine pushed back; try to eliminate the hollow in the lower back. If possible, elevate the knees higher than hips while sitting in an automobile. Secretaries should adjust posture chairs accordingly. Sit all the way back in the chair with your back erect.

Lifting

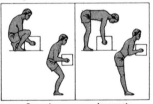

Correct   Incorrect

Bend your knees; squat and lift with your thigh muscles, not your back. Never bend over with your knees straight and lift with the upper torso.

Move slowly and avoid sudden movements. Try to avoid lifting loads in front of you above the waist line. Avoid bending over to lift heavy objects from car trunks, as this places a strain on low back muscles.

Sleeping

Correct

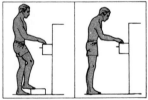

Incorrect

Sleep on a firm mattress; a ¾ inch plywood bed board is helpful and should be used with all but a very firm orthopedic mattress. With acute back pain, sleep with a pillow or blanket rolled under the knees and a pillow under the head. Keep your knees and hips bent when sleeping on your side.

Driving

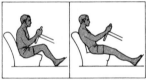

Correct   Incorrect

Use a firm seat with a padded plywood or special seat support. Sit close to the wheel with knees bent. On long trips, stop every one to two hours and walk to relieve tension and relax muscles.

Working

Correct   Incorrect

Try to avoid fatigue caused by work requiring long standing. Flex hips and knees by occasionally placing a foot on a stool or bench. Take exercise breaks from desk work by getting up, moving around and performing a few back exercises in the standing position.

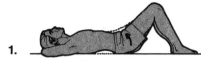

1.

Lie on your back with knees bent and hands clasped behind neck. Feet flat on the floor. Take a deep breath and relax. Press the small of your back against the floor and tighten your stomach and buttock muscles. This should cause the lower end of the pelvis to rotate forward and flatten your back against the floor. Hold for five seconds. Relax.

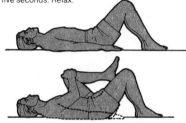

2.

Lie on your back with knees bent. Feet flat on the floor. Take a deep breath and relax. Grasp one knee with both hands and pull as close to your chest as possible. Return to starting position. Straighten leg. Return to starting position. Repeat with alternate leg.

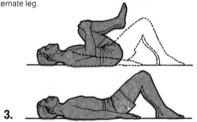

3.

Lie on your back with knees bent. Feet on the floor. Take a deep breath and relax. Grasp *both* knees and pull them as close to your chest as possible. Hold for three seconds, then return to starting position. Straighten legs and relax.

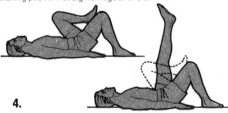

4.

Lie on your back with knees bent. Feet flat on the floor. Take a deep breath and relax. Draw one knee to chest. Then point leg upward as far as possible. Return to starting position. Relax. Repeat with alternate leg.

NOTE: This exercise is useful in stretching tight hamstring muscles, but is not recommended for patients with sciatic pain associated with a herniated disc.

5.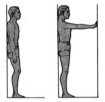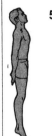

a. Lie on your stomach with hands clasped behind back. Pull shoulders back and down by pushing hands downward towards feet, pinching shoulder blades together, and lift head from floor. Take a deep breath. Hold for two seconds. Relax.

b. Stand erect. With one hand grasp the thumb of other hand behind the back, then pull downwards toward the floor; stand on toes and look at the ceiling while exerting the downward pull. Hold momentarily, then relax. Repeat 10 times at intervals of two hours during the working day. Take an exercise break instead of a coffee break!

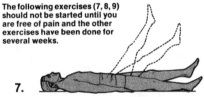

6. Stand with your back against doorway. Place heels four inches away from frame. Take a deep breath and relax. Press the small of your back against doorway. Tighten your stomach and buttock muscles, allowing your knees to bend slightly. This should cause the lower end of the pelvis to rotate forward (as in Exercise 1). Press your neck up against doorway. Press both hands against opposite side of doorway and straighten both knees. Hold for two seconds. Relax.

The following exercises (7, 8, 9) should not be started until you are free of pain and the other exercises have been done for several weeks.

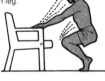

7.

Lie on your back with your legs straight out, knees unbent and arms at your sides. Take a deep breath and relax. Raise legs one at a time as high as is comfortable and lower to floor as slowly as possible. Repeat five times for each leg.

8.

May be done holding onto a chair or table. After squatting, flex head forward, bounce up and down two or three times, then assume erect position.

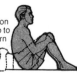

9.

Lie on your back with knees bent. Feet flat on floor. Take a deep breath and relax. Pull up to a sitting position keeping knees bent. Return to starting position. Relax. Having someone hold your feet down facilitates this exercise.

A SERVICE OF RIKER LABORATORIES.

443

APPENDIX 7

THE CHILDREN'S MEDICAL CENTER, BOSTON - ANTHROPOMETRIC CHART

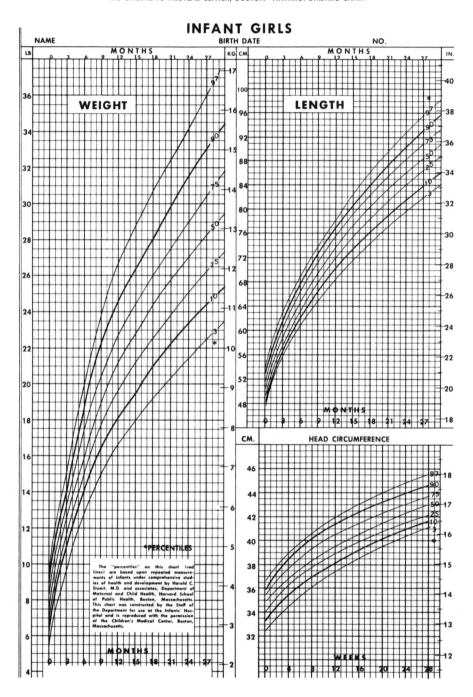

INFANT GIRLS

The "percentiles" on this chart (red lines) are based upon repeated measurements of infants under comprehensive studies of health and development by Harold C. Stuart, M.D. and associates, Department of Maternal and Child Health, Harvard School of Public Health, Boston, Massachusetts. This chart was constructed by the Staff of the Department for use at the Infants' Hospital and is reproduced with the permission of the Children's Medical Center, Boston, Massachusetts.

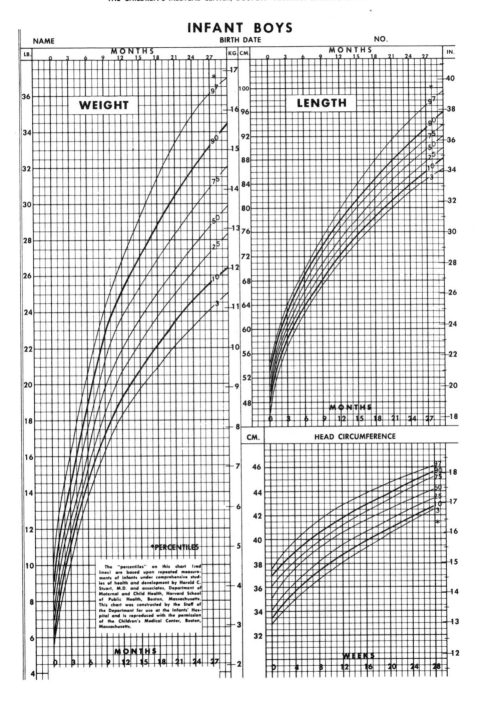

THE CHILDREN'S MEDICAL CENTER, BOSTON - ANTHROPOMETRIC CHART

INFANT BOYS

445

THE CHILDREN'S MEDICAL CENTER, BOSTON - ANTHROPOMETRIC CHART

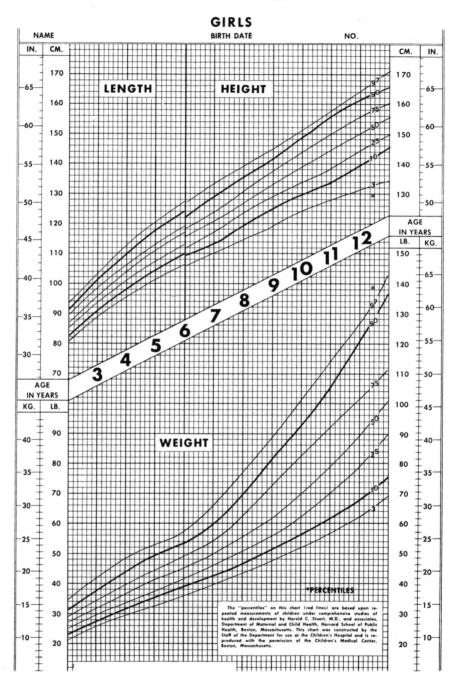

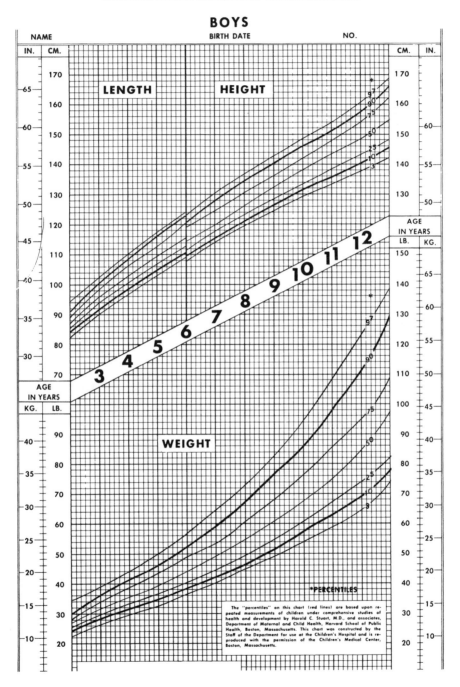

THE CHILDREN'S MEDICAL CENTER, BOSTON - ANTHROPOMETRIC CHART

BOYS

NAME   BIRTH DATE   NO.

LENGTH   HEIGHT

WEIGHT

*PERCENTILES

The "percentiles" on this chart (red lines) are based upon re-peated measurements of children under comprehensive studies of health and development by Harold C. Stuart, M.D., and associates, Department of Maternal and Child Health, Harvard School of Public Health, Boston, Massachusetts. This chart was constructed by the Staff of the Department for use at the Children's Hospital and is re-produced with the permission of the Children's Medical Center, Boston, Massachusetts.

Table 9. Desirable Weights for Men and Women Aged 25 and Over*

Weight in Pounds According to Frame (In Indoor Clothing)

MEN

Height Feet	Inches	Small Frame	Medium Frame	Large Frame
5	2	112-120	118-129	126-141
5	3	115-123	121-133	129-144
5	4	118-126	124-136	132-148
5	5	121-129	127-139	135-152
5	6	124-133	130-143	138-156
5	7	128-137	134-147	142-161
5	8	132-141	138-152	147-166
5	9	136-145	142-156	151-170
5	10	140-150	146-160	155-174
5	11	144-154	150-165	159-179
6	0	148-158	154-170	164-184
6	1	152-162	158-175	168-189
6	2	156-167	162-180	173-194
6	3	160-171	167-185	178-199
6	4	164-175	172-190	182-204

WOMEN†

Height Feet	Inches	Small Frame	Medium Frame	Large Frame
4	10	92- 98	96-107	104-119
4	11	94-101	98-110	106-122
5	0	96-104	101-113	109-125
5	1	99-107	104-116	112-128
5	2	102-110	107-119	115-131
5	3	105-113	110-122	118-134
5	4	108-116	113-126	121-138
5	5	111-119	116-130	125-142
5	6	114-123	120-135	129-146
5	7	118-127	124-139	133-150
5	8	122-131	128-143	137-154
5	9	126-135	132-147	141-158
5	10	130-140	136-151	145-163
5	11	134-144	140-155	149-168
6	0	138-148	144-159	153-173

* Metropolitan Life Insurance Company.

† For girls between 18 and 25, subtract 1 pound for each year under 25.

YOUR CHILD'S HEALTH RECORD

Name of Child_____

Date of Birth_____

Vaccine	Doctor or Clinic	Date	Repeat Date	Repeat Date	Repeat Date
Diphtheria or **DPT**					
Pneumonia					
Tetanus					
Polio					
Hepatitis B					
Measles or **MMR**					
Hepatitis B					

DISEASE AND ACCIDENT RECORD

Disease or Accident	Exposure Date	Contraction Date	Recovery Date	After-effects	Doctor

INDEX

A